TENTH EDITION

LANGE Q&A™

PHARMACY

Gary D. Hall, MS
Professor of Pharmaceutics
Albany College of Pharmacy
Union University
Albany, New York

Barry S. Reiss, PhD
Professor Emeritus
Albany College of Pharmacy
Union University
Albany, New York

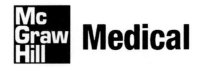

Medical

New York   Chicago   San Francisco   Lisbon   London   Madrid   Mexico City
Milan   New Delhi   San Juan   Seoul   Singapore   Sydney   Toronto

Lange Q&A™ Pharmacy, Tenth Edition

1 2 3 4 5 6 7 8 9 0   QDB/QDB   14 13 12 11

Set ISBN 978-0-07-174067-8; MHID 0-07-174067-8
Book ISBN 978-0-07-174065-4; MHID 0-07-174065-1
CD ISBN 978-0-07-174066-1; MHID 0-07-174066-X

Notice

Medicine is an ever-changing science. As new research and clinical experience broaden our knowledge, changes in treatment and drug therapy are required. The authors and the publisher of this work have checked with sources believed to be reliable in their efforts to provide information that is complete and generally in accord with the standards accepted at the time of publication. However, in view of the possibility of human error or changes in medical sciences, neither the authors nor the publisher nor any other party who has been involved in the preparation or publication of this work warrants that the information contained herein is in every respect accurate or complete, and they disclaim all responsibility for any errors or omissions or for the results obtained from use of the information contained in this work. Readers are encouraged to confirm the information contained herein with other sources. For example and in particular, readers are advised to check the product information sheet included in the package of each drug they plan to administer to be certain that the information contained in this work is accurate and that changes have not been made in the recommended dose or in the contraindications for administration. This recommendation is of particular importance in connection with new or infrequently used drugs.

This book was set in Palatino by Aptara, Inc.
The editors were Michael Weitz and Christine Diedrich.
The production supervisor was Catherine Saggese.
Project management was provided by Shikha Sharma, Aptara, Inc.
The cover designer was The Gazillion Group.
Quad/Graphics was printer and binder.

This book is printed on acid-free paper.

Library of Congress Cataloging-in-Publication Data

Hall, Gary D., author.
    Lange Q & A pharmacy / Gary D. Hall, MS, Professor of Pharmaceutics, Albany College of Pharmacy,
Union University, Albany, New York, Barry S. Reiss, PhD, Professor Emeritus, Albany College of Pharmacy,
Union University, Albany, New York. – Tenth Edition.
        p. ; cm.
    Includes bibliographical references.
    Summary: "1500 questions and answers deliver unmatched preparation for the NAPLEX NEW COMPANION CD-ROM
includes 12 patient profiles and a more! LANGE Q&A Pharmacy, 10e is the most effective and comprehensive review available for
the NAPLEX. The book features 1500 questions and answers with detailed answer explanations along with tried-and-proven tips
for boosting exam performance. The questions cover all major testing areas, including pharmacy, pharmacology, pharmaceutical
calculations and compounding, biopharmaceutics and pharmacokinetics, and health equipment and supplies. Features companion
CD includes 12 patient profiles; a listing of more than 200 drugs by generic name that the author considers the most likely to be
dispensed by pharmacists; and a cross-reference of trade and generic drug names. Herbal and dietary supplements are included.
Helps you recognize all frequently dispensed drugs, including top sellers and newly licensed ones." – Provided by publisher.
    ISBN-13: 978-0-07-174067-8 (alk. paper)
    ISBN-10: 0-07-174065-1 (alk. paper)
    1. Pharmacy–Examinations, questions, etc. I. Reiss, Barry S., 1944- author. II. Title. III. Title: Lange Q and A pharmacy.
IV. Title: Q & A pharmacy.
    [DNLM: 1. Pharmacological Phenomena–Examination Questions. 2. Pharmacy–Examination Questions.
3. Technology, Pharmaceutical–Examination Questions. QV 18.2]
    RS97.H35 2011
    615'.1076—dc22

                                                                                                    2010053300

McGraw-Hill books are available at special quantity discounts to use as premiums and sales promotions, or for use in corporate training programs. To contact a representative please e-mail us at bulksales@mcgraw-hill.com.

The 10th edition of our review book is dedicated to two outstanding individuals—our wives.

For ten editions, Doris and Naomi have stood behind us with patience, text suggestions, critical evaluation of material, and accurate proofreading. Without their help and encouragement, this revision would have been far more difficult and tedious to complete. THANK YOU BOTH.

The pharmacy profession has undergone significant changes over the past 20 years, resulting in pharmacists who are more attuned to the health needs of communities. We wish to acknowledge the efforts of pharmacy college clinical faculties throughout the country in improving pharmaceutical education.

Contents

Preface

Pharmacy licensing examinations are designed to determine whether a candidate has the minimum competencies required to enter and then carry out the responsibilities of the profession. A candidate preparing for the licensing examination must be prepared to demonstrate competence in many areas, any one of which may be the subject for in-depth questioning.

This book is designed as a self-testing tool for the pharmacy student to identify individual areas of strength and weakness, to suggest areas for further review, and to impart new concepts and other information useful to both the student and the practicing pharmacist. Students, especially those approaching graduation and the NAPLEX will find the book useful for review purposes. The practicing pharmacist will be able to refresh his/her knowledge of many topics.

The book consists of three major sections: Chapters 1 through 7 concentrate on specific disciplines in order to improve the student's competence in each. Within each chapter, some questions dealing with related subject matter have been grouped together, whereas others have intentionally not been categorized. Immediately following each chapter is an Answers and Explanations section, which we think is the keystone of our book. Some comments are quite extensive and represent miniature reviews, whereas others are limited to brief specifics. In every instance, the cited references offer a way for more extensive review.

Chapter 8 consists of patient profiles, each accompanied by a series of related questions. Information obtained from the questions and commentaries in Chapters 1 through 7 will probably aid in answering some of the questions in Chapter 8.

A self-assessment DVD is included in this tenth edition to help in preparing for the computerized format of the NAPLEX. A description of the computer-based examination is provided on page xii.

There are also two appendices: the first lists more than 200 drugs by generic names that the authors consider most likely to be dispensed by pharmacists. Included in the table are trade or brand names, manufacturing companies, a brief description of therapeutic uses, and common dosage forms and strengths. It is *not* necessary to memorize the name of the company manufacturing a certain product, especially with the numerous company name changes; however, many individuals find it easier to relate a trade name to a company. The second appendix serves as a cross-reference of trade names with generic names.

We trust that this book will not be viewed as simply a means to review material for the licensing examination. Passing this examination does not guarantee continued competence throughout a long professional career. Practicing pharmacists must not only retain their previously acquired knowledge and skill, but must remain up to date on contemporary modes of practice. We hope that this book will serve both as a means for self-assessment of competence to practice as well as a valuable guided review. A statement listing professional competency in pharmacy originally prepared by the California State Board of Pharmacy appears on page xi. Many of the test items in this book relate to these competencies.

How to Use This Book

Professional Competence in Pharmacy

A competent pharmacist is one who is able to confer with a physician about the care and treatment of his or her patient. The pharmacist should appreciate the essentials of the clinical diagnosis and understand the medical management of the patient. He or she should also be informed about the drugs that may be used in the treatment of the patient—their mechanism of action; their combinations and dosage forms; the fate and disposition of the drugs (if known); the factors that may influence the physiological availability and biological activity of the drugs from their dosage forms; how age, sex, or secondary disease states might influence the course of treatment; and how other drugs, foods, and diagnostic procedures may interact to modify the activity of the drug.

A competent pharmacist is one whose overall function is to ensure optimum drug therapy. He or she should know the appropriate indications and dosage regimen for the drug therapy being undertaken as well as the contraindications and potential untoward reactions that may result during therapy. He or she should also be informed as to the proprietary products that might interact adversely with or be useful adjuncts to drug therapy, facilitating administration or improving overall patient care.

A competent pharmacist must be aware of the proposed therapeutic actions of proprietary medications, their composition, and any unique applications or potential limitations of their dosage forms. He or she should be able to objectively appraise advertising claims. At the patient's request, he or she should be able to ascertain the probable therapeutic usefulness of a certain drug in resolving the patient's complaints.

A competent pharmacist should be able to review a scientific publication and summarize the practical implications of the findings as they may relate to the clinical use of drugs. He or she should be able to analyze a published report of a clinical trial in terms of the appropriateness of the study design and the validity of the statistical analysis, and should be able to prepare an objective summary of the significance of the data and the authors' conclusions.

A competent pharmacist is a specialist as to the stability characteristics and storage requirements of drugs and drug products, the factors that influence the release of drugs from dosage forms, and the effect of the site of administration or its environment within the body on the absorption of a drug from the administered dosage form. Most importantly, the pharmacist understands the effect of the interaction of all these factors on the onset, intensity, or duration of therapeutic action.

A competent pharmacist should be precisely informed as to the legal limitations on procurement, storage, distribution, and sale of drugs; the approved use of a drug as specified by federal authorities and acceptable medical practice; and his or her legal responsibilities to the patient when drugs are used in experimental therapeutic procedures.

A competent pharmacist should be able to recommend the drug and dosage form that are most likely to fulfill a particular therapeutic need, supporting his or her choice objectively with appropriate source material. In addition, he or she should be capable of identifying a drug, within a reasonable period of time, on the basis of its color, shape, and proposed use, as described in reference books or other sources.

On the basis of symptoms described in an interview with the patient, a competent pharmacist should know what additional information he or she must obtain from the patient. Based on this information, he or she should be able to refer the patient to the proper medical practitioner, specialist, or agency that would be of most help.

vi

A competent pharmacist should be aware of drug toxicities, as well as the most effective means of treatment for them.

A competent pharmacist should be able to instruct patients on the proper administration of prescription and proprietary drugs. He or she should know which restrictions should be placed on food intake, other medication, and physical activity.

A competent pharmacist should be able to communicate with other health care professionals or laymen on appropriate subjects, ensuring that the recipient understands the contents of the message being communicated.

A competent pharmacist should be capable of compounding appropriate drugs or drug combinations in acceptable dosage forms.

Finally, a competent pharmacist is a person who takes appropriate measures to maintain his or her level of competency in each of the areas described above.

Computer-Based Examinations

Following the lead of the nursing profession, many professions have reorganized their entry-level professional examinations to a computer-adaptive test (CAT) format. Qualified candidates have the opportunity to take their examination anytime during the year at a geographical location convenient for them. The actual examination format for pharmacy consists mainly of patient profiles followed by a series of questions that may or may not require reviewing the patient's profile. Using the computer keyboard or mouse, the candidate can scroll back to the profile for any needed information to answer a specific question. The questions will be presented one at a time and must be answered in sequence—that is, one may not skip or skim questions with the intention of returning to them later. Also, once the candidate has selected an answer and entered it into the computer, it is NOT possible to retrieve the answer and make changes. Be sure that you are satisfied with your answer before entering it into the computer. Once entered, forget about that question even if later questions lead you to believe that you gave a wrong answer.

Remember that no one is expected to answer all questions correctly. Instead, the examining body has set reasonable goals based on both easy and more difficult questions or concepts. The examination is designated as a CAT because the system evaluates each individual candidate by varying the question difficulty depending on the candidate's response to previous questions. Thus, different candidates at the same testing site may be answering different questions of varying difficulty. The scoring will be based at least partially on the number of questions answered correctly and the relative level of question difficulty.

When preparing for computer-based examinations, the candidate should review material in the exact manner as for any other examination. It is suggested that the candidate participate in any tutorial session offered at the examination site just prior to the actual examination. These sessions will include instruction in the mechanics of operating the computer system being used. However, any anxiety about the use of the computer will soon be overcome once the examination has started. In addition, you are likely to benefit by receiving your grade and pharmacist license much earlier!

Helpful Hints

There are several ways to maximize learning from this review book. For example, the reader could answer a short series of questions before looking for the answers at the end of each chapter. Keeping score will make these chapters function as miniature tests. Unfortunately, when challenged by multiple-choice questions, even in the nonthreatening environment of a self-learning program, our behavioral response is often predictable. When more than 75% of the questions are answered correctly, satisfaction and confidence dominate. As the percentage of missed questions increases, frustration and even panic develop. Such reactions lead to a self-limiting response: namely, the quick memorization of answers. Keep in mind, however, that although you may have increased your knowledge by one fact, you may not have maximized your learning experience. Do you really expect to see the same question on another examination? Do you realize why the other answer choices are not correct? Have you read the explanations of all the questions, even those you answered correctly? Hopefully, these explanations will contain additional tidbits of information that will increase your knowledge base. If the question mentions a drug with which you are not familiar, be sure to look up the drug in one of the reference sources at your disposal. The next time you see that drug may be when it is the subject of a question. Some questions may concern topics with which you are not familiar. This is a perfect opportunity for learning!

Rather than blindly guessing at the answers, seek information in the cited reference or other sources and then attempt to answer the question. If your answer does not agree with the one given in this book, check further in another source. Keep digging—learning cannot be passive. Recognize that a question stating "which of these does *not*" or "all of these *except*" gives you four positive facts or statements. These, in themselves, have expanded your knowledge base.

References

The references listed represent a small number of sources available in most pharmacy libraries. The individual pharmacist or pharmacy could accumulate a collection to fit their needs but economically the cost would be high. Instead, many pharmacists now depend on the internet for information to supplant their private collections. References 31 and 32 are especially valuable for up-to-date information.

Because of the increasing costs and frequent issuing of new editions, the authors of *Lange Q&A Pharmacy, 10th edition,* have attempted to limit the total number of books cited but realize that there are many other textbooks containing similar material. To maintain an up-to-date personal library, the reader should obtain at least a general pharmaceutical science book (eg, Ref. 1 or 24), a pharmacology book (Ref. 6 being the classic), a book with a clinical pharmacy orientation, and a book devoted to discussions of drug therapy in managing certain disease states (Refs. 5 and 16). To keep current with new drugs, drug products, and recent developments in drug therapy, it is necessary to have publications that are updated periodically (monthly for Ref. 3 and yearly for Refs. 9 and 25). Monthly journals, such as *U.S. Pharmacist, Drug Topics,* and *American Druggist,* offer both current information and continuing education programs.

1. Troy DB. *Remington: The Science and Practice of Pharmacy,* 21st ed. Philadelphia, PA: Lippincott Williams & Wilkins, 2006.
2. Bernardi R. *Handbook of Nonprescription Drugs: An Interactive Approach to Self-Care,* 16th ed. Washington, DC: American Pharmacists Association, 2009.
3. *Facts and Comparisons Loose-leaf with monthly updates or online.* St. Louis, MO: Wolters Kluwer Health, Inc., 2010.
4. Thompson JE. *A Practical Guide to Contemporary Pharmacy Practice.* 3rd ed. Baltimore, MD: Lippincott Williams & Wilkins, 2009.
5. Dipiro JT, et al. *Pharmacotherapy. A Pathophysiologic Approach,* 7th ed. New York: McGraw-Hill, 2008.
6. Brunton LL. *Goodman and Gilman's Pharmacological Basis of Therapeutics,* 11th ed. New York: McGraw-Hill, 2006.
7. Koda-Kimble MA, et al. *Applied Therapeutics,* 9th ed. Baltimore, MD: Wolters Kluwer, 2008.
8. Tatro DS. *Drug Interactions Facts 2009.* St. Louis, MO: Facts & Comparisons, Wolters Kluwer Health, Inc., 2009.
9. *AHFS Drug Information 10.* Bethesda, MD: American Society of Health-System Pharmacists, 2010.
10. Product literature drug package inserts current in 2010.
11. Pray WS. *Nonprescription Product Therapeutics,* 2nd ed. Philadelphia, PA: Lippincott Williams & Wilkins, 2005.
12. Sinko PJ. *Martin's Physical Pharmacy and Pharmaceutical Sciences,* 6th ed. Lippincott Williams & Wilkins, 2010.
13. Turco SJ. *Sterile Dosage Forms,* 4th ed. Philadelphia, PA: Lippincott Williams & Wilkins, 1994.
14. Kasper DL, et al. *Harrison's Principles of Internal Medicine.* New York: McGraw-Hill, 2005.
15. Winter ME. *Basic Clinical Pharmacokinetics,* 5th ed. Baltimore, MD: Lippincott Williams & Wilkins, 2009.
16. Beers MH, Berkow R. *The Merck Manual of Diagnosis and Therapy,* 18th ed. Whitehouse Station, NJ: Merck Research Labs, 2006.
17. Shargel L, et al. *Applied Biopharmaceutics and Pharmacokinetics,* 5th ed. New York: McGraw-Hill, 2005.

18a. USP Convention Inc. *USP DI Volume I—Drug Information for the Health Care Professional*, 26th ed. Rockville, MD: Thomson Micromedex USPC Inc., 2007.

18b. USP Convention Inc. *USP DI Volume II—Advice for the Patient*, 26th ed. Rockville, MD: Thomson Micromedex USPC Inc., 2007.

18c. USP Convention Inc. *USP DI Volume III—Approved Drug Products and Legal Requirements*, 26th ed. Rockville, MD: Thomson Micromedex USPC Inc., 2007.

19. Allen, LV. *The Art, Science, and Technology of Pharmaceutical Compounding*, 2nd ed. Washington, DC: American Pharmacists Association, 2002.

20. Trissel LA. *Stability of Compounded Formulations*, 3rd ed. Washington, DC: American Pharmacists Association, 2005.

21. Trissel LA. *Handbook on Injectable Drugs*, 15th ed. Bethesda, MD: American Society of Health-System Pharmacists, 2009.

22. Catania PN, Rosner M. *Home Health Care Practice*, 2nd ed. Palo Alto, CA: Health Market Research, 1994.

23. Ansel HC. *Pharmaceutical Calculations*, 13th ed. Philadelphia, PA: Wolters Kluwer, 2009.

24. Allen LV, Popovich NG, Ansel HC. *Ansel's Pharmaceutical Dosage Forms and Drug Delivery Systems*, 7th ed. Baltimore, MD: Lippincott Williams & Wilkins, 2005.

25. *Physician's Desk Reference*, 63th ed. Montvale, NJ: Medical Economics Co., 2010.

26. Sweetman S, et al. *Martindale—The Complete Drug Reference*, 36th ed. Grayslake, IL: Pharmaceutical Press, 2009.

27. Venes D, et al. *Taber's Cyclopedic Medical Dictionary*, 21st ed. Philadelphia, PA: F.A. Davis Co., 2009.

28. *U.S. Pharmacist*. New York: Jobson Publishing.

29. DiPiro JT, et al: *Concepts in Clinical Pharmacokinetics*, 5th ed. American Society of Health Systems Pharmacists, Washington DC, 2010.

30. *The Medical Letter on Drugs and Therapeutics*. New Rochelle, NY: The Medical Letter, Inc., cited as Volume, page, year.

31. RxList Inc. RxList - The Internet Drug Index. http://www.rxlist.com, 2010.

32. Drugs.com. FDA Professional Drug Information. http://www.drugs.com/pro/.

CHAPTER 1

Pharmacology

Pharmacology has been said to be the cornerstone of modern pharmacy practice. Simply put, it is the study of how medicinal substances interact with living systems. Pharmacology encompasses drug composition and properties, absorption, distribution, biotransformation, elimination, interactions, toxicology, and therapeutic applications. The test items in this chapter deal with some of these areas of pharmacology. Related questions may be found in chapters on biopharmaceutics and pharmacokinetics and on pharmaceutical care.

Questions

DIRECTIONS (Questions 1 through 190): Each of the numbered items or incomplete statements in this section is followed by answers or completions of the statement. Select the one lettered answer or completion that is most correct in each case.

1. Zanamivir is indicated for which of the following?

   I. treatment of influenza
   II. prophylaxis of influenza
   III. treatment of respiratory syncytial virus (RSV)

   (A) I only
   (B) III only
   (C) I and II only
   (D) II and III only
   (E) I, II, and III

2. As an antiarrhythmic drug, lidocaine is most similar in action to which one of the following agents?

   (A) phenytoin
   (B) propafenone
   (C) digoxin
   (D) verapamil
   (E) sotalol

3. What is the liothyronine sodium USP dose that is approximately equivalent to 100 μg of levothyroxine sodium?

   (A) 25 μg
   (B) 0.4 μg
   (C) 250 μg
   (D) 120 μg
   (E) 100 μg

4. Which of the following are expected effects of inhaling the smoke of cannabis (marijuana)?

   I. vascular congestion of the eye
   II. perceptual changes
   III. decreased pulse rate

   (A) I only
   (B) III only
   (C) I and II only
   (D) II and III only
   (E) I, II, and III

5. How does hydralazine, an antihypertensive agent, work?

   (A) blocks alpha-adrenergic receptors
   (B) directly dilates peripheral blood vessels
   (C) inhibits angiotensin-converting enzyme (ACE)
   (D) inhibits catechol-O-methyltransferase (COMT)
   (E) blocks beta-adrenergic receptors

6. Which agent would be MOST likely to cause drug-induced bronchospasm?

   (A) salmeterol
   (B) zileuton
   (C) miglitol
   (D) carvedilol
   (E) levalbuterol

7. Respiratory damage is most likely to occur with the use of which of the following anti-neoplastic agents?

(A) vincristine
(B) cytarabine
(C) doxorubicin
(D) bleomycin
(E) flutamide

8. The anti-inflammatory effect of nonsteroidal anti-inflammatory drugs (NSAIDs) is due to their ability to do which of the following?

I. inhibit prostaglandin synthesis
II. inhibit the stimulation of the chemoreceptor trigger zone (CTZ)
III. reset the hypothalamic "setpoint"

(A) I only
(B) III only
(C) I and II only
(D) II and III only
(E) I, II, and III

9. Which one of the following drugs is indicated for the treatment of primary nocturnal enuresis?

(A) bimatoprost (Latisse)
(B) desmopressin acetate (DDAVP)
(C) dicyclomine (Bentyl)
(D) metolazone (Zaroxolyn)
(E) mannitol (Osmitrol)

10. Which of the following statements is (are) true of "crack"?

I. It is a central nervous system depressant.
II. It is a free-base form of cocaine.
III. It is generally smoked.

(A) I only
(B) III only
(C) I and II only
(D) II and III only
(E) I, II, and III

11. Which of the following statements is (are) true of insulin glargine?

I. It should never be administered IV.
II. It has a longer duration than insulin lispro.
III. It has an alkaline pH.

(A) I only
(B) III only
(C) I and II only
(D) II and III only
(E) I, II, and III

12. A patient is told that one of the medications he is using is cilastatin. How is cilastatin best described?

(A) urinary anti-infective
(B) beta-lactamase inhibitor
(C) renal dipeptidase inhibitor
(D) rapid-onset hypnotic
(E) NSAID

13. Which of the following agents are classified as macrolides?

I. azithromycin
II. clarithromycin
III. tobramycin

(A) I only
(B) III only
(C) I and II only
(D) II and III only
(E) I, II, and III

14. Which of the following hormones are considered to be posterior pituitary hormones?

I. human growth hormone
II. vasopressin
III. oxytocin

(A) I only
(B) III only
(C) I and II only
(D) II and III only
(E) I, II, and III

15. Which one of the following statements is true of tenecteplase (TNKase)?

    (A) It is an anticoagulant.
    (B) It is administered intramuscularly.
    (C) It is derived from porcine tissue.
    (D) It is a thrombolytic agent.
    (E) It is derived from bovine tissue.

16. Valacyclovir is indicated for the treatment of which of the following?

    (A) multiple sclerosis
    (B) shingles
    (C) HIV infection
    (D) mononucleosis
    (E) psoriasis

17. A female patient with irritable bowel syndrome (IBS) is prescribed tegaserod (Zelnorm) for her condition. How is this drug best classified?

    (A) $5HT_3$-receptor antagonist
    (B) anti-inflammatory agent
    (C) $5HT_4$-receptor agonist
    (D) H_2-receptor antagonist
    (E) anticholinergic

18. Which of the following is (are) true of dutasteride?

    I.   It is useful in treating benign prostatic hyperplasia (BPH).
    II. It is a prostaglandin.
    III. It has estrogenic properties.

    (A) I only
    (B) III only
    (C) I and II only
    (D) II and III only
    (E) I, II, and III only

19. Which of the following is (are) true of ritonavir (Norvir)?

    I.   It is a non-nucleoside reverse transcriptase inhibitor (NNRTI).
    II. It is indicated for the treatment of herpes simplex infections.
    III. It is an enzyme inhibitor.

    (A) I only
    (B) III only
    (C) I and II only
    (D) II and III only
    (E) I, II, and III

20. Which of the following agents is (are) indicated for the treatment of convulsive disorders?

    I.   clonidine
    II. tiagabine
    III. topiramate

    (A) I only
    (B) III only
    (C) I and II only
    (D) II and III only
    (E) I, II, and III

21. Which of the following is (are) TRUE of mifepristone?

    I.   It blocks progesterone activity.
    II. It is often used in combination with misoprostol.
    III. It may cause multiple pregnancies.

    (A) I only
    (B) III only
    (C) I and II only
    (D) II and III only
    (E) I, II, and III

22. Michael is a 9-year-old boy who has been diagnosed with attention-deficit hyperactivity disorder (ADHD). He has been using Ritalin 5 mg tablets BID for the past 6 months but is embarrassed about taking one of his tablets at noon when his classmates and teachers are present. Which of the following might be a better choice for Michael?

    I.   Lialda
    II. Daytrana
    III. Concerta

(A) I only

(B) III only

(C) I and II only

(D) II and III only

(E) I, II, and III

23. The anxiolytic action of benzodiazepines is usually attributed to their ability to do which of the following?

(A) alter the sodium ion influx into the central nervous system

(B) potentiate the effects of GABA

(C) alter the calcium ion influx into the central nervous system

(D) interfere with the amine pump

(E) inhibit the action of monoamine oxidase

24. TB testing should be performed before a patient starts receiving which of the following?

(A) gold

(B) valsartan

(C) infliximab

(D) amphotericin B

(E) clozapine

25. Transfusional hemosiderosis can best be treated with the administration of which of the following?

(A) ferrous sulfate

(B) ferrous gluconate

(C) anagrelide

(D) defasirox

(E) erythropoetin

26. What is (are) true of lactulose (Cephulac, Chronulac)?

I. It is an artificial sweetener.

II. It is a laxative.

III. It decreases blood ammonia levels.

(A) I only

(B) III only

(C) I and II only

(D) II and III only

(E) I, II, and III

27. Which of the following morphine derivatives is most likely to cause dependence?

(A) diacetylmorphine

(B) hydromorphone

(C) codeine

(D) hydrocodone

(E) oxycodone

28. Grapefruit juice should be avoided in patients using which of the following drugs?

I. valsartan

II. buspirone

III. felodipine

(A) I only

(B) III only

(C) I and II only

(D) II and III only

(E) I, II, and III

29. Which of the following is (are) true of almotriptan (Axert)?

I. It is a $5-HT_1$-receptor agonist.

II. It must be used regularly to prevent migraines.

III. It is available orally or as a nasal spray.

(A) I only

(B) III only

(C) I and II only

(D) II and III only

(E) I, II, and III

30. Colestipol can best be classified as which of the following?

(A) bile acid sequestrant

(B) HMG-CoA reductase inhibitor

(C) potassium-sparing diuretic

(D) lipase inhibitor

(E) alpha-glucosidase inhibitor

31. Which of the following agents decreases the production of hydrochloric acid in the stomach?

    I. esomeprazole
    II. magnesium hydroxide
    III. olsalazine

    (A) I only
    (B) III only
    (C) I and II only
    (D) II and III only
    (E) I, II, and III

32. Which of the following is an active metabolite of primidone (Mysoline)?

    I. COMT
    II. GABA
    III. PEMA

    (A) I only
    (B) III only
    (C) I and II only
    (D) II and III only
    (E) I, II, and III

33. Which of the following is (are) an indication for the use of metoclopramide?

    I. IBS
    II. Symptomatic gastroesophageal reflux
    III. Diabetic gastroparesis

    (A) I only
    (B) III only
    (C) I and II only
    (D) II and III only
    (E) I, II, and III

34. Lactase enzyme is commercially available for the treatment of which of the following?

    (A) Crohn's disease
    (B) galactokinase deficiency
    (C) lactose intolerance
    (D) phenylketonuria
    (E) G6PD deficiency

35. Prolonged use of organic nitrates (eg, nitroglycerin) is likely to result in the development of which of the following?

    (A) urinary retention
    (B) nephrotoxicity
    (C) tolerance
    (D) hepatotoxicity
    (E) megaloblastic anemia

36. Timothy is a 14-year-old asthmatic. He has heard about several drugs that are used in treating asthma and wishes to know which one(s) could be used to treat an acute asthma attack. Which of the following drugs is (are) indicated for the treatment of an acute attack?

    I. formoterol
    II. terbutaline
    III. pirbuterol

    (A) I only
    (B) III only
    (C) I and II only
    (D) II and III only
    (E) I, II, and III

37. Which one of the following antimicrobial agents would be MOST useful in the treatment of an infection caused by beta-lactamase-producing staphylococci?

    (A) cephalexin
    (B) imipenem
    (C) cefepime
    (D) ticarcillin
    (E) cephapirin

38. Aspirin is believed to inhibit clotting by its action on which of the following endogenous substances?

    (A) serotonin
    (B) cyclooxygenase
    (C) fibrinogen
    (D) endorphin A
    (E) xanthine oxidase

39. Quetiapine is used for the same indication as which of the following drugs?

(A) duloxetine
(B) mirtazapine
(C) atomoxetine
(D) ziprazidone
(E) chlorpromazine

40. How can tamoxifen citrate be best characterized?

(A) gonadotropin-releasing hormone analog
(B) posterior pituitary hormone
(C) progestin
(D) selective estrogen receptor modulator (SERM)
(E) antiestrogen

41. Which of the following beta-adrenergic blocking agents also exhibit alpha$_1$-adrenergic blocking action?

  I. timolol
 II. sotalol
III. labetalol

(A) I only
(B) III only
(C) I and II only
(D) II and III only
(E) I, II, and III

42. Which of the following drugs may be classified as an alpha-glucosidase inhibitor?

(A) acetazolamide
(B) acarbose
(C) sitagliptin
(D) glyburide
(E) glucagon

43. Moxifloxacin is an example of a drug in which of the following categories?

(A) macrolide
(B) glycoside
(C) aminoglycoside
(D) fluoroquinolone
(E) monobactam

44. How can soriatane (Acitretin) be best classified?

(A) psoriasis treatment
(B) estrogen
(C) progestin
(D) ovulatory stimulant
(E) anabolic steroid

45. Most drugs used in treating Alzheimer's disease are designed to produce which of the following effects?

(A) dopaminergic
(B) cholinergic
(C) anticholinergic
(D) sympathetic
(E) COMT inhibition

46. Which of the following agents is indicated for the treatment of chronic inflammatory bowel disease?

(A) misoprostol (Cytotec)
(B) tegaserod (Zelnorm)
(C) mesalamine (Lialda)
(D) metoclopramide (Reglan)
(E) ibuprofen (Advil)

47. Kineret (Anakinra) is employed in the treatment of which of the following?

(A) rheumatoid arthritis
(B) multiple sclerosis
(C) ulcerative colitis
(D) recalcitrant cystic acne
(E) ear infections

48. Which one of the following agents is most similar in action to dicloxacillin?

(A) amoxicillin
(B) amphotericin B
(C) penicillin V potassium
(D) nafcillin
(E) ticarcillin

49. Retinol is equivalent to which of the following?

    (A) betaseron
    (B) beta interferon
    (C) vitamin E
    (D) tocopherol
    (E) vitamin A

50. Which of the following is (are) an example of a pure narcotic antagonist?

    I. naltrexone (ReVia)
    II. nalbuphine (Nubain)
    III. buprenorphine (Subutex)

    (A) I only
    (B) III only
    (C) I and II only
    (D) II and III only
    (E) I, II, and III

51. Which of the following is indicated for the prevention of thrombotic stroke?

    (A) oprelvekin
    (B) filgrastim
    (C) ticlopidine
    (D) cilostazol
    (E) sargramostim

52. The development of which of the following has been associated with clozapine (Clozaril) use?

    (A) thrombocytopenia
    (B) agranulocytosis
    (C) hypercalcemia
    (D) hypocalcemia
    (E) thrombotic thrombocytopenic purpura

53. A pharmacist prepares a product containing 400 mg of penicillin VK per dose. This is equivalent to approximately how many units of penicillin VK activity?

    (A) 480,000
    (B) 1,600
    (C) 320,000
    (D) 32,000
    (E) 640,000

54. Morphine administration is associated with which of the following pharmacological effects?

    I. pupillary dilation
    II. constipation
    III. respiratory depression

    (A) I only
    (B) III only
    (C) I and II only
    (D) II and III only
    (E) I, II, and III

55. What should a patient who has experienced urticaria and allergic-type reactions when using aspirin avoid?

    I. nabumetone
    II. oxaprozin
    III. naproxen

    (A) I only
    (B) III only
    (C) I and II only
    (D) II and III only
    (E) I, II, and III

56. Prolonged activity (8–10 h) is an advantage in the use of which of the following topical decongestants?

    I. oxymetazoline
    II. xylometazoline
    III. naphazoline

    (A) I only
    (B) III only
    (C) I and II only
    (D) II and III only
    (E) I, II, and III

57. What is eplerenone most similar in action to?

    (A) metolazone
    (B) hydrochlorthiazide
    (C) spironolactone
    (D) bumetanide
    (E) torsemide

58. Which of the following is (are) true of pentamidine isethionate?

    I. It may be administered by inhalation.

    II. It may be administered parenterally.

    III. It may be used to treat MAC.

    (A) I only

    (B) III only

    (C) I and II only

    (D) II and III only

    (E) I, II, and III

59. How does haloperidol (Haldol) differ from chlorpromazine (Thorazine)?

    I. It is not a phenothiazine.

    II. It does not produce extrapyramidal effects.

    III. It cannot be administered parenterally.

    (A) I only

    (B) III only

    (C) I and II only

    (D) II and III only

    (E) I, II, and III

60. How does neteglinide (Starlix) work?

    (A) decreases hepatic gluconeogenesis

    (B) stimulates the release of insulin from the pancreas

    (C) reduces glucagon secretion from the pancreas

    (D) increases hepatic gluconeogenesis

    (E) decreases the absorption of carbohydrates

61. Which of the following is (are) true of permethrin?

    I. It is used to treat topical fungal infections.

    II. It is a natural product.

    III. Only used topically.

    (A) I only

    (B) III only

    (C) I and II only

    (D) II and III only

    (E) I, II, and III

62. How can enalapril be best classified?

    (A) angiotensin II antagonist

    (B) H_2-receptor antagonist

    (C) calcium channel blocker

    (D) ACE inhibitor

    (E) alpha-adrenergic blocking agent

63. Which of the following agents are classified as antiseptics or germicides?

    I. povidone-iodine

    II. chlorhexidine gluconate

    III. cetylpyridinium chloride

    (A) I only

    (B) III only

    (C) I and II only

    (D) II and III only

    (E) I, II, and III

64. Which of the following statements is (are) true of buprenorphine?

    I. It is used in the treatment of narcotic dependence.

    II. It has opioid agonist—antagonist properties.

    III. It is available in a transdermal dosage form.

    (A) I only

    (B) III only

    (C) I and II only

    (D) II and III only

    (E) I, II, and III

65. In the treatment of cardiac arrhythmias, amiodarone (Cordarone) is most similar in action to which of the following drugs?

    (A) tocainide

    (B) verapamil

    (C) sotalol

    (D) digoxin

    (E) flecainide

66. After oral administration, the greatest amount of iron absorption occurs in which area?

    (A) transverse colon
    (B) stomach
    (C) ascending colon
    (D) duodenum
    (E) enterohepatic system

67. Which of the following is (are) classified as a monoamine oxidase inhibitor?

    I. gemcitabine
    II. selegeline
    III. tranylcypromine

    (A) I only
    (B) III only
    (C) I and II only
    (D) II and III only
    (E) I, II, and III only

68. How is rasagiline best described?

    (A) COMT inhibitor
    (B) anticholinergic
    (C) alpha$_1$ agonist
    (D) dopamine antagonist
    (E) MAO-B inhibitor

69. Which of the following is (are) true of irbesartan (Avapro)?

    I. It is an ACE inhibitor.
    II. It is indicated for the treatment of diabetic nephropathy.
    III. It should NOT be used in women during the second or third trimester of pregnancy.

    (A) I only
    (B) III only
    (C) I and II only
    (D) II and III only
    (E) I, II, and III

70. A pharmacist is about to dispense bumetanide 1 mg tablets. Which of the following concerns should be considered in using this product?

    I. Ototoxicity may occur.
    II. Potassium supplementation may be required.
    III. Patients with sulfonylurea hypersensitivity should not use this product.

    (A) I only
    (B) III only
    (C) I and II only
    (D) II and III only
    (E) I, II, and III

71. Which one of the following drugs is employed in treating acute attacks of gout?

    (A) zoledronic acid (Reclast)
    (B) ergonovine maleate (Ergotrate)
    (C) naproxen (Anaprox)
    (D) tramadol (Ultram)
    (E) allopurinol (Zyloprim)

72. Which one of the following antimicrobial agents would be the BEST choice for the treatment of a systemic *Pseudomonas* infection?

    (A) ceftizoxime
    (B) cefoxitin
    (C) cephradine
    (D) cefprozil
    (E) cefazolin

73. Which of the following drugs is (are) NOT indicated for the abortive treatment of migraine headaches?

    I. naratriptan
    II. methysergide
    III. raloxifene

    (A) I only
    (B) III only
    (C) I and II only
    (D) II and III only
    (E) I, II, and III

74. Which of the following is (are) indicated for the treatment of hypoparathyroidism?

    I. dihydrotachysterol
    II. propylthiouracil
    III. levothyroxine

(A) I only
(B) III only
(C) I and II only
(D) II and III only
(E) I, II, and III

75. A pharmacist is about to dispense tiotropium bromide (Spiriva) to a COPD patient. Which of the following is (are) true of this product?

    I. It is available as an inhalation powder.

    II. The patient should be advised not to eat, drink, or rinse his mouth for 30 minutes after the drug has been administered.

    III. It is indicated for the treatment of acute asthma attacks.

(A) I only
(B) III only
(C) I and II only
(D) II and III only
(E) I, II, and III

76. What is the purpose of ardeparin sodium?

(A) regulate menstrual activity
(B) prevent blood clot formation
(C) inhibit thyroid function
(D) dissolve blood clots
(E) manage preterm labor

77. The "first-dose" effect is characterized by marked hypotension and syncope upon taking the first few doses of certain medications. Which of the following drug(s) are likely to cause this effect?

    I. terazosin (Hytrin)

    II. nisoldipine (Sular)

    III. acebutolol (Sectral)

(A) I only
(B) III only
(C) I and II only
(D) II and III only
(E) I, II, and III only

78. Mr. Harris has just begun treatment with metformin. He should be monitored for the development of which of the following?

    I. lactic acidosis

    II. respiratory alkalosis

    III. hyperuricemia

(A) I only
(B) III only
(C) I and II only
(D) II and III only
(E) I, II, and III

79. Which of the products listed below is a vaccine?

    I. Tamiflu

    II. Engerix-B

    III. Tripedia

(A) I only
(B) III only
(C) I and II only
(D) II and III only
(E) I, II, and III

80. Which of the following is likely to have the shortest duration of hypnotic action?

(A) zaleplon
(B) melatonin
(C) estazolam
(D) eszopiclone
(E) temazepam

81. Which of the following is (are) classified as an antiviral agent?

    I. docosanol

    II. enfuviritide

    III. rimantadine

(A) I only
(B) III only
(C) I and II only
(D) II and III only
(E) I, II, and III

82. Which of the following is (are) best described as a selective norepinephrine reuptake inhibitor?

    I. atomoxetine
    II. escitalopram
    III. amoxapine

    (A) I only
    (B) III only
    (C) I and II only
    (D) II and III only
    (E) I, II, and III

83. Which one of the following statements best describes the mechanism of action of nizatidine (Axid)?

    (A) interferes with the synthesis of histamine in the body
    (B) forms an inactive complex with histamine
    (C) stimulates the metabolism of endogenous histamine
    (D) blocks the receptor sites on which histamine acts
    (E) inhibits the proton pump in the stomach

84. Which of the following is (are) true of pramlintide (Symlin)?

    I. for type I and type II diabetes mellitus
    II. administered subcutaneously
    III. a synthetic analog of human amylin

    (A) I only
    (B) III only
    (C) I and II only
    (D) II and III only
    (E) I, II, and III

85. Which of the following forms of erythromycin may be given parenterally?

    I. ethylsuccinate
    II. base
    III. lactobionate

    (A) I only
    (B) III only
    (C) I and II only

    (D) II and III only
    (E) I, II, and III

86. Which of the following agents is (are) an anabolic steroid?

    I. stanozolol
    II. oxandrolone
    III. fluorometholone

    (A) I only
    (B) III only
    (C) I and II only
    (D) II and III only
    (E) I, II, and III

87. What is a common adverse effect associated with the use of antacids containing calcium carbonate?

    (A) nausea and vomiting
    (B) flatulence
    (C) diarrhea
    (D) GI bleeding
    (E) hypoparathyroidism

88. Which is the most correct description of endorphins?

    (A) endogenous neurotransmitters
    (B) a new class of topical anti-inflammatory agents
    (C) endogenous monoclonal antibodies
    (D) biogenic amines believed to cause schizophrenia
    (E) endogenous opioid peptides

89. Which of the following is (are) useful in the eradication of *Tinea* organisms?

    I. butoconazole
    II. griseofulvin
    III. terbinafine

    (A) I only
    (B) III only
    (C) I and II only
    (D) II and III only
    (E) I, II, and III

90. Which of the following is (are) true of dobutamine (Dobutrex)?

    I. beta$_1$ agonist
    II. only administered parenterally
    III. has a positive inotropic effect

    (A) I only
    (B) III only
    (C) I and II only
    (D) II and III only
    (E) I, II, and III

91. Which of the following drugs are H$_1$-histamine receptor antagonists?

    I. cetirizine
    II. fexofenadine
    III. dexloratadine

    (A) I only
    (B) III only
    (C) I and II only
    (D) II and III only
    (E) I, II, and III

92. Which of the following agents have cortical stimulant action?

    I. methylphenidate
    II. cocaine
    III. pemoline

    (A) I only
    (B) III only
    (C) I and II only
    (D) II and III only
    (E) I, II, and III

93. Which property is a disadvantage in the use of cimetidine (Tagamet)?

    (A) enzyme induction
    (B) aplastic anemia
    (C) gastric hyperparesis
    (D) inhibition of hepatic enzyme activity
    (E) decreased prolactin secretion

94. A physician calls a pharmacist and asks which of the following drugs are likely to cause dry mouth. Which of the following would you choose?

    I. donepezil
    II. darifenacin
    III. ipratropium bromide

    (A) I only
    (B) III only
    (C) I and II only
    (D) II and III only
    (E) I, II, and III

95. Which of the following anti-anxiety agents causes the least sedation?

    (A) buspirone (Buspar)
    (B) lorazepam (Ativan)
    (C) alprazolam (Xanax)
    (D) oxazepam (Serax)
    (E) chlordiazepoxide (Librium)

96. A pharmacist dispenses Ortho Tri-Cyclen to Janice, a 19-year-old new user of this product. The patient reads the patient package insert and asks how the norgestimate component of this product works. Which of the following would be an appropriate response by the pharmacist?

    I. It prevents implantation of a fertilized egg onto the endometrial surface.
    II. It increases the viscosity of cervical mucus.
    III. It prevents ovulation.

    (A) I only
    (B) III only
    (C) I and II only
    (D) II and III only
    (E) I, II, and III

97. Which of the following is (are) true of insulin glulisine (Apidra)?

    I. may be used in insulin pump devices
    II. clear
    III. may be given IV

    (A) I only
    (B) III only
    (C) I and II only
    (D) II and III only
    (E) I, II, and III

98. Which of the following is an action of inamrinone?

    (A) antiparkinson effects
    (B) antidepressant action
    (C) control of focal seizures
    (D) narcotic antagonism
    (E) positive inotropism

99. Which of the following calcium channel blockers may be employed parenterally in the treatment of cardiac arrhythmias?

    I. verapamil (Isoptin, Calan)
    II. isradipine (DynaCirc)
    III. amlodipine (Norvasc)

    (A) I only
    (B) III only
    (C) I and II only
    (D) II and III only
    (E) I, II, and III

100. Which of the following statements is (are) true of ticlopidine HCl (Ticlid)?

    I. inhibits platelet aggregation
    II. it is a glycoprotein IIb/IIIa inhibitor
    III. dissolves blood clots

    (A) I only
    (B) III only
    (C) I and II only
    (D) II and III only
    (E) I, II, and III

101. Sulfonamides exert their antimicrobial effect by competitively inhibiting the action of which of the following?

    (A) renal dipeptidase
    (B) DNA polymerase
    (C) gamma aminobutyric acid
    (D) p-aminobenzoic acid (PABA)
    (E) beta lactamase

102. Which of the following agents is (are) likely to reduce blood sugar in a patient with type II diabetes mellitus?

    I. glucagon
    II. saxagliptin
    III. miglitol

    (A) I only
    (B) III only
    (C) I and II only
    (D) II and III only
    (E) I, II, and III

103. Which of the following is in a different pharmacological class than all of the others?

    (A) saquinavir
    (B) nelfinavir
    (C) ritonavir
    (D) amprenavir
    (E) abacavir

104. Which of the following is (are) considered to be prokinetic agents?

    I. Lotronex
    II. Prokine
    III. Reglan

    (A) I only
    (B) III only
    (C) I and II only
    (D) II and III only
    (E) I, II, and III

105. Which of the following statements is (are) TRUE of beclomethasone dipropionate (Beclovent, Vanceril) aerosol?

    I.   It should only be used in the treatment of an acute asthmatic attack.
    II. It should not be used in children younger than 18 years.
    III. If used in conjunction with a bronchodilator administered by inhalation, the bronchodilator should be used first.

    (A) I only
    (B) III only
    (C) I and II only
    (D) II and III only
    (E) I, II, and III

106. Zosyn is a product that contains piperacillin sodium and tazobactam sodium. Which statement describes tazobactam sodium?

    (A) It is a renal dipeptidase inhibitor.
    (B) It prevents the urinary excretion of piperacillin sodium.
    (C) It is a beta-lactamase inhibitor.
    (D) It is an antimicrobial agent that potentiates piperacillin activity.
    (E) It is an enzyme inducer.

107. Isotretinoin (Accutane) is a drug employed in the treatment of severe recalcitrant cystic acne. Which one of the following is NOT an adverse effect associated with its use?

    (A) conjunctivitis
    (B) fetal abnormalities
    (C) pseudotumor cerebri
    (D) hyponatremia
    (E) hypertriglyceridemia

108. Rosuvastatin (Crestor) is contraindicated for use in which patients?

    I.   patients with type I diabetics
    II. patients with active liver disease
    III. patients who are pregnant

    (A) I only
    (B) III only
    (C) I and II only
    (D) II and III only
    (E) I, II, and III

109. Which of the following is (are) true of butenafine?

    I.   It must be refrigerated.
    II. It is used in treating serious burns.
    III. It is only used topically.

    (A) I only
    (B) III only
    (C) I and II only
    (D) II and III only
    (E) I, II, and III

110. Which of the following is (are) a fat-soluble vitamin?

    I.   phytonadione
    II. tocopherol
    III. retinol

    (A) I only
    (B) III only
    (C) I and II only
    (D) II and III only
    (E) I, II, and III

111. Which of the following drugs is (are) indicated for the treatment of alopecia?

    I.   minoxidil
    II. finasteride
    III. chlorhexidine

    (A) I only
    (B) III only
    (C) I and II only
    (D) II and III only
    (E) I, II, and III

112. Methadone is a(n)

    I.   narcotic antagonist
    II. analgesic drug
    III. controlled substance

    (A) I only
    (B) III only
    (C) I and II only
    (D) II and III only
    (E) I, II, and III

113. Iron is required by the body to maintain normal functioning of which of the following?

    (A) oxygen transport
    (B) ascorbic acid absorption
    (C) bone growth
    (D) visual acuity
    (E) leukocyte development

114. Which of the following is a product of sulfasalazine metabolism?

    (A) aspirin
    (B) pyridium
    (C) mesalamine
    (D) salicylic acid
    (E) salicylamide

115. Which of the following drugs is (are) available in a transdermal dosage form?

    I.   fentanyl
    II. clonidine
    III. selegiline

    (A) I only
    (B) III only
    (C) I and II only
    (D) II and III only
    (E) I, II, and III

116. Which one of the following beta-adrenergic blocking agents is MOST likely to cause central nervous system adverse effects?

    (A) acebutolol (Sectral)
    (B) atenolol (Tenormin)
    (C) pindolol (Visken)
    (D) propranolol HCl (Inderal)
    (E) esmolol (Brevibloc)

117. Fosfomycin is used specifically for the treatment of infections of the

    (A) urinary tract
    (B) lower respiratory tract
    (C) skin
    (D) bone
    (E) eye

118. Which of the following is (are) true of infliximab (Remicade)?

    I.   administered intravenously
    II. used in treating Crohn's disease
    III. a monoclonal antibody

    (A) I only
    (B) III only
    (C) I and II only
    (D) II and III only
    (E) I, II, and III

119. Patients who recieve amiodarone (Cordarone) should be monitored for the development of which of the following?

    (A) pseudomembranous enterocolitis
    (B) pulmonary toxicity
    (C) ptosis
    (D) cardiomyopathy
    (E) tinnitus

120. Which of the following is a bronchodilator that acts by inhibiting phosphodiesterase?

    I.   dyphylline (Lufyllin)
    II. pentoxifylline (Trental)
    III. nedocromil sodium (Tilade)

    (A) I only
    (B) III only
    (C) I and II only
    (D) II and III only
    (E) I, II, and III

121. Which of the following is (are) true of Simvastatin (Zocor)?

I. It should be administered in the morning.

II. It enhances HMG-CoA reductase activity.

III. It may cause myopathy.

(A) I only

(B) III only

(C) I and II only

(D) II and III only

(E) I, II, and III

122. Which of the following agents is (are) classified as a leukotriene receptor antagonist?

I. omalizumab

II. tiotropium bromide

III. zileuton

(A) I only

(B) III only

(C) I and II only

(D) II and III only

(E) I, II, and III only

123. Of the following glucocorticoids, which one has the GREATEST anti-inflammatory potency when administered systemically?

(A) hydrocortisone (Cortef)

(B) prednisone (Meticorten)

(C) triamcinolone (Aristocort)

(D) betamethasone (Celestone)

(E) cortisone (Cortone)

124. Which of the following antacids may be used in treating hyperphosphatemia?

I. calcium carbonate

II. sodium bicarbonate

III. aluminum hydroxide

(A) I only

(B) III only

(C) I and II only

(D) II and III only

(E) I, II, and III

125. The primary function of simethicone in antacid products is to act as which of the following?

(A) suspending agent

(B) antiflatulent

(C) H_2-receptor antagonist

(D) adsorbent

(E) emulsifying agent

126. How can the drug carbidopa be best described?

(A) exerts an anticholinergic action

(B) dopa-decarboxylase inhibitor

(C) dopaminergic agent

(D) prevents the wearing-off effect

(E) COMT inhibitor

127. How can the drug didanosine be best described?

(A) NNRTI

(B) nucleoside reverse transcriptase inhibitor (NRTI)

(C) protease inhibitor

(D) fusion inhibitor

(E) entry inhibitor

128. Cardioselectivity is a property of which of the following ophthalmic beta-adrenergic blocking agents?

I. timolol (Timoptic)

II. metipranolol HCl (OptiPranolol)

III. levobetaxolol (Betaxon)

(A) I only

(B) III only

(C) I and II only

(D) II and III only

(E) I, II, and III

129. Vidarabine (Vira-A) is an antiviral agent indicated for the treatment of which of the following?

(A) rubella

(B) AIDS

(C) influenza

(D) herpes simplex encephalitis

(E) PCP

130. Methimazole is used for the same therapeutic indication as which drug?

    (A) propylthiouracil
    (B) danazol
    (C) methoxsalen
    (D) fluorouracil
    (E) azathioprine

131. Liotrix is a thyroid preparation that contains which of the following?

    I.   liothyronine sodium
    II. levothyroxine sodium
    III. desiccated thyroid

    (A) I only
    (B) III only
    (C) I and II only
    (D) II and III only
    (E) I, II, and III

132. Which of the following is (are) classified as a broad-spectrum antifungal agent?

    I.   caspofungin
    II. ciclopirox
    III. clotrimazole

    (A) I only
    (B) III only
    (C) I and II only
    (D) II and III only
    (E) I, II, and III

133. Which of the following is (are) TRUE of sildenafil?

    I.   phosphodiesterase inhibitor
    II. may cause priapism
    III. used to treat pulmonary hypertension

    (A) I only
    (B) III only
    (C) I and II only
    (D) II and III only
    (E) I, II, and III

134. Which of the following is (are) classified as an osmotic laxative?

    I.   polyethylene glycol
    II. lactulose
    III. magnesium hydroxide

    (A) I only
    (B) III only
    (C) I and II only
    (D) II and III only
    (E) I, II, and III

135. Which of the following is (are) TRUE of the use of bupropion?

    I.   indicated for seasonal affective disorder
    II. indicated for smoking cessation treatment
    III. not likely to cause sexual dysfunction

    (A) I only
    (B) III only
    (C) I and II only
    (D) II and III only
    (E) I, II, and III

136. Which of the following agents is (are) indicated for use in the treatment of emesis?

    I.   granisetron
    II. dronabinol
    III. aprepitant

    (A) I only
    (B) III only
    (C) I and II only
    (D) II and III only
    (E) I, II, and III

137. Helene T. is a 45-year-old female who is 5 ft 6 in tall and weighs 185 lb. She has failed to lose weight on several "crash" diets. Which of the following would be appropriate to prescribe for Helene?

    I.   paroxetine
    II. atomoxetine
    III. phentermine

(A) I only

(B) III only

(C) I and II only

(D) II and III only

(E) I, II, and III

138. Which of the following drugs is (are) classified as a protease inhibitor?

 I. cidofovir

 II. ritonavir

 III. nelfinavir

(A) I only

(B) III only

(C) I and II only

(D) II and III only

(E) I, II, and III

139. Which of the following drugs is a sulfonamide?

(A) busulfan

(B) tacrolimus

(C) tramadol

(D) milrinone

(E) mafenide

140. Unoprostone (Rescula) is a drug used in the treatment of glaucoma. Which one of the following best describes its pharmacological action?

(A) miotic

(B) prostaglandin antagonist

(C) carbonic anhydrase inhibitor

(D) mydriatic

(E) prostaglandin agonist

141. Gastric intrinsic factor is a glycoprotein that is required for the GI absorption of which of the following?

(A) cyanocobalamin

(B) folic acid

(C) iron

(D) pyridoxine

(E) ascorbic acid

142. Most antipsychotic drugs can be said to have which of the following actions?

(A) dopamine antagonist

(B) alpha$_1$-adrenergic agonist

(C) dopamine agonist

(D) cholinergic

(E) COMT antagonist

143. Sulfones such as dapsone are indicated for the treatment of which of the following?

(A) Hansen's disease

(B) ADHD

(C) Bright's disease

(D) acetaminophen toxicity

(E) psoriasis

144. Which of the following antimicrobial products are prodrug(s)?

 I. fesoterodine

 II. valacyclovir

 III. clindamycin palmitate ester

(A) I only

(B) III only

(C) I and II only

(D) II and III only

(E) I, II, and III

145. What is the primary site of action of triamterene (Dyrenium) and spironolactone (Aldactone)?

(A) glomerulus

(B) descending loop of Henle

(C) ascending loop of Henle

(D) proximal tubule

(E) distal tubule

146. How can clonidine be best described?

(A) alpha-adrenergic agonist

(B) beta-adrenergic blocker

(C) COMT inhibitor

(D) alpha-adrenergic blocker

(E) beta-adrenergic agonist

147. Which of the following is an anticholinergic antiParkinson agent?

   I. ropinirole (Requip)
   II. pergolide (Permax)
   III. benztropine (Cogentin)

   (A) I only
   (B) III only
   (C) I and II only
   (D) II and III only
   (E) I, II, and III

148. Tretinoin is commonly employed in the treatment of which of the following?

   (A) multiple sclerosis
   (B) psoriasis
   (C) seborrheic dermatitis
   (D) trichomoniasis
   (E) acne

149. A patient with allergic rhinitis may be treated with a topical nasal corticosteroid such as which drug?

   (A) triamcinolone
   (B) cetirizine
   (C) budesonide
   (D) zafirlukast
   (E) prednisone

150. Gabapentin is indicated for the treatment of which of the following?

   I. epilepsy
   II. postherpetic neuralgia
   III. nocturnal enuresis

   (A) I only
   (B) III only
   (C) I and II only
   (D) II and III only
   (E) I, II, and III

151. Which of the following is (are) true of tinidazole?

   I. interacts with ethanol
   II. is an antiprotozoal drug
   III. may cause Stevens–Johnson syndrome

   (A) I only
   (B) III only
   (C) I and II only
   (D) II and III only
   (E) I, II, and III

152. What is the most serious potential consequence of ingestion of a liquid hydrocarbon such as kerosene or gasoline?

   (A) inactivation of hepatic enzymes
   (B) the corrosive action of the poison on the stomach lining
   (C) the aspiration of the poison into the respiratory tract
   (D) dissolution of the mucus coat of the esophagus
   (E) the paralysis of peristaltic motion of the GI tract

153. Which of the following drugs may interfere with ethanol metabolism?

   I. cephalothin (Keflin)
   II. chlorpropamide (Diabinese)
   III. metronidazole (Flagyl)

   (A) I only
   (B) III only
   (C) I and II only
   (D) II and III only
   (E) I, II, and III only

154. Which of the following is (are) true of vitamin B-3?

   I. Administration of high doses may cause flushing.
   II. A deficiency may result in beriberi.
   III. Should be supplemented to patients on long-term isoniazid

   (A) I only
   (B) III only
   (C) I and II only
   (D) II and III only
   (E) I, II, and III

155. Oprelvekin (Neumega) would be appropriate to use in order to raise levels of which of the following?

   I. RBCs

  II. hematocrit

 III. platelets

(A) I only

(B) III only

(C) I and II only

(D) II and III only

(E) I, II, and III

156. Which of the following is (are) true of fentanyl?

   I. more potent than morphine

  II. available as a transdermal dosage form

 III. available as a transmucosal dosage form

(A) I only

(B) III only

(C) I and II only

(D) II and III only

(E) I, II, and III

157. Xenical (Orlistat) works by acting as which of the following?

(A) bile acid sequestrant

(B) HMG-CoA reductase inhibitor

(C) central nervous system stimulant

(D) lipase inhibitor

(E) amylase inhibitor

158. Cinchonism is an adverse effect associated with which drug?

(A) quinidine

(B) procainamide

(C) clozapine

(D) vinblastine

(E) clindamycin

159. Which of the following describes the properties of glargine insulin?

   I. more acidic than other insulins

  II. binds to plasma protein

 III. contains PEG as an adjuvant

(A) I only

(B) III only

(C) I and II only

(D) II and III only

(E) I, II, and III only

160. Which of the following is a COMT inhibitor?

(A) selegiline

(B) clozapine

(C) pramipexole

(D) ropinerole

(E) entacapone

161. Which of the following is a drug indicated for the treatment of both diarrhea and constipation?

(A) polycarbophil

(B) lactulose

(C) polyethylene glycol

(D) sodium phosphate

(E) magnesium hydroxide

162. Thiazide diuretics DECREASE the excretion of which of the following?

   I. uric acid

  II. calcium

 III. chloride

(A) I only

(B) III only

(C) I and II only

(D) II and III only

(E) I, II, and III only

163. Which of the following statements is (are) true of potassium?

   I. It is a monovalent cation.

  II. It facilitates the utilization of glucose by cells.

 III. It is the principal extracellular ion.

(A) I only

(B) III only

(C) I and II only

(D) II and III only

(E) I, II, and III

164. Which one of the following antihistamines would be LEAST likely to cause sedation?

(A) azatadine (Optimine)

(B) dimenhydrinate (Dramamine)

(C) clemastine (Tavist)

(D) desloratidine (Clarinex)

(E) doxylamine

165. Urinary alkalinization can decrease the renal excretion of amphetamines. Which of the following would tend to diminish the excretion rate of amphetamine sulfate?

   I. potassium citrate

  II. ammonium chloride

 III. methenamine hippurate

(A) I only

(B) III only

(C) I and II only

(D) II and III only

(E) I, II, and III only

166. Olsalazine sodium is employed in the treatment of which of the following?

(A) psoriasis

(B) duodenal ulcers

(C) urinary tract infections

(D) diabetes insipidus

(E) ulcerative colitis

167. Which of the following cancer chemotherapeutic agents is (are) classified as an antimetabolite?

   I. cladribine (Leustatin)

  II. fluorouracil (Adrucil)

 III. fludarabine (Fludara)

(A) I only

(B) III only

(C) I and II only

(D) II and III only

(E) I, II, and III

168. Which of the following statements is (are) true of metronidazole?

   I. It is used to treat CDAD.

  II. It has disulfiram-like activity.

 III. It has antiprotozoal activity.

(A) I only

(B) III only

(C) I and II only

(D) II and III only

(E) I, II, and III

169. How is mifepristone primarily used?

(A) gastric protectant

(B) sunscreen

(C) DMARD

(D) abortifacient

(E) antipsoriatic agent

170. During ovulation, peak plasma concentration(s) of which of the following hormone(s) will be reached?

   I. progesterone

  II. luteinizing hormone (LH)

 III. follicle-stimulating hormone (FSH)

(A) I only

(B) III only

(C) I and II only

(D) II and III only

(E) I, II, and III supplement

171. Cyclosporine would most likely be found as an ingredient in which of the following products?

(A) drops for dry eyes

(B) topical antifungal

(C) topical nasal decongestant

(D) psoriasis product

(E) systemic antifungal

172. Which of the following is (are) true of latanoprost?

   I. reduces intraocular pressure

  II. promotes growth of eyelashes

 III. ocular decongestant

(A) I only
(B) III only
(C) I and II only
(D) II and III only
(E) I, II, and III

173. Reduced clotting ability of the blood is associated with the administration of which of the following?

  I. prasugrel
  II. abciximab
  III. pegfilgrastim

(A) I only
(B) III only
(C) I and II only
(D) II and III only
(E) I, II, and III

174. Which of the following analgesics has (have) opioid agonist and antagonist action?

  I. naloxone
  II. pentazocine
  III. butorphanol

(A) I only
(B) III only
(C) I and II only
(D) II and III only
(E) I, II, and III only

175. Which of the following agents are classified pharmacologically as carbonic anhydrase inhibitors?

  I. dorzolamide
  II. torsemide
  III. nilutamide

(A) I only
(B) III only
(C) I and II only
(D) II and III only
(E) I, II, and III only

176. Which of the following agents would be most appropriate to use in the treatment of narcolepsy?

(A) modafinil
(B) buspirone
(C) bupropion
(D) ziprasidone
(E) rivastigmine

177. Reflex tachycardia is an adverse effect most likely to be associated with the use of which of the following drug(s)?

  I. nesiritide (Natrecor)
  II. hydralazine (Apresoline)
  III. minoxidil (Loniten)

(A) I only
(B) III only
(C) I and II only
(D) II and III only
(E) I, II, and III only

178. Cyclophosphamide (Cytoxan) is an example of which of the following?

(A) alkylating agent
(B) estrogen antagonist
(C) purine analog
(D) pyrimidine analog
(E) prostaglandin inhibitor

179. A patient being treated for cancer inadvertently takes an overdose of methotrexate. Which of the following would be the BEST agent to treat this overdose?

(A) physostigmine salicylate
(B) leucovorin calcium
(C) mesna
(D) flumazenil
(E) naltrexone

180. How is fesoterodine best described?

(A) androgen inhibitor
(B) antispasmodic
(C) bleaching agent
(D) sedative
(E) urinary antiseptic

181. Tiludronate disodium is indicated for the treatment of

(A) Hansen's disease
(B) Meniere's syndrome
(C) Crohn's disease
(D) Paget's disease
(E) Parkinson's disease

182. Which one of the following is not a progestin?

(A) norethynodrel
(B) mestranol
(C) ethynodiol diacetate
(D) norethindrone
(E) levonorgestrel

183. Which one of the following antibiotics is a third-generation cephalosporin?

(A) cefixime (Suprax)
(B) cefonicid (Monocid)
(C) cefoxitin (Mefoxin)
(D) cephalexin (Keflex)
(E) cefaclor (Ceclor)

184. The pharmacological properties of which one of the following agents is similar to amphetamine?

(A) haloperidol
(B) lithium carbonate
(C) zonisamide
(D) methylphenidate
(E) atomoxetine

185. Which of the following drugs used in treating Alzheimer's disease is DIFFERENT in mechanism of action from all of the others?

(A) tacrine
(B) donepezil
(C) rivastigmine
(D) galantamine
(E) memantine

186. Which of the following tetracyclines is (are) eliminated by nonrenal pathways?

I. doxycycline
II. minocyline
III. demeclocycline

(A) I only
(B) III only
(C) I and II only
(D) II and III only
(E) I, II, and III only

187. Which drug would MOST effectively treat thrombocythemia?

(A) anagrelide (Agrylin)
(B) filgrastim (Neupogen)
(C) oprelvekin (Neumega)
(D) eptifibatide (Integrelin)
(E) pentoxifylline (Trental)

188. How is ramelteon (Rozerem) best described?

(A) COMT inhibitor
(B) melatonin receptor agonist
(C) antipsychotic drug
(D) selective serotonin reuptake inhibitor (SSRI)
(E) product for ADHD

189. Which of the following drugs is (are) associated with pulmonary toxicity?

(A) flutamide
(B) bleomycin
(C) doxorubicin
(D) mitoxantrone
(E) cisplatin

190. A patient who has overdosed on diazepam would best be treated with which of the following agents?

(A) flumazenil
(B) fomepizole
(C) mesna
(D) naloxone
(E) pralidoxime chloride

Answers and Explanations

Numbers within parentheses at the end of the answers refer to the numbered references that are listed in the front matter.

1. **(C)** Zanamivir (Relenza) is an antiviral compound that is used to treat illness caused by influenza A or B in patients 7 years or older. It is only effective if used within 48 hours of symptom outbreak. The drug is also indicated for the prophylaxis of influenza in patients 5 years or older. The product is a powder for inhalation, which utilizes a Rotadisk and Diskhaler device. *(10)*

2. **(A)** Lidocaine is most similar to phenytoin. Both are classified as Group IB antiarrhythmic drugs. These are agents that slightly depress phase 0 and may shorten the duration of the action potential. They are most commonly used for the treatment of ventricular arrhythmias. *(6)*

3. **(A)** Levothyroxine sodium (Synthroid) is a synthetic form of the natural thyroid hormone T4. Approximately 25 μg of liothyronine sodium (T3) is equivalent to 100 μg of levothyroxine sodium (T4). *(6)*

4. **(C)** Upon inhaling the smoke of cannabis (marijuana) perceptual changes, vascular congestion of the eye, and increased heart rate generally occur. These effects generally continue for approximately 1 to 2 hours after smoke inhalation; however, one of cannabis' active components, tetrahydrocannabinol (THC), may remain in the body for as long as 10 days. *(6)*

5. **(B)** Hydralazine is a direct-acting peripheral vasodilator. Because of its potential for producing a number of serious adverse effects, hydralazine is not a first-choice antihypertensive agent. Its use has been associated with causing reflex tachycardia and/or lupus-like effects in some patients. *(6)*

6. **(D)** Carvedilol is a nonselective beta-adrenergic and alpha$_1$-blocking agent used for the treatment of hypertension. As is the case with all other beta-adrenergic blockers, carvedilol should not generally be used in patients with a history of bronchospastic disease. *(3)*

7. **(D)** Bleomycin (Blenoxane) is an antineoplastic drug in the antibiotic group. The most serious adverse effect associated with this drug is pulmonary fibrosis. Approximately 10% of patients on this drug experience some form of pulmonary toxicity. *(6)*

8. **(A)** The anti-inflammatory and analgesic action of NSAIDs is believed to result from inhibition of prostaglandin synthesis. *(6)*

9. **(B)** Desmopressin acetate is the synthetic analog of naturally occurring human antidiuretic hormone (ADH) produced by the posterior pituitary gland. It is administered intranasally (Stimate) or orally (DDAVP) for the treatment of primary nocturnal enuresis. A single dose of the drug will produce an antidiuretic effect lasting from 8 to 20 hours. *(6)*

10. **(D)** Crack is a free-base form of cocaine. It is generally smoked and rapidly absorbed through the respiratory membranes. Within seconds, it reaches the brain and produces central nervous system stimulation and euphoria.

Dependence may occur with only a single dose of the drug. (6)

11. **(C)** Insulin glargine (Lantus) is a long-acting insulin analog that is made by recombinant DNA (rDNA) technology. It should only be administered by subcutaneous injection and may be used in the treatment of type I or type II diabetes mellitus. It has a pH of approximately 4. Insulin lispro is a rapid-acting insulin that is normally administered within 15 minutes of mealtime. (3)

12. **(C)** Cilastatin is a renal dipeptidase inhibitor that is combined with imipenem, an antimicrobial, in order to protect imipenem from destruction. (6)

13. **(C)** Azithromycin (Zithromax) and clarithromycin (Biaxin) are both macrolide antimicrobial agents related to erythromycin. Tobramycin (Nebcin) is an aminoglycoside antimicrobial agent. (6)

14. **(D)** Oxytocin and vasopressin are endogenous hormones produced by the posterior pituitary gland. Vasopressin is an ADH that is primarily used for the treatment of diabetes insipidus. Oxytocin is a uterine stimulant that promotes uterine contractions, particularly during labor. Human growth hormone is released by the anterior pituitary gland. (6)

15. **(D)** Tenecteplase (TNKase) is a tissue plasminogen activator produced by rDNA technology. It is used intravenously in the management of acute myocardial infarction (AMI) patients in order to lyse thrombi that are obstructing coronary arteries. It is administered as soon as possible after the onset of an AMI. (6)

16. **(B)** Valacyclovir (Valtrex) is an antiviral agent used in the treatment of shingles, a painful disorder caused by the herpes zoster virus. It is also indicated for use in treating genital herpes. (3)

17. **(C)** Tegaserod (Zelnorm) is an agent that acts as a $5HT_4$-receptor agonist. This agent tends to increase the motility of the GI tract, increase intestinal secretions, and inhibit sensitivity of the GI lining. This drug is specifically indicated for the treatment of IBS in women whose primary IBS symptom is constipation. (3)

18. **(A)** Dutasteride (Avodart) is an androgen hormone inhibitor used to treat BPH. It is in pregnancy category X. Women who may be pregnant or become pregnant should avoid coming in contact with the capsules. (3)

19. **(B)** Ritonavir (Norvir) is a protease inhibitor antiviral agent used in treating patients with HIV. Because of its ability to inhibit a wide array of metabolic enzymes, it may elevate the blood levels of other drugs and increase their toxicity. This enzyme inhibition is also used beneficially to increase blood levels and effectiveness of other antiviral drugs such as saquinavir. (3)

20. **(D)** Tiagabine (Gabitril) and topiramate (Topamax) are anticonvulsants primarily utilized for the treatment of partial seizures. Clonidine is primarily used as an antihypertensive. (6)

21. **(C)** Mifepristone (Mifeprex) is an anti-progesterone drug that competes with progesterone at receptor sites. It is indicated for the medical termination of early pregnancy. It is only indicated for use if less than 49 days have elapsed since the first day of the patient's last menstrual period. If a complete abortion has not occurred within 2 days of taking three 200 mg tablets of Mifeprex, the patient must take 200 μg of misoprostol (Cytotec) to facilitate abortion. (3)

22. **(D)** Concerta would be a better choice because it is a sustained-release form of methylphenidate, the active ingredient in Ritalin. The use of a single dose of Concerta in the morning, before leaving for school, would provide action throughout the school day and diminish the need for an additional dose during school hours. Daytrana would also be a possible alternative to oral Ritalin since this is a transdermal form of methylphenidate, which needs only to be applied in the morning and produces activity throughout the school day. Lialda is a long-acting form of mesalamine, a drug used for treating ulcerative colitis. (3)

23. **(B)** Benzodiazepines are believed to act by potentiating the effects of GABA, an inhibitory amino acid in the central nervous system. Some benzodiazepines are also used for the treatment of muscle spasms and convulsive disorders. *(6)*

24. **(C)** Infliximab (Remicade) is a monoclonal antibody that neutralizes the biological activity of tumor necrosis factor alpha (TNF-α). It is used in treating chronic rheumatoid arthritis, Crohn's disease, ulcerative colitis, and ankylosing spondylitis. Because it suppresses immune function, underlying cases of tuberculosis may be exacerbated when this drug is used. The use of the drug may also increase the likelihood of a variety of opportunistic fungal and bacterial disorders. *(3)*

25. **(D)** Defasirox (Exjade) is an orally administered iron-chelating agent that is used to treat chronic iron overload caused by blood transfusions (transfusional hemosiderosis). *(3)*

26. **(D)** Lactulose (Cephulac, Chronulac), a synthetic disaccharide, is an analog of lactose. Unlike lactose, which is hydrolyzed enzymatically to its monosaccharide components, oral doses of lactulose pass to the colon virtually unchanged. In the colon, bacteria chemically convert the lactulose to low-molecular-weight acids and carbon dioxide. The acids produce an osmotic effect that draws water into the colon and makes the stools more watery. They also permit ammonia in the body to be converted to ammonium ion in the acidic colon and allow it to be eliminated in the stool. *(3)*

27. **(A)** Diacetylmorphine is another name for heroin. Because of its great ability to cause dependence, diacetylmorphine may not be legally prescribed in the United States. *(6)*

28. **(D)** Grapefruit juice has been shown to increase the oral bioavailability of many drugs by decreasing the expression of cytochrome P450 3A4 (CYP3A4) in the intestinal wall. Drugs such as buspirone, felodipine, carbamazepine, amiodarone, and many others are affected in this way. Because the effect of grapefruit juice may be as long as 24 hours, patients should be advised to avoid grapefruit juice when taking these drugs. *(6)*

29. **(A)** Almotriptan (Axert) is a 5-HT$_1$-receptor agonist used orally to abort acute migraine headaches. It is not used prophylactically. *(3)*

30. **(A)** Colestipol (Colestid) is an anion exchange resin that binds bile acids, particularly glycocholic acid, the major bile acid in humans, causing them to be removed in the feces. This causes further breakdown of cholesterol to bile acids, as well as a decrease in low-density lipoproteins and serum cholesterol levels. *(3)*

31. **(A)** Esomeprazole (Nexium) is a proton pump inhibitor that dramatically reduces the secretion of hydrochloric acid in the stomach. Magnesium hydroxide is an antacid that neutralizes existing hydrochloric acid. *(3)*

32. **(B)** Primidone (Mysoline) is an anticonvulsant drug used in grand mal, psychomotor, and focal epileptic seizures. Primidone, as well as its two active metabolites, phenobarbital and phenylethylmalonamide (PEMA), have anticonvulsant activity. *(6)*

33. **(D)** Metoclopramide (Reglan) is a prokinetic agent that increases the motility of the upper GI tract without stimulating gastric, biliary, or pancreatic secretions. It is indicated for the treatment of diabetic gastroparesis and symptomatic gastroesophageal reflux. *(6)*

34. **(C)** Lactase enzyme is effective in treating symptoms of lactose intolerance. These symptoms are most evident shortly after consuming a lactose-containing food and may include bloating and diarrhea. Lactase enzyme is available as a liquid or, caplets (LactAid), capsules (Lactrase), or as chewable tablets (Dairy Ease). It is also added to some commercial dairy products. *(11)*

35. **(C)** The development of tolerance to the action of nitroglycerin and other organic nitrates may occur with repeated use or with

the use of sustained-release products. Sensitivity to the action of nitroglycerin is generally restored after several hours of withdrawal from the drug. *(6)*

36. **(D)** Terbutaline (Brethine) and pirbuterol (Maxair) are rapidly acting selective beta$_2$-agonist bronchodilators. Because of their rapid action, their use is suitable for the treatment of acute asthma attacks as well as for the prevention of attacks. Formoterol (Foradil) is also a selective beta$_2$ agonist; however, it has a relatively slower onset and longer duration of action. Formoterol would, therefore, not be appropriate to use in treating an acute asthma attack but would be useful in the prevention of asthma attacks. *(3)*

37. **(C)** Cefepime (Maxipime) is a beta-lactamase-resistant cephalosporin that would be suitable for treating an infection caused by beta-lactamase-producing staphylococci. Other antimicrobial agents that would also be suitable include oxacillin, nafcillin, and others. *(6)*

38. **(B)** Single aspirin doses are known to inhibit platelet aggregation. This is believed to occur by the acetylation of platelet cyclooxygenase by aspirin. This, in turn, prevents the synthesis of thromboxane A$_2$, a prostaglandin that is a potent vasoconstrictor, and an inducer of platelet aggregation. *(6)*

39. **(D)** Quetiapine (Seroquel) is an atypical antipsychotic drug that is chemically classified as a dibenzothiazepine. The only choice provided that is also an antipsychotic drug is ziprasidone (Geodon), another atypical antipsychotic agent. *(3)*

40. **(E)** Tamoxifen citrate is an agent that has potent antiestrogenic effects because of its ability to compete with estrogen for binding sites in target tissues such as the breast. It is used in the treatment of metastatic breast cancer in women, particularly in patients with tumors that are estrogen receptor positive. It is also used to reduce the incidence of breast cancer in high-risk women. *(6)*

41. **(B)** Labetalol (Trandate) is a nonselective beta-adrenergic blocking agent primarily used for the management of hypertension. In addition to its beta-blocking action, labetalol is also able to block alpha$_1$-adrenergic receptors. This lowers standing blood pressure and may result in hypotension and syncope. *(3)*

42. **(B)** Acarbose (Precose) is an alpha-glucosidase inhibitor that delays the absorption of dietary carbohydrates, thereby resulting in a smaller rise in blood glucose concentrations after mealtime. It is indicated for the treatment of patients with noninsulin-dependent diabetes mellitus. *(6)*

43. **(D)** Moxifloxacin (Avelox) and other "floxacin" drugs such as ciprofloxacin, ofloxacin, and levofloxacin are considered to be fluoroquinolones. These agents are particularly useful in the treatment of urinary tract infections, gonorrhea, and respiratory infections. *(3)*

44. **(A)** Soriatane (Acitretin) is an oral retinoid drug used to treat moderate psoriasis. Because it can cause serious birth defects, it is essential that soriatane not be used in women of childbearing age unless they have had two negative pregnancy tests immediately before taking soriatane and that they use two effective forms of birth control for at least 1 month prior to starting the drug and for 3 years after stopping soriatane treatment. *(10)*

45. **(B)** Alzheimer's disease is characterized by findings of brain atrophy and neuronal changes that coincide with diminished levels of choline acetyltransferase. This results in a substantial reduction in acetylcholine production. Most drugs used to treat this disease, therefore, are aimed at increasing the production of acetylcholine or preventing its breakdown. *(6)*

46. **(C)** Mesalamine (Lialda) or 5-aminosalicylic acid (5-ASA) is a metabolite of sulfasalazine. It is believed to be useful in treating chronic ulcerative colitis. Although its mechanism is unclear, it may act as a free radical scavenger and/or by inhibiting TNF. *(6)*

47. **(A)** Kineret (Anakinra) is an interleukin antagonist that is used to reduce the pain and swelling associated with rheumatoid arthritis. The drug is generally administered subcutaneously once daily and should be stored in the refrigerator. *(3)*

48. **(D)** Nafcillin and dicloxacillin are both beta-lactamase-resistant penicillins. They are employed primarily in treating infections caused by beta-lactamase-producing staphylococci. *(3)*

49. **(E)** Retinol is a synonym for vitamin A. It is one of several compounds collectively called retinoids. *(11)*

50. **(A)** A pure narcotic antagonist is one that reverses the effects of opioids without producing agonist action of its own. Naltrexone (ReVia) is an example of a pure narcotic antagonist. Other drugs listed have agonist and some antagonist activity. *(3)*

51. **(C)** Ticlopidine (Ticlid) is an inhibitor of platelet aggregation that is administered orally, with food, in doses of 250 mg twice daily. Patients using this drug should have a complete blood count with differential performed every 2 weeks for 3 months to detect neutropenia (decreased number of WBCs). The drug's antiplatelet effects are not maximal until at least 8 to 11 days of therapy have been completed. *(3)*

52. **(B)** Clozapine (Clozaril) is an atypical antipsychotic agent indicated for use in patients who do not respond to typical antipsychotic therapy (phenothiazines, etc). Use of clozapine has been associated with the development of agranulocytosis, a potentially life-threatening blood disorder. Patients being treated with clozapine must have a baseline WBC and an absolute neutrophil count performed before initiating treatment, as well as every week during the first 6 months of treatment. If the results of these blood tests have been within normal limits for the first 6 months they should be performed every 2 to 4 weeks thereafter. *(3)*

53. **(E)** The strength of penicillin VK is usually measured in milligrams or units. Each milligram of the pure drug is equivalent to 1,600 units of activity. Thus, 400 mg of penicillin VK is approximately equivalent to 640,000 units of activity. *(6)*

54. **(D)** Constipation is a common effect because morphine decreases peristaltic activity in the GI tract. Constriction of the pupils, central nervous system and respiratory depression, and nausea and vomiting are also effects associated with morphine use. *(6)*

55. **(E)** Nabumetone (Relafen), oxaprozin (Daypro), and naproxen (Anaprox, Aleve) are NSAIDs. They should be avoided in patients who are sensitive to aspirin because of possible crosssensitivity reactions. *(3)*

56. **(C)** Oxymetazoline (Afrin, Duration) and xylometazoline (Otrivin), when used as topical nasal decongestants, produce an effect that may persist for 8 to 12 hours. This is in sharp contrast to other topical nasal decongestant drugs such as phenylephrine, naphazoline, and tetrahydrozoline, which normally require dosing at 3- to 4-hour intervals. *(6)*

57. **(C)** Spironolactone (Aldactone) and eplerenone (Inspra) are diuretics that antagonize aldosterone activity and promote the excretion of sodium and water while causing the retention of potassium. The other choices are all potassium-depleting diuretics. *(3)*

58. **(C)** Pentamidine isethionate (Pentam, NebuPent) is an agent that has activity against *Pneumocystis carinii*, the cause of PCP. It is administered by inhalation to prevent PCP in high-risk HIV patients. It is administered parenterally to treat PCP. *(3)*

59. **(A)** Haloperidol (Haldol) is an antipsychotic agent available in oral and parenteral forms. It has pharmacological actions similar to the phenothiazines (sedation, extrapyramidal effects, etc). Chemically, haloperidol is a butyrophenone. *(6)*

60. **(B)** Repaglinide (Prandin) acts by stimulating the release of insulin from the pancreas. It is sometimes referred to as a "secretagogue". *(6)*

61. **(B)** Permethrin (Nix, Elimite) is a topical scabicide and pediculocide. It acts by disrupting the nerve cell membranes of parasites, resulting in their paralysis. It is a synthetic derivative of pyrethrins, which are plant derivatives. *(11)*

62. **(D)** Enalapril (Vasotec) is an ACE inhibitor indicated for the treatment of hypertension. When administered orally, antihypertensive action generally occurs within 1 to 2 hours. The drug's action persists for 24 hours. This permits single daily dosing. *(6)*

63. **(E)** Chlorhexidine gluconate (Hibiclens, Betasept), cetylpyridinium chloride (Cepacol), and povidone-iodine (Betadine) are antiseptic agents used either as surgical scrubs or for the disinfection of surgical and dental equipments. *(6)*

64. **(E)** Buprenorphine (Buprenex, Subutex, Butrans) is an opioid narcotic agonist—antagonist. As an analgesic, it is approximately 30 times as potent as morphine. It is administered intramuscularly, intravenously, and transdermally (Butrans) for the relief of moderate to severe pain. It is also used sublingually for the treatment of narcotic dependence. A combination of buprenorphine and naloxone (Suboxone) for sublingual use is also available for the treatment of opioid dependence. *(6)*

65. **(C)** Sotalol (Betapace) and amiodarone (Cordarone) are both Group III antiarrhythmic agents. This means that they both act to prolong the repolarization phase (phase 3). *(6)*

66. **(D)** Iron is primarily absorbed in the duodenum and the jejunum by an active transport mechanism. The ferrous salt form is absorbed approximately three times more readily than the ferric form. The presence of food, particularly dairy products, eggs, coffee, and tea, in the GI tract may decrease the absorption of iron significantly, although the concurrent administration of vitamin C maintains iron in the ferrous state, thereby enhancing its absorption from the GI tract. *(6)*

67. **(D)** Tranylcypromine (Parnate) and selegeline (Eldepryl) are MAO inhibitors. Patients using them should avoid tyramine-containing foods as well as most cold and allergy products. *(3)*

68. **(E)** Rasagiline (Azilect) and selegeline (Eldepryl) are MAO-B inhibitors that are used in the adjunctive treatment of Parkinson's disease. *(3)*

69. **(D)** Irbesartan (Avapro) is an angiotensin II-receptor blocker. It should not be administered to women during the second and third trimester of pregnancy because of the potential for fetal harm during that period. This drug is also indicated for the treatment of diabetic nephropathy in patients with elevated serum creatinine and proteinuria. *(3)*

70. **(E)** Bumetanide (Bumex) is a loop diuretic that is similar in action to furosemide (Lasix), ethacrynic acid (Edecrin), and torsemide (Demadex). Loop diuretics inhibit the reabsorption of sodium, chloride, and potassium ions in the ascending loop of Henle and may, therefore, cause hypokalemia and other electrolyte disturbances. They may also cause ototoxicity. All of these drugs are chemically related to the sulfonylureas and may cause adverse reactions in patients who have a history of sulfonylurea hypersensitivity. *(6)*

71. **(C)** NSAIDs reduce the inflammation caused by deposits of uric acid crystals seen in gout but have no effect on the amount of uric acid in the body. The NSAIDs most commonly prescribed for gout are indomethacin (Indocin) and naproxen (Anaprox, Naprosyn), which are taken orally every day. *(6)*

72. **(A)** Ceftizoxime (Cefizox) is a parenterally administered third generation cephalosporin. Third generation cephalosporins are usually good choices for the treatment of systemic *Proteus* and *Pseudomonas* infections. The other cephalosporins listed are either first- or second-generation cephalosporins. *(6)*

73. **(B)** Raloxifene (Evista) is a SERM that is used to treat symptoms of menopause. Naratriptan (Amerge) is a 5-hydroxytryptamine-1 (sero-

tonin) agonist used for treating acute migraine attacks. It is typical of the "triptan" group of drugs. Methysergide (Sansert) is an ergot alkaloid used to prevent migraine attacks, but not for aborting an existing acute migraine attack. *(6)*

74. **(A)** Dihydrotachysterol is a synthetic product of tachysterol, a substance similar to vitamin D. It is used in combination with calcium supplements in the treatment of hypoparathyroidism. *(6)*

75. **(A)** Tiotropium bromide (Spiriva) is an anticholinergic agent that is useful in opening up bronchiolar passages to assist breathing in patients with chronic obstructive pulmonary disorders such as chronic bronchitis or emphysema. It is an inhalational powder that requires the use of a special inhaler. Patients using this product are advised to rinse their mouth with water in order to reduce dryness or throat irritation caused by the drug. *(3)*

76. **(B)** Ardeparin sodium (Normiflo) is a low-molecular-weight heparin derivative most commonly used in preventing deep vein thrombosis. It is administered subcutaneously. *(6)*

77. **(A)** Terazosin (Hytrin) is an alpha$_1$-adrenergic blocking agent used in the treatment of hypertension. By causing dilation of arterioles and veins, the drug causes the lowering of both supine and standing blood pressures. The "first-dose" effect is the development of marked hypotension and syncope (fainting) on administration of the first few doses of the drug. Administering low initial doses of the drug at bedtime can minimize this effect. Dosage may be increased gradually until the drug is better tolerated. Terazosin is also indicated for the treatment of benign prostatic hypertrophy (BPH), a condition associated with an enlarged prostate gland in males. *(6)*

78. **(A)** Metformin (Glucophage, Glumetza) is part of the chemical group known as the biguanides. Metformin is used as an adjunct to diet and exercise in controlling blood glucose levels in patients with type II diabetes. It is be-

lieved to work by reducing hepatic glucose production, reducing the absorption of glucose from the intestinal tract and improving insulin sensitivity. Biguanides are associated with the development of lactic acidosis. *(6)*

79. **(D)** Engerix-B (Glaxo Smith Kline) is a hepatitis-B vaccine. Tripedia (Sanofi Pasteur) is a diphtheria, tetanus, and acellular pertussis vaccine. Tamiflu is an antiviral drug used orally in the prevention and treatment of influenza A and B. *(10)*

80. **(A)** Zaleplon (Sonata) is a short-acting (peak concentration occurs in approximately 1 hour) hypnotic agent. It is particularly useful for decreasing the time to sleep onset. It is not useful for prolonging total sleep time or for decreasing the number of awakenings. *(3)*

81. **(E)** Docosanol (Abreva) is a topically applied antiviral medication used to treat cold sore infections caused by the herpes simplex virus. Enfuviritide (Fuzeon) interferes with the fusion of HIV-1 with CD4$^+$ cells. Rimantadine (Flumadine) is an antiviral agent used in the treatment of influenza A viral infections. *(3)*

82. **(A)** Atomoxetine (Strattera) is a selective norepinephrine reuptake inhibitor (SNRI). Amoxapine (Asendin) is a tricyclic antidepressant and escitalopram (Lexapro) is a SSRI. *(3)*

83. **(D)** Nizatidine (Axid) and other histamine H$_2$-receptor antagonists competitively block H$_2$-receptor sites, particularly those found in gastric parietal cells. These agents do not block histamine release, antibody production, or antigen–antibody reactions and they do not bind histamine. *(6)*

84. **(E)** Pramlintide (Symlin) is synthetic analog of human amylin that is administered subcutaneously for the treatment of type I and type II diabetes mellitus. It works by slowing the passage of glucose to the intestine from the stomach, it reduces the production of glucose by the liver, and it increases the feeling of fullness after a meal and, therefore, helps to control appetite. *(10)*

85. **(B)** Erythromycin lactobionate is the only form of erythromycin that is suitable for parenteral use. Erythromycin base and ethylsuccinate are generally used orally. *(6)*

86. **(C)** Anabolic steroids are related to androgens. Their use results in enhanced tissue building. They are used in the treatment of certain types of anemia and in treating metastatic breast cancer in women. Fluorometholone is an anti-inflammatory corticosteroid often used ophthalmically after laser-based refractive surgery. *(6)*

87. **(B)** Calcium carbonate-containing antacids may cause flatulence because when carbonate comes in contact with the acid pH of the stomach, carbon dioxide gas is formed. *(11)*

88. **(E)** Endorphins are endogenous (naturally found in the body) opioid peptides that are released in response to stress. *(6)*

89. **(D)** *Tinea* fungi often cause finger or toenails to become thickened, discolored, disfigured, and/or split. Griseofulvin is an antifungal drug that binds to *tubulin*, interfering with *microtubule* function, thus inhibiting *mitosis* of fungal cells. It is primarily used in treating tinea infections. Terbinafine (Lamisil) is an antifungal compound that may be administered orally or topically in treating *tinea* infections. Its antifungal action is believed to be the result of its ability to inhibit a key enzyme needed in the sterol synthesis of fungi. Butoconazole is an agent primarily used to treat fungal infections caused by *Candida albicans*. *(3)*

90. **(E)** Dobutamine (Dobutrex) is a parenterally administered agent that is chemically related to dopamine. It acts by stimulating primarily beta$_1$-adrenergic receptors to produce an inotropic effect. It is commonly employed in the treatment of shock syndrome. Unlike dopamine, dobutamine does not cause the endogenous release of norepinephrine. *(3)*

91. **(E)** Cetirizine (Zyrtec), dexloratadine (Clarinex), and fexofenadine (Allegra) are histamine H$_1$-receptor antagonists used for the treatment of seasonal allergic rhinitis. Unlike older H$_1$-receptor antagonists such as chlorpheniramine or diphenhydramine, these drugs tend to be less sedating and are better tolerated. *(3)*

92. **(E)** Pemoline (Cylert), methylphenidate (Ritalin), and cocaine stimulate the central nervous system and increase alertness and a heightened awareness of surroundings. High doses may produce hyperactivity, autonomic effects on the heart, and muscle tremor. *(6)*

93. **(D)** Cimetidine (Tagamet) is an H$_2$-histamine-receptor antagonist used to decrease gastric acid secretion in patients with peptic ulcer disease. It has been shown to inhibit the hepatic metabolism of drugs metabolized via the cytochrome P450 pathway, thereby delaying metabolism and increasing serum levels. Cimetidine may affect the metabolism of drugs such as theophylline, some benzodiazepines, phenytoin, and warfarin. *(6)*

94. **(D)** Ipratropium bromide (Atrovent) is an anticholinergic compound that produces a bronchodilator effect when administered by inhalation. It is used either alone or with beta-adrenergic compounds to treat bronchospasm associated with COPD. Darifenacin (Enablex) is an anticholinergic drug that is used in treating patients with an overactive bladder. Because of their anticholinergic effects these drugs can be expected to produce dry mouth and constipation in some patients. Donepezil (Aricept) is a drug used for treating dementia. Because it increases cholinergic activity it may cause salivation. *(3)*

95. **(A)** Buspirone (Buspar) is an anti-anxiety agent that unlike the other choices provided, which are benzodiazepines, does not produce significant sedative, muscle relaxant, or anticonvulsant effects. *(6)*

96. **(C)** Norgestimate is a progestin compound. Although estrogens tend to work by preventing ovulation, progestins work primarily by increasing the viscosity of cervical mucous and by altering the endometrial lining (the inner lining of the uterus) to prevent implantation of a fertilized egg. *(6)*

97. **(C)** Insulin glulisine (Apidra) is a clear, rapid-acting insulin analog that is only administered subcutaneously, generally within 15 to 20 minutes of mealtime. It may be injected directly or used in an insulin pump device. It is similar to other insulin analogs such as insulin aspart and insulin lispro. *(3)*

98. **(E)** Inamrinone (Inocor) is an agent that produces a positive inotropic effect as well as vasodilation. It is used to treat congestive heart failure (CHF) in patients who have not responded adequately to digitalis glycosides, diuretics, or vasodilators. It was formerly called "amrinone," but its name was changed to avoid confusion with amiodarone. *(3)*

99. **(A)** Verapamil (Calan, Isoptin) is a calcium channel blocking agent used orally and parenterally in the treatment of cardiac arrhythmias. The other calcium channel blocking agents listed are used in the treatment of angina pectoris and/or essential hypertension. Oral verapamil is also used for these indications. *(10)*

100. **(A)** Ticlopidine HCl (Ticlid) is an orally administered platelet aggregation inhibitor, which prolongs bleeding time. It acts by inhibiting ADP-induced platelet-fibrinogen binding and subsequent platelet–platelet adhesion. The effect on platelet function is irreversible for the life of the platelet. Ticlopidine is indicated for reducing risk of thrombotic stroke (fatal or nonfatal) in patients who have experienced stroke precursor symptoms and in patients who have had a completed thrombotic stroke. *(6)*

101. **(D)** Sulfonamides exert their antimicrobial action by competitively antagonizing PABA. Sulfonamide resistance may occur if an organism produces excessive amounts of PABA, or if PABA-containing products are used concurrently with a sulfonamide drug. *(6)*

102. **(D)** Saxagliptin (Onglyza) is a dipeptidyl peptidase-4 (DPP-4) inhibitor used to treat patients with type II diabetes. Miglitol (Glyset) is an alpha-glucosidase inhibitor that reduces the absorption of carbohydrates from the GI tract and, thereby, reduces blood sugar levels. Glucagon is a polypeptide secreted by the pancreas. It acts to enhance gluconeogenesis and glycogenolysis, thereby causing higher levels of glucose in the blood. Glucagon is used to treat severe hypoglycemia. It is generally administered intramuscularly or intravenously. *(5)*

103. **(E)** Abacavir (Ziagen) is an NRTI. The other agents are protease inhibitors. All are used in treating HIV-positive patients. *(3)*

104. **(B)** Metoclopramide (Reglan) is a prokinetic agent, that is, it stimulates the motility of the upper GI tract, thereby increasing duodenal and jejunal peristalsis as well as the rate of stomach emptying. It is used for the short-term treatment of gastroesophageal reflux and for the treatment of diabetic gastroparesis. It may also be useful in controlling nausea and vomiting in postoperative patients and in those receiving emetogenic cancer chemotherapy. Olosetron (Lotronex) is used to modulate GI motion in patients with IBD, and sargramostim (Prokine) is a hematological stimulant that increases the formation of WBCs. *(3)*

105. **(B)** Beclomethasone dipropionate (Beclovent, Vanceril) is a synthetic corticosteroid used by inhalation in children and adults to control bronchial asthma. It is generally reserved for patients in whom bronchodilators and other nonsteroidal medications have not been totally successful in controlling asthmatic attacks. When used with a bronchodilator administered by inhalation, the beclomethasone dipropionate should be administered several minutes after the bronchodilator in order to enhance the penetration of the beclomethasone into the bronchial tree. *(6)*

106. **(C)** Tazobactam sodium is a broad-spectrum beta-lactamase inhibitor. It is used in combination with penicillins such as piperacillin sodium in order to enhance the activity of the penicillin to include the treatment of infection caused by beta-lactamase-producing organisms. *(6)*

107. (D) Hyponatremia is not a problem commonly associated with the use of isotretinoin (Accutane). Cheilitis (cracked margins of the lips), conjunctivitis, and dry mouth occur in a large proportion of patients receiving this drug. Hypertriglyceridemia and pseudotumor cerebri have also been reported. Isotretinoin is classified in pregnancy category X and will, therefore, potentially cause fetal abnormalities if used by a pregnant woman. *(6)*

108. (D) Rosuvastatin (Crestor) is a cholesterol-lowering agent in the "statin" group of drugs. It is contraindicated for use during pregnancy because of its great potential for causing fetal harm. The drug is in FDA pregnancy category X. Its use is also contraindicated in active liver disease because of its potential for elevating liver enzyme concentrations. *(3)*

109. (B) Butenafine (Mentax, Lotrimin Ultra) is an antifungal drug useful in the topical treatment of superficial dermatophyte infections, including tinea pedis (athlete's foot), tinea corporis (ringworm), and tinea cruris (jock itch). It should be stored at controlled room temperature. It also has some activity against topical fungal infections caused by *Candida* organisms. *(3)*

110. (E) Phytonadione is a form of vitamin K, tocopherol is a form of vitamin E, and retinol is a form of vitamin A. All are fat-soluble vitamins. *(6)*

111. (C) Finasteride (Propecia) is an anti-androgen drug that is used orally for the treatment of alopecia. It is also available as Proscar, an orally administered product indicated for the treatment of BPH. Minoxidil (Rogaine) is used topically for the treatment of alopecia. It is also available orally for the treatment of hypertension. Chlorhexidine is a chemical antiseptic. *(3)*

112. (D) Methadone (Dolophine, Methadose) is a narcotic agonist analgesic, which is a controlled substance with actions similar to those of morphine. It is twice as potent when used parenterally as when used orally. It is employed in the treatment of severe pain and in maintenance treatment of narcotic addiction. *(6)*

113. (A) Iron is an essential component of hemoglobin, myoglobin, and several enzymes. Approximately two-thirds of total body iron is in the circulating RBCs as part of hemoglobin, the most important carrier of oxygen in the body. *(6)*

114. (C) When sulfasalazine (Azulfidine) is metabolized, the by-products are sulfapyridine (a sulfonamide) and mesalamine. Although sulfasalazine is useful in treating ulcerative colitis, mesalamine alone may also be effective, and is particularly useful in patients who have a history of sulfa allergy. Mesalamine is available alone in such products as Asacol, Rowasa, Pentasa, and Lialda. *(3)*

115. (E) Transdermal dosage forms are generally formulated from potent, low-dose drugs that will easily pass through the skin. Fentanyl (Duragesic), a potent opioid analgesic, is available in a transdermal form that has a duration of action of approximately 72 hours. Clonidine (Catapres TTS) is a transdermal product that exerts a centrally acting alpha$_2$-adrenergic-agonist action that will provide an antihypertensive effect that will have about a 1-week duration. Selegiline (Emsam) is the first transdermal product used in the treatment of depression. Selegiline is an MAO-B inhibitor. The patch is designed to provide 24 hours of medication. *(10)*

116. (D) Propranolol (Inderal) is a nonspecific beta-adrenergic blocking agent that exhibits a high degree of lipid solubility. As a result, it is more likely than other beta-blockers to enter the central nervous system and produce central nervous system adverse effects. *(6)*

117. (A) Fosfomycin (Monurol) is an antimicrobial agent that is indicated only for the treatment of uncomplicated urinary tract infections in women caused by susceptible strains of *Escherichia coli* and *Enterococcus faecalis*. This is a single-dose treatment that requires a single packet of fosfomycin to be dissolved in approximately 4 oz. of cool water and then consumed. *(3)*

118. **(E)** Infliximab (Remicade) is a monoclonal antibody produced by recombinant technology. It acts by inhibiting the binding of TNF (specifically TNF-α) to its receptor sites, thereby reducing inflammation within the colon. It is administered intravenously as a single dose in the treatment of moderate to severe Crohn's disease. *(10)*

119. **(B)** Amiodarone (Cordarone) is an antiarrhythmic agent used in treating ventricular arrhythmias. It may cause a number of serious adverse effects, the most serious being pulmonary toxicity. Baseline chest x-rays and pulmonary function studies should be performed before therapy begins. Studies should be repeated at 3- to 6-month intervals. *(6)*

120. **(A)** Dyphylline is a theophylline derivative. It exerts its effect by competitively inhibiting the enzyme phosphodiesterase, thereby increasing cyclic-AMP levels and producing bronchodilation. Pentoxyfylline (Trental) is a phosphodiesterase inhibitor that acts to decrease the viscosity of the blood. It is used primarily for the treatment of intermittent claudication. Nedocromil sodium (Tilade) is an inhibitor of histamine release from mast cells in the respiratory tract, thereby inhibiting bronchoconstriction. It is used prophylactically in the treatment of bronchial asthma. *(3)*

121. **(B)** Simvastatin (Zocor) is an HMG-CoA reductase inhibitor. This and similar agents such as fluvastatin, lovastatin, atorvastatin, pravastatin, and rosuvastatin inhibit HMG-CoA reductase, an enzyme that catalyzes an early step in the synthesis of cholesterol in the body. These drugs have also been associated with causing myopathy, rhabdomyolysis, hepatotoxicity, and fetal abnormalities. They are all in pregnancy category X. *(3)*

122. **(B)** Zileuton (Zyflo) is a leukotriene receptor antagonist. Since leukotrienes are associated with causing asthmatic symptoms, the use of such drugs reduces the likelihood of asthma attacks. They are, therefore, used to prevent attacks, not to treat an acute attack. Tiotropium bromide (Spiriva) is a long-acting anticholinergic bronchodilator. Omalizumab (Xolair) is a monoclonal antibody that inhibits the binding of IgE antibodies to IgE receptors on mast cells and basophils. It is administered SC every 2 to 4 weeks to prevent asthma attacks. *(3)*

123. **(D)** Betamethasone is approximately 25 times as potent as hydrocortisone, 5 to 6 times as potent as prednisone, 4 to 6 times as potent as triamcinolone, and approximately 30 times as potent as cortisone. *(6)*

124. **(B)** Aluminum hydroxide combines with phosphate ion in the intestine to form insoluble aluminum phosphate, which is eliminated in the feces. This may be of value in treating hyperphosphatemia associated with chronic renal failure. *(11)*

125. **(B)** Simethicone is a mixture of inert silicon polymers. It is employed as an ingredient in antacid products because of its defoaming action in the GI tract. It acts to reduce the surface tension of gas bubbles, thereby causing them to break and release their entrapped gases. *(11)*

126. **(B)** Carbidopa is a dopa-decarboxylase inhibitor that prevents peripheral decarboxylation of levodopa in the body. This reduces the adverse effects associated with peripheral dopa decarboxylation and reduces the dose of levodopa required to control a patient with Parkinson's disease. Carbidopa is available alone (Lodosyn) or in combination with levodopa (Sinemet). *(6)*

127. **(B)** Didanosine (Videx) is an NRTI that is active against HIV. Its use has been associated with the development of peripheral neuropathy and pancreatitis. *(6)*

128. **(B)** Levobetaxolol (Betaxon) is a beta-adrenergic blocking agent used to reduce intraocular pressure in the eye, particularly, in patients with chronic open-angle glaucoma. Levobetaxolol and betaxolol are ophthalmic beta-blockers

that are more selective for beta₁-adrenergic receptors than for beta₂-receptors, making them less likely to affect respiratory function. *(3)*

129. **(D)** Vidarabine (Vira-A) is an antiviral agent that possesses activity against herpes simplex virus. It is administered by slow IV infusion for the treatment of herpes simplex encephalitis. It may also be used ophthalmically for the treatment of herpes simplex infections of the eye. *(6)*

130. **(A)** Propylthiouracil and methimazole (Tapazole) are antithyroid agents that inhibit the synthesis of thyroid hormone and are, therefore, useful in the treatment of hyperthyroidism. *(6)*

131. **(C)** Liotrix consists of a uniform mixture of synthetic levothyroxine sodium (T4) and liothyronine sodium (T3) in a ratio of 4:1 by weight. It is used in products such as Euthroid and Thyrolar as a thyroid hormone supplement. *(3)*

132. **(B)** Clotrimazole (Fungoid Solution, Gyne-Lotrimin) is a broad-spectrum antifungal agent effective against yeast infections (*Candida albicans*) as well as dermatophyte infections (*Tinea cruris, Tinea corporis*). Ciclopirox (Penlac) is primarily used for the topical treatment of onychomycosis and caspofungin (Cancidas) and is indicated only for the treatment of invasive aspergillosis. *(3)*

133. **(E)** Sildenafil (Viagra, Revatio) is a phosphodiesterase-5 inhibitor that is indicated for the treatment of erectile dysfunction. One possible adverse effect associated with its use is priapism, a condition characterized by painful erections that last more than 6 hours. Sildenafil (Revatio) and tadalafil (Adcirca) are products that are also indicated for the treatment of pulmonary hypertension. These drugs should not be used with nitrates because of the possibility of potentiating the hypotensive effects of the nitrates. *(3)*

134. **(E)** Each of these choices is considered to be an osmotic laxative. Magnesium hydroxide is the active ingredient in Milk of Magnesia. Lactulose is available as Chronulac and Duphalac,

etc. Polyethylene glycol is the primary active ingredient in MiraLax and in bowel-prep products such as Go-LYTELY and NuLYTELY. *(3)*

135. **(C)** Bupropion (Wellbutrin, Zyban) is an antidepressant that is the first drug approved for the treatment of seasonal affective disorder. It is also indicated for use as an adjunct in smoking cessation programs. It appears to reduce the symptoms of nicotine withdrawal and reduces the craving for nicotine. It is one of the least likely antidepressants to cause sexual dysfunction. *(3)*

136. **(E)** Aprepitant (Emend) is a neurokinin receptor antagonist used to reduce emesis in highly emetogenic regimens such as high-dose cisplatin therapy. Dronabinol (Marinol) is a marijuana derivative and granisetron (Kytril) is a selective 5HT₃ antagonist used for the prevention of nausea and vomiting associated with cancer chemotherapy. *(3)*

137. **(B)** Phentermine (Fastin, Adipex-P) is a central nervous system stimulant used as an anorexiant, that is, to reduce appetite. Paroxetine (Paxil) is an SSRI antidepressant, which is associated with causing weight gain. Atomoxetine (Strattera) is an SNRI used in treating ADHD. *(3)*

138. **(D)** Ritonavir (Norvir) and nelfinavir (Viracept) are both protease inhibitors. Cidofovir is an inhibitor of DNA polymerase that is used for the treatment of CMV retinitis. *(3)*

139. **(E)** Mafenide (Sulfamylon) is a bacteriostatic agent that is active against many gram-positive and gram-negative organisms. Topical products containing mafenide are applied to second and third degree burns in order to reduce the chance of infection and increase the speed of healing. *(6)*

140. **(E)** Unoprostone (Rescula) is a prostaglandin analog that reduces intraocular pressure by increasing the outflow of aqueous humor. *(3)*

141. **(A)** Cyanocobalamin, or vitamin B₁₂, is essential for proper growth, cell reproduction, formation of blood components, and many other functions. In order for cyanocobalamin to be

absorbed properly from the GI tract, it must combine with a glycoprotein called intrinsic factor. In the absence of proper levels of intrinsic factor, cyanocobalamin is administered parenterally or intranasally. *(3)*

142. **(A)** Most antipsychotic agents are believed to act by antagonizing dopamine D_2 receptors. They may also cause some blockade of cholinergic, alpha$_1$-adrenergic, and histamine receptors. *(6)*

143. **(A)** Dapsone is a sulfone that is bactericidal and bacteriostatic against *Mycobacterium leprae*, the organism believed to be the cause of leprosy (Hansen's disease). *(6)*

144. **(E)** Fesoterodine (Toviaz) is a drug for overactive bladder. Valacyclovir (Valtrex) is an antiviral drug for treating herpes simplex and herpes zoster infections. Clindamycin palmitate ester is a lincosamide antimicrobial. All of these drugs are prodrugs that are converted into an active form once they are metabolized in the body. *(3)*

145. **(E)** Both triamterene (Dyrenium) and spironolactone (Aldactone) inhibit sodium reabsorption in the distal tubule. Spironolactone is an aldosterone antagonist that prevents the formation of a protein important for sodium transport in the distal tubule. Triamterene inhibits sodium reabsorption induced by aldosterone and inhibits basal sodium reabsorption. Triamterene is not an aldosterone antagonist. *(3)*

146. **(A)** Clonidine is a central alpha-adrenergic stimulant. Its primary action is to stimulate alpha$_2$-adrenergic receptors to reduce sympathetic outflow from the central nervous system, thereby reducing peripheral vascular resistance and reducing heart rate and blood pressure. *(6)*

147. **(B)** Benztropine (Cogentin) is an anticholinergic drug used to treat Parkinson's disease. Ropinirole (Requip) and pergolide (Permax) are dopaminergic agents that enhance dopamine activity and provide palliative treatment of Parkinson's disease. *(3)*

148. **(E)** Tretinoin (Retin-A) is a derivative of vitamin A. It is used in the treatment of mild to moderate acne. It is believed that tretinoin acts by irritating the skin and causing the skin cells in the area to which it is applied to turn over more rapidly. This causes removal of comedones and prevents their reoccurrence. Tretinoin (Vesanoid) has also been used to treat acute promyelocytic leukemia (APL). *(3)*

149. **(C)** Budesonide (Rhinocort) is a corticosteroid that is used intranasally either as a nasal inhaler or spray. Either may be used for the treatment of allergic rhinitis. Side effects may include epistaxis (nosebleed), cough, or nasal and throat irritation. *(3)*

150. **(C)** Gabapentin (Neurontin) is an anticonvulsant that is structurally related to the neurotransmitter GABA. It is indicated as an adjunct in the treatment of partial seizures in adults and for the management of postherpetic neuralgia. *(14)*

151. **(E)** Tinidazole (Tindamax) is an antiprotozoal agent used in treating trichomoniasis, giardiasis, and amebiasis. Patients using tinidazole should avoid ethanol use because of the possibility of a disulfiram reaction. The use of this drug has also been associated with the development of Stevens–Johnson syndrome. In some cases it can be successfully administered as a single dose. *(6)*

152. **(C)** Aspiration of a liquid hydrocarbon, such as gasoline or kerosene, may result in severe inflammation of pulmonary tissues, interference with gas exchange, pneumonitis, and possible death. Emesis or gastric lavage is avoided in such patients to avoid aspiration. Catharsis using magnesium or sodium sulfate may be attempted. Supportive therapy is generally recommended for such patients. *(14)*

153. **(D)** Chlorpropamide (Diabinese) and metronidazole (Flagyl) have aldehyde dehydrogenase inhibition activity. They cause intolerance to alcohol so that consumption of even a small amount may produce a broad array of unpleasant effects. These include flushing,

throbbing headaches, nausea, sweating, and palpitations. Cephalothin (Keflin) is a cephalosporin antimicrobial agent that appears not to interact with alcohol. *(6)*

154. **(C)** Vitamin B-3, also called niacin or nicotinic acid, when used in large doses, is useful in the treatment of certain hyperlipidemias. The most common adverse effect of such high doses is flushing. A deficiency of this vitamin may result in the development of pellagra. *(6)*

155. **(B)** Oprelvekin (Neumega) is a thrombopoietic growth factor that increases the formation of platelets. It is useful in the treatment of thrombocytopenia. *(3)*

156. **(E)** Fentanyl is a potent narcotic agonist analgesic used IM or IV to promote analgesia during anesthesia. It is also available in a transmucosal (Fentanyl Oralet, Actiq) and transdermal (Duragesic) dosage form. It does not have narcotic antagonist activity. *(6)*

157. **(D)** Xenical (Orlistat, Alli) is a lipase inhibitor that reduces the amount of dietary fat that is absorbed from the GI tract by binding some of the gut lipase. If the use of this drug is accompanied by a reduction in fat intake, the combination can result in weight loss. Consumption of high amounts of dietary fat while taking this drug may cause diarrhea and other adverse GI effects. *(3)*

158. **(A)** Quinidine is an antiarrhythmic agent derived from the bark of the cinchona tree. As does quinine, quinidine may cause an array of adverse effects collectively referred to as cinchonism. *(6)*

159. **(A)** Glargine insulin (Lantus) is a long-acting insulin that has a pH of 4. When this acidic formulation is injected subcutaneously, microcrystals of insulin are formed that slowly dissolve and release insulin over a 20 to 24-hour period. Because of its acidity, glargine insulin should never be mixed with any other insulin. *(6)*

160. **(E)** Entacapone (Comtan) is a reversible inhibitor of (COMT) used as an adjunct to levodopa/carbidopa in the treatment of Parkinson's disease. When used with a combination of levodopa and carbidopa (eg, Sinemet) entacapone increases the AUC of levodopa by approximately 35% and the elimination half-life of levodopa is almost doubled. Entacapone has no significant antiparkinson effects when used alone. Entacapone should not be used with nonspecific MAO inhibitors, such as tranylcypromine or phenelzine, but may be used with selective MAO-B inhibitors such as selegiline. *(3)*

161. **(A)** Polycarbophil (Mitrolan, Equalactin, Polycarb) is a synthetic hydrophilic compound that is capable of absorbing large amounts of water. It is indicated for use as a bulk laxative in the treatment of constipation. It is also employed in the treatment of diarrhea, in which it absorbs excess free fecal water and helps create formed stools. *(11)*

162. **(C)** Thiazide diuretics such as hydrochlorothiazide increase the renal excretion of sodium, chloride, and potassium while decreasing the excretion of calcium and uric acid. These drugs compete with uric acid for secretion in the kidney. *(6)*

163. **(C)** Potassium monovalent cation is the principal intracellular ion of the body. It is essential for proper transmission of nerve impulses; contraction of cardiac, skeletal, and smooth muscles; and in the transport of glucose across cell membranes. *(6)*

164. **(D)** Desloratidine (Clarinex), loratadine (Claritin), cetirizine (Zyrtec), fexofenadine (Allegra), and levocetirizine (Xyzal) are peripherally selective antihistamines that produce a low degree of sedation. The other agents are much more likely to produce sedation as an adverse effect. *(3)*

165. **(A)** Potassium citrate (Urocit-K) and sodium bicarbonate are urinary alkalinizers. Ammonium chloride and ascorbic acid are urinary acidifiers. Methenamine hippurate is a urinary antiseptic that requires acid urine to be effective. *(6)*

166. **(E)** Olsalazine sodium (Dipentum) is a salicylate compound that is converted to 5-ASA in the colon. This exerts an anti-inflammatory effect useful in treating ulcerative colitis. Because it does not contain a sulfa component, it is particularly useful in treating patients who cannot tolerate sulfasalazine. *(3)*

167. **(E)** Antimetabolites are a diverse group of compounds that interfere with normal metabolic processes and thereby disrupt nucleic acid synthesis and normal cell function. Cladribine (Leustatin) and fludarabine (Fludara) are purine analogs, and fluorouracil (Adrucil) is a pyrimidine analog. *(3)*

168. **(E)** Metronidazole (Flagyl) is an agent that is primarily used because of its antiprotozoal activity, particularly, in the treatment of trichomoniasis. It is also employed as an antibacterial in treating certain anaerobic bacterial infections such as *Clostridium difficile*. Patients using metronidazole should avoid alcoholic beverages to avoid disulfiram-like effects when the combination is used. *(6)*

169. **(D)**. Mifepristone (Mifeprex) is an antiprogestational drug that is used to terminate early pregnancies in women who had the first day of their last menstrual period less than 49 days ago. It may be used with misoprostol (Cytotec) to enhance the abortifacient effects. *(6)*

170. **(D)** During the menstrual cycle, levels of FSH and LH vary widely. At the time of ovulation, the plasma concentration of each of these hormones reaches a peak, coinciding with the release of the ovum and the complete development of a mature endometrial wall. The plasma level of progesterone generally reaches a peak much later in the menstrual cycle. *(14)*

171. **(A)** Cyclosporine has been used for many years under the names Neoral and Sandimmune as an antirejection drug when a patient has received an organ transplant. More recently, cyclosporine has been formulated into an ophthalmic product (Restasis), which is designed to increase tear production in patients with dry eyes. It appears to work by de-creasing swelling in the eye, thereby increasing tear flow from the tear ducts.*(11)*

172. **(C)** Latanoprost is a prostaglandin used as an ophthalmic product (Xalatan) for the treatment of elevated intraocular pressure. Because it was shown to cause growth of eyelashes in patients who used it, the drug was marketed as another product called Latisse, specifically to promote eyelash growth. *(3)*

173. **(C)** Prasugrel (Effient) and abciximab (ReoPro) are platelet aggregation inhibitors. Pegfilgrastim (Neulasta) is a human granulocyte colony-stimulating factor. The use of PEG in the product results in longer acting activity than is seen with filgrastim (Neupogen). *(3)*

174. **(D)** Pentazocine and butorphanol (Stadol) are analgesic agents that have both narcotic agonist and antagonist action. They should be used with caution in patients who have been on long-term opiate therapy to avoid acute withdrawal symptoms. Naloxone (Narcan) is a pure narcotic antagonist, that is, it does not produce any agonist activity. *(6)*

175. **(A)** Dorzolamide (Trusopt) is a carbonic anhydrase inhibitor used clinically in the treatment of chronic open-angle glaucoma. Systemically used carbonic anhydrase inhibitors increase the excretion of sodium, potassium, bicarbonate, and water, and may cause the alkalinization of the urine. Torsemide (Demadex) is a loop diuretic and nilutamide (Nilandron) is an anti-androgen drug used to treat patients with prostate cancer. *(3)*

176. **(A)** Modafinil (Provigil) is a drug that is useful in promoting wakefulness in patients with excessive daytime sleepiness associated with narcolepsy. Its mechanism of action is not clear. *(10)*

177. **(D)** Reflex tachycardia is commonly seen with the use of peripheral vasodilators such as minoxidil (Loniten) and hydralazine (Apresoline). The drop in blood pressure produced by the use of these agents causes increased renin secretion, heart rate, and output as well as sodium and water retention. This may

worsen both angina and CHF. These adverse effects observed with the use of peripheral vasodilators may be managed by the concurrent administration of a beta-adrenergic blocking agent and/or a diuretic. Nesiritide (Natrecor) is a cardiac hormone used in the treatment of acutely decompensated CHF. *(6)*

178. **(A)** Cyclophosphamide (Cytoxan) is an alkylating agent related to the nitrogen mustards. Patients using this agent should be advised to take the drug on an empty stomach. Since hemorrhagic cystitis may occur with the use of this drug, patients should be advised to drink lots of fluids. *(6)*

179. **(B)** Leucovorin calcium, a derivative of folic acid, is indicated after high-dose methotrexate (a folic acid antagonist) therapy to diminish the toxicity of methotrexate. *(6)*

180. **(B).** Fesoterodine (Toviaz) is an antispasmodic most commonly used to decrease muscle spasms of the bladder and the frequent urge to urinate caused by such spasms, that is, overactive bladder. The drug exerts a direct antispasmodic effect on smooth muscle and inhibits the muscarinic action of acetylcholine on smooth muscle. *(3)*

181. **(D)** Tiludronate (Skelid) is an agent used in treating Paget's disease of the bone, a condition characterized by abnormal bone resorption and the development of fractures. The use of the drug seems to decrease the dissolution of hydroxyapatite crystals, the building blocks of bone tissue. *(6)*

182. **(B)** Mestranol is an estrogen commonly employed in several oral contraceptive products (eg, Norinyl, Ortho-Novum). *(3)*

183. **(A)** Cefixime (Suprax) is a third-generation cephalosporin. Third-generation cephalosporins generally have greater gram-negative activity, less gram-positive activity, greater efficacy against resistant organisms, and higher cost than cephalosporins in first- or second-generation groups. *(6)*

184. **(D)** Methylphenidate (Ritalin) is an amphetamine-like cortical stimulant employed in treating attention deficit disorder as well as narcolepsy. Nervousness and insomnia are common adverse effects associated with methylphenidate use. *(3)*

185. **(E)** Memantine (Namenda) is indicated for the treatment of dementia associated with Alzheimer's disease. Unlike the other Alzheimer's drugs listed, which act as cholinesterase inhibitors, memantine is an *N*-methyl-D-aspartate receptor antagonist. *(3)*

186. **(C)** Doxycycline (Vibramycin) and minocycline (Minocin) are the only tetracycline drugs that are eliminated by nonrenal pathways. These are, therefore, preferable to use in patients with renal impairment. *(6)*

187. **(A)** Anagrelide (Agrylin) is used to decrease platelet levels and is, therefore, useful in treating thrombocythemia. Oprelvekin (Neumega) is a thrombopoietic growth factor that increases the production of platelets and is, therefore, useful in preventing and treating thrombocytopenia. Filgrastim (Neupogen) is used to increase granulocyte production, eftifibatide (Integrelin) is a IIb/IIIa inhibitor that is used after stent placement or angioplasty, and pentoxyfylline (Trental) is used in treating intermittent claudication. *(3)*

188. **(B)** Ramelteon (Rozerem) is a melatonin receptor agonist that is designed to target the wake–sleep cycle to treat insomnia. Unlike most hypnotics, ramelteon is not a controlled substance and has no apparent abuse potential. *(10)*

189. **(B)** Bleomycin (Blenoxane) is an antitumor antibiotic that has the potential for causing severe pulmonary toxicity. *(6)*

190. **(A)** Flumazenil (Romazicon) is a specific benzodiazepine receptor antagonist that is used to treat benzodiazepine overdose. Patients who have been on high doses of benzodiazepines or have used them for a prolonged period may develop seizures when flumazenil is administered to them. *(6)*

CHAPTER 2

Pharmaceutical Calculations

Although the number of prescriptions being compounded in community and institutional settings has diminished during the past decade, the importance of pharmaceutical calculations has not declined. There is a continued necessity for accurate compounding of some prescriptions and medical orders, especially for pharmacists preparing parenteral admixtures in both institutional and community settings. The concern over medication errors has made it imperative that the pharmacist be competent in handling pharmaceutical calculations. In addition, the pharmacist must be able to comprehend and evaluate the mathematics included in the scientific literature.

There are several textbooks dealing with pharmaceutical calculations that present the reader with many problems to solve. We have attempted to present this topic with a sampling of pharmaceutical calculations relevant to current pharmacy practice. Following the lead of the USP/NF, the metric system is the basis for this chapter. Any problems from previous editions that involved the apothecary system have been dropped. Obviously, units that are commonly referred to as "household measures" have been retained.

Questions

DIRECTIONS (Questions 1 through 83): Each of the numbered items or incomplete statements in this section is followed by answers or completions of the statement. Select the one lettered answer or completion that is most correct in each case.

1. Micro, nano, atto, and mega are prefixes associated with which of the following measuring systems?

    I. avoirdupois
    II. metric
    III. Système International

    (A) I only
    (B) III only
    (C) I and II only
    (D) II and III only
    (E) I, II, and III

2. What does 100 μg equal?

    I. 100,000 ng
    II. 0.1 mg
    III. 0.001 g

    (A) I only
    (B) III only
    (C) I and II only
    (D) II and III only
    (E) I, II, and III

3. A nurse adds a 4-mL syringe unit of 2.4 M units penicillin suspension to a 20-mL vial containing 10 mL of normal saline. What is the new concentration of penicillin expressed as units/mL?

    (A) 170
    (B) 240
    (C) 170,000
    (D) 240,000
    (E) 600,000

4. A patient's serum cholesterol value is reported as 4 mM/L. What is this concentration expressed in terms of mg/dL? (mol. wt. of cholesterol = 386)

    (A) 0.154 mg/dL
    (B) 1.54 mg/dL
    (C) 154 mg/dL
    (D) 596 mg/dL
    (E) 1,540 mg/dL

5. What is the minimum amount of a potent drug that may be weighed on a prescription balance with a sensitivity requirement of 6 mg if at least 95% accuracy is required?

    (A) 6 mg
    (B) 120 mg
    (C) 180 mg
    (D) 200 mg
    (E) 300 mg

6. A popular vitamin complex contains 250 μg of lutein. How much stronger is a lutein capsule labeled 6 mg?

    (A) 10×
    (B) 24×
    (C) 250×
    (D) same strength
    (E) lower strength

7. Which one of the following values is most accurate when determining an appropriate dose for a child?

   (A) age in rounded years
   (B) age in months
   (C) height compared to an adult
   (D) surface area
   (E) weight compared to an adult

8. The patient weighs 140 lb. What drug dose should be administered if the dosing regimen is listed as 2 mg/kg/d?

   (A) 65 mg
   (B) 130 mg
   (C) 300 mg
   (D) 350 mg
   (E) 600 mg

9. A package insert lists a drug dose for a neonate as being 10 μg/kg/d. What is the age range for a neonate?

   (A) birth to 1 month
   (B) 1 month to 6 months
   (C) 1 month to 1 year
   (D) birth to 1 week
   (E) 1 year through 5 years

10. A child's dose of a drug is reported as 1.2 mg/kg body weight. What is the appropriate dose for a child weighing 60 lb?

    (A) 6 mg
    (B) 9 mg
    (C) 32 mg
    (D) 72 mg
    (E) 126 mg

11. The patient weighs 175 lb. An injection is labeled "20 mg/mL." How many milliliters should be added to 50 mL D_5W if the usual dose is 0.5 mg/kg?

    (A) 0.2
    (B) 0.5
    (C) 1
    (D) 2
    (E) 4

12. The hospital protocol calls for additional dosing when the trough level of tobramycin (mol. wt. = 470) approaches 2 μg/mL. The concentration may also be expressed as how many μmol/L?

    (A) 2.1
    (B) 4.2
    (C) 6.4
    (D) 8.5
    (E) 0.04

13. A hospital pharmacy technician adds by syringe 20 mL of a concentrated sterile 2% w/v dye solution to a 250-mL commercial bag of sterile normal saline. What is the concentration of the dye in the final solution?

    (A) 0.15%
    (B) 0.3%
    (C) 0.8%
    (D) 1.6%
    (E) 8.0%

14. A very accurate assay of the above solution will probably result in the solution being which of the following?

    (A) slightly stronger than that calculated
    (B) significantly stronger than calculated
    (C) exactly as calculated
    (D) slightly weaker than desired
    (E) significantly lower than desired

15. How many milligrams of codeine phosphate is being consumed daily by a patient taking the following prescription as directed?

Rx	
Codeine phosphate	200 mg
Dimetapp Elix	qs 120 mL
Sig: 1 tsp t.i.d. p.c. and h.s.	

    (A) 6.25
    (B) 8.25
    (C) 19
    (D) 25
    (E) 33

16. How many milligrams of codeine base is in each dose of the cough product used in Question 15? (mol. wt.: codeine = 299; codeine phosphate = 406)

    (A) 6
    (B) 8
    (C) 11
    (D) 16
    (E) 24

17. The adult dose of a drug is 250 mg. What would be the approximate dose for a 6-year-old child weighing 60 lb? (Use Young's rule.)

    (A) 60 mg
    (B) 85 mg
    (C) 100 mg
    (D) 125 mg
    (E) 180 mg

18. The USP contains nomograms for estimating body surface area (BSA) for both children and adults. Which of the following measurements must be known in order to use these nomograms?

    (A) age and height
    (B) age and weight
    (C) height and creatinine clearance
    (D) height and weight
    (E) weight and sex

19. The adult dose of a drug is 200 mg. What is the appropriate dose for an 8-year-old child whose BSA is calculated to be 0.6 m²?

    (A) 25 mg
    (B) 40 mg
    (C) 50 mg
    (D) 70 mg
    (E) 80 mg

20. The usual dose for paclitaxel intravenous (IV) is 135 mg/m². How many milligrams should be administered to a 40-year-old female weighing 120 lb if her BSA was calculated to be 1.5 m²?

    (A) 110
    (B) 120
    (C) 135
    (D) 180
    (E) 200

21. A hospital pharmacy technician has written the following formula for inclusion into the master manufacturing formula book. When reviewing this formula, the pharmacist should comment upon which of the following expressions?

    | Codeine sulfate | 0.5 g |
    | Aspirin | 1.6 g |
    | Hydrocortisone | 120 mg |
    | Lactose | qs 6 grams |
    | Mix and make 30 capsules | |

    I. 0.5
    II. gr
    III. qs

    (A) I only
    (B) III only
    (C) I and II only
    (D) II and III only
    (E) I, II, and III

22. Blood pressure measurements were made for 1 week on five patients with the following averages:

Patient	1	2	3	4	5
B.P.	140/70	160/84	180/88	190/90	150/70

    What is the median systolic pressure?

    (A) 80
    (B) 83
    (C) 84
    (D) 160
    (E) 164

23. Using the data in Question 22, what is the approximate mean diastolic blood pressure value?

    (A) 80
    (B) 84
    (C) 100
    (D) 115
    (E) 160

24. After 1 month of therapy, all of the patients listed in Question 22 had a systolic blood pressure reduction of 10 mm with a standard deviation (SD) of ±5 mm. What percentage of patients had a reduction between 5 and 15 mm?

    (A) 20
    (B) 40
    (C) 50
    (D) 70
    (E) 90

Questions 25 through 26

A pharmacist in a clinical setting is asked to evaluate a new blood test that has been developed to detect a specific disease. Available data include the following:

Number of subjects (*n* = 910)

Results	Disease Present	Disease Not Present
Testing positive	80	20
Testing negative	10	800

25. Based on the above values, what is the sensitivity of this test?

    (A) 67%
    (B) 88%
    (C) 90%
    (D) 93%
    (E) 98%

26. Based on the previous data, what is the prevalence of this disease in the population tested?

    (A) 9%
    (B) 10%
    (C) 12%
    (D) 13%
    (E) >13%

27. A vial containing 1,000 units of an expensive drug powder is labeled "add 9 mL SWFI to obtain 100 units/mL." How many milliliters of diluent is needed if the nursing staff requests a concentration of 120 units/mL?

    (A) 7.3
    (B) 8.3
    (C) 9.0
    (D) 10
    (E) 11

28. A pharmacy technician adds 10 mL of diluent instead of 9 mL to the powder described in Question 27. How many milliliters of the new dilution must the nurse administer to obtain 120 units of drug?

    (A) 0.88
    (B) 0.96
    (C) 1.1
    (D) 1.2
    (E) 1.3

29. A hospital pharmacist adds 200 mL of alcohol USP to sufficient mouthwash formula to make 1 L of final product. What is the new percentage of ethanol present if the original mouthwash was labeled as 12% v/v ethanol?

    (A) 10
    (B) 19
    (C) 23
    (D) 29
    (E) 36

30. A prescription calls for the dispensing of a 4% Pilocar solution with the directions of "gtt i OU TID." Assume that the dropper is calibrated to deliver 20 drops per milliliter. How many milligrams of pilocarpine hydrochloride is being used per day?

    (A) 4
    (B) 6
    (C) 12
    (D) 24
    (E) 60

31. The infusion rate of theophylline established for an infant is 0.08 mg/kg/h. How many milligrams of drug is needed for a 12-hour infusion bottle if the body weight is 16 lb?

    (A) 0.58
    (B) 14
    (C) 30
    (D) 150
    (E) 7

32. The adult IV dose of zidovudine is 2 mg/kg q4h six times daily. How many milligrams will a 180-lb patient receive daily?

    (A) 12
    (B) 164
    (C) 650
    (D) 980
    (E) 2,160

33. A pharmacist dilutes 100 mL of Clorox with sufficient water to make 1 qt of solution. Commercial Clorox contains 5.25% w/v sodium hypochlorite. What is the concentration of sodium hypochlorite in the final dilution as a w/v ratio?

    (A) 1/10
    (B) 1/90
    (C) 1/100
    (D) 1/180
    (E) 1/200

Questions 34 and 35 relate to the following hospital formula for T-A-C solution.

Cocaine HCl	4%
Tetracaine HCl 2%	0.5 mL
Epinephrine HCl	1/2,000
Sodium Chloride Injection q.s.	4 mL

34. How many milligrams of cocaine HCl is in the final solution?

    (A) 4
    (B) 8
    (C) 20

(D) 40
(E) 160

35. How many milliliters of Epinephrine HCl solution (0.1%) may be used to prepare the solution?

    (A) 0.002
    (B) 0.04
    (C) 1
    (D) 2
    (E) 5

Questions 36 and 37 relate to the following hospital order.

Parenteral admixture order	
For: Alex Sanders	Room: M 704
Cefazolin sodium	400 mg in 100 mL normal saline
Infuse over 20 min q6h ATC for 3 days	

Available in the pharmacy are cefazolin sodium 1-g vials with reconstitution directions of "addition of 2.5 mL SWFI will give 3.0 mL of solution."

36. How many milliliters of the reconstituted solution is required for each day of therapy?

    (A) 1.2
    (B) 4.8
    (C) 3
    (D) 6
    (E) 12

37. What infusion rate in mL/min should the nurse establish for each bottle?

    (A) 0.15
    (B) 0.28
    (C) 1.1
    (D) 2
    (E) 5

38. An ICU medical order reads "KCl 40 mEq in 1 L N/S. Infuse at 0.5 mEq/min." How many minutes will this bottle last on the patient?

   (A) 20
   (B) 80
   (C) 500
   (D) 1,000
   (E) 2,000

39. The attending physician changes the flow rate of the above solution (KCl 40 mEq/1 L normal saline) to 2 mEq/h. What will be the approximate flow rate in mL/min?

   (A) 0.8
   (B) 1.5
   (C) 8
   (D) 10
   (E) 50

40. How many milliliters of normal saline should be mixed in a syringe with 1 mL of a 1:1,000 strength solution in order to obtain a 1:2,500 dilution?

   (A) 1.0
   (B) 1.5
   (C) 2.0
   (D) 2.5
   (E) 4.5

41. Dopamine (intropin) 200 mg in 500 mL normal saline at 5 μg/kg/min is ordered for a 155-lb patient. What is the final concentration of solution in μg/mL?

   (A) 0.4
   (B) 2.5
   (C) 40
   (D) 400
   (E) 25

42. Referring to Question 41, at what rate (mL/min) should the solution be infused to deliver the desired dose of 5 μg/kg/min?

   (A) 0.35
   (B) 0.40

   (C) 0.88
   (D) 2.0
   (E) 5.0

43. A floor nurse requests a 50-mL minibottle to contain heparin injection 100 units/mL. How many milliliters of heparin injection 10,000 units/mL is needed for this order?

   (A) 0.1
   (B) 0.5
   (C) 1
   (D) 2.5
   (E) 5

44. A medication order reads "Aclovate Oint. 0.05% 15 g. Dilute to 0.02% with white pet and apply to hands t.i.d." How many grams of white petrolatum should the pharmacist use?

   (A) 15
   (B) 20
   (C) 22.5
   (D) 37.5
   (E) 360

Questions 45 through 47 relate to the following order received by a home infusion pharmacy.

> Morphine sulfate 500 mg in a 100-mL PCA unit to deliver 0.05 mg/min
>
> Dosing to start at 08:00 AM tomorrow.

45. How many milliliters of a commercial morphine sulfate vial (25 mg/mL) is needed to fill this order?

   (A) 10
   (B) 20
   (C) 25
   (D) 30
   (E) 50

46. What flow rate must be programmed into the PCA unit to obtain the desired amount of morphine per minute?

    (A) 0.01 mL/min
    (B) 0.05 mL/min
    (C) 0.1 mL/min
    (D) 0.1 mL/h
    (E) 1.0 mL/min

47. Upon consultation, the prescriber decides to allow bolus PRN dosing of 2 mg with a lockout of 1-hour intervals. Assuming that the patient uses all bolus-dosing intervals, approximately how long will the PCA last?

    (A) <2.5 days
    (B) 4 days
    (C) 7 days
    (D) 10 days
    (E) >14 days

Questions 48 through 52 relate to the following formula for a psoriasis lotion.

Coal tar solution	5 mL
Salicylic acid	
Urea	aa 5%
Triamcinolone acetonide	0.25 g
Alcohol USP	20 mL
Propylene glycol	qs 120 mL

48. What weight of salicylic acid is needed to prepare 1 pt of the formula listed?

    (A) 11.8 g
    (B) 12 g
    (C) 23.7 g
    (D) 24 g
    (E) 25 g

49. What % v/v concentration of alcohol would be listed on the label?

    (A) 8
    (B) 15.8
    (C) 16.7
    (D) 19
    (E) 20

50. The community pharmacy does not have a permit for grain alcohol. Which of the following may be reasonable sources for the 20 mL of alcohol needed for the topical solution?

    I.   38 mL SDA alcohol 50% v/v
    II. 20 mL isopropyl alcohol
    III. 47.5 mL 80 Proof (prf) Vodka

    (A) I only
    (B) III only
    (C) I and II only
    (D) II and III only
    (E) I, II, and III

51. How many milliliters of triamcinolone acetonide aqueous injection (40 mg/mL) could be used to prepare 240 mL of the formula?

    (A) 6.3
    (B) 12.5
    (C) 1.2
    (D) 10
    (E) 15

52. Propylene glycol was purchased at a cost of $24.00 per pound. What is the cost of 100 mL of the liquid? (Specific gravity = 1.04)

    (A) $2.60
    (B) $2.64
    (C) $2.75
    (D) $5.50
    (E) $13.00

53. A pharmacist adds 2 mL of tobramycin injection (40 mg/mL) to 4 mL of tobramycin ophthalmic solution 0.3%. What is the concentration of tobramycin in the final mixture?

    (A) 0.012 g/mL
    (B) 0.015 g/mL
    (C) 0.03 g/mL
    (D) 0.052 g/mL
    (E) 0.092 g/mL

54. A physician requests 1 lb of bacitracin ointment containing 200 U of bacitracin per gram. How many grams of bacitracin ointment (500 U/g) must be used to make this ointment?

(A) 182
(B) 200
(C) 227
(D) 362
(E) 400

55. A total parenteral nutrition (TPN) order requires 500 mL of $D_{30}W$. How many milliliters of $D_{50}W$ should be used if the $D_{30}W$ is not available?

(A) 125
(B) 300
(C) 375
(D) 400
(E) 200

56. How many grams of 1% hydrocortisone (HC) cream must be mixed with 0.5% HC cream if one wishes to prepare 60 g of a 0.8% w/w preparation?

(A) 6
(B) 12
(C) 24
(D) 36
(E) 48

57. How many grams of pure HC powder must be mixed with 60 g of 0.5% HC cream if one wishes to prepare a 2.0% w/w preparation?

(A) 0.90
(B) 0.92
(C) 0.30
(D) 1.2
(E) 1.53

58. How much sodium chloride is needed to adjust the following prescription to isotonicity? (E value for sodium thiosulfate is 0.31.)

Rx	
Sodium thiosulfate	1.2%
Sodium chloride	qs
Purified water	qs 100 mL

(A) 0.37 g
(B) 0.45 g
(C) 0.53 g
(D) 0.31 g
(E) 0.90 g

59. How many milligrams of sodium chloride should be added to the following medication order to maintain isotonicity? "Atrovent Inhalation Solution 0.02% 5 mL + SWF Injection 25 mL. Place in nebulizer ut dict" (Note: Atrovent inhalation solution is isotonic.)

(A) 45
(B) 225
(C) 270
(D) 900
(E) 0 (since sterile water for injection is already isotonic)

60. What is the dissociation factor of calcium chloride in an aqueous solution if only 70% ionization occurs? (Mol. wt. calcium chloride, anhydrous = 111; monohydrate = 147; calcium = 40; chloride = 35.5)

(A) 0.7
(B) 1.4
(C) 2.0
(D) 2.4
(E) 3

61. What is the estimate of the milliosmolarity (mOsm/L) for normal saline (Na = 23, Cl = 35.5)?

(A) 150 mOsm/L
(B) 300 mOsm/L
(C) 350 mOsm/L
(D) 400 mOsm/L
(E) 600 mOsm/L

62. A pharmacist adds 2 g of potassium chloride to 1 L of $D_5W/1/2$ normal saline. What is the estimate of the osmolarity (mOsm/L) of this solution assuming the final volume is 1 L (atomic wt.: sodium = 23, potassium = 39, chloride = 35.5, dextrose = 198)?

    (A) 54 mOsm/L
    (B) 300 mOsm/L
    (C) 405 mOsm/L
    (D) 460 mOsm/L
    (E) 477 mOsm/L

63. A nurse in a nursing home setting mixes 240 mL of a dietary supplement formula (400 mOsm/L) with 250 mL of $D_{10}W$ and 200 mL of water containing 5 g calcium chloride. What is the osmolarity of this solution? (mol. wt. = 111; mol. wt. of dextrose = 180.)

    (A) 280 mOsm/L
    (B) 370 mOsm/L
    (C) 410 mOsm/L
    (D) 470 mOsm/L
    (E) 540 mOsm/L

64. A nursing home patient is experiencing diarrhea from his enteral nutritional solution, which has an osmolarity of 520 mOsm/L. How many milliliters of purified water is needed to reduce 500 mL of this solution to an osmolarity of 300 mOsm/L?

    (A) 290
    (B) 310
    (C) 360
    (D) 500
    (E) 870

65. A 250-mL infusion container contains 5.86 g of potassium chloride (KCl). How many milliequivalents (mEq) of KCl is present? (Mol. wt. of KCl = 74.6)

    (A) 12.7
    (B) 20
    (C) 78.5
    (D) 150
    (E) 157

66. How much elemental iron is present in every 300 mg of ferrous sulfate ($FeSO_4 \cdot 7H_2O$)? (Atomic wt.: Fe = 55.9, S = 32, O = 16, H = 1. Iron has valences of 2 and 3.)

    (A) 30 mg
    (B) 60 mg
    (C) 110 mg
    (D) 120 mg
    (E) 164 mg

67. Approximately how many mEq of iron is present in every 300 mg of ferrous sulfate ($FeSO_4 \cdot 7H_2O$)? (Atomic wt.: Fe = 55.9, S = 32, O = 16, H = 1. Iron has valences of 2 and 3.)

    (A) 1
    (B) 2
    (C) 3
    (D) 4
    (E) 6

68. Calcium chloride ($CaCl_2 \cdot 2H_2O$) has a formula weight of 147. What weight of the chemical is needed to obtain 40 mEq of calcium? (Ca = 40.1; Cl = 35.5; H_2O = 18)

    (A) 0.80 g
    (B) 1.47 g
    (C) 2.22 g
    (D) 2.94 g
    (E) 5.88 g

Questions 69 and 70 relate to the following formula for citrate of magnesia.

Rx	
Magnesium carbonate	15 g
Citric acid (anhydrous)	27.4 g
Syrup	60 mL
Purified water	qs 350 mL

69. How many grams of magnesium is present in every 350 mL dose? (Mg = 24.3, carbonate = 60)

    (A) 2.5
    (B) 4.32
    (C) 6.08

(D) 6.7

(E) 8.6

70. What % w/v of hydrated citric acid could be listed in a formula if the anhydrous citric acid is not available? The hydrated form of citric acid contains 10% water. (Mol. wt.: citric acid anhydrous = 192 g/mol; water = 18 g/mol)

(A) 7.0

(B) 7.8

(C) 8.7

(D) 24.7

(E) 30.4

71. The level of iron impurities in a water sample is 2 mg/L. How is this concentration in terms of ppm expressed?

(A) 0.2

(B) 2

(C) 20

(D) 200

(E) 2,000

72. The concentration of mercury in a water sample is reported as 5 ppm. How is this concentration expressed as a percentage?

(A) 0.00005

(B) 0.0005

(C) 0.005

(D) 0.05

(E) 0.5

73. A medication order in CCU reads "Heparin 20,000 units in normal saline 250 mL. Infuse at 20 units/min." What flow rate in drops per minute should be established if a Buretrol delivering 60 drops per milliliter is used?

(A) 15

(B) 20

(C) 25

(D) 30

(E) 60

74. A pharmacist places 200 mg of a drug into 500 mL of normal saline solution. What is the resulting concentration in terms of μg/mL?

(A) 0.4

(B) 4

(C) 40

(D) 400

(E) 4,000

75. How many grams of glacial acetic acid (99.9% w/w) must be added to 1 gal purified water to prepare an irrigation solution containing 0.25% wt./vol. acetic acid?

(A) 1.2

(B) 9.5

(C) 12

(D) 20

(E) 95

76. A hospital clinic requests 2 lb of 2% HC ointment. How many grams of 5% HC ointment should be diluted with white petrolatum to prepare this order?

(A) 18.2

(B) 27.5

(C) 45.4

(D) 363

(E) 545

77. For how many days will a 20-mL vial of morphine injection (4 mg/mL) last if the home patient is ordered on 3 mg q6h ATC?

(A) 4

(B) 6

(C) 8

(D) 9

(E) 12

78. What is the decay constant (k) of the radioisotope ^{32}P if its half-life is 14.3 days? Assume that radiopharmaceutical decay follows first-order kinetics.

(A) 0.048/d
(B) 0.07/d
(C) 0.097/d
(D) 0.1/d
(E) 0.15/d

79. A radiopharmacist prepares a solution of ^{99m}Tc (40 mCi/mL) at 06:00 AM. If the solution is intended for administration at 12:00 PM at a dose of 20 mCi, how many milliliters of the original solution is needed? The half-life of the radioisotope is 6 hours.

(A) 0.5
(B) 1.0
(C) 1.5
(D) 2.0
(E) 5.0

80. What concentration of the original ^{99m}Tc solution described in Question 79 will remain 24 hours after its original preparation?

(A) 15 mCi
(B) 10 mCi
(C) 7.5 mCi
(D) 5.0 mCi
(E) 2.5 mCi

81. An ointment contains 2,000 units of an enzyme per gram. What will be the drug's half-life if the decomposition rate is calculated to be 50 units per month?

(A) 10 months
(B) 20 months
(C) 28 months
(D) 36 months
(E) 40 months

82. The manufacturer decides to market the above enzyme ointment at the higher strength of 4,000 units per gram. What is the approximate expiration date if a standard of "not less than 90% of labeled claim" is established?

(A) 4 months
(B) 8 months
(C) 10 months
(D) 20 months
(E) 40 months

83. The upper therapeutic drug concentration for a drug is considered to be 40 µg/mL. How is this value in terms of mg/dL expressed?

(A) 0.04
(B) 0.4
(C) 4
(D) 40
(E) 400

Answers and Explanations

Numbers within parentheses at the end of the answers refer to the numbered references that are listed in the front matter.

1. **(D)** The metric system is used exclusively in most nations in the world except the United States. The prefixes in the metric system are based on increasing or decreasing magnitudes of 10, 100, or 1,000. Converting from one set of quantities to another simply requires the movement of decimal points. For example, converting 1 kg to g requires moving the decimal point three places to the right. The metric system has been expanded into the Système International (SI) measuring system that encompasses all types of measures. The major prefixes in the order of magnitude are as follows:

Prefix	Magnitude	Example
mega	$1,000,000 \times$	megagram
kilo	$1,000 \times$	kilogram
—	$1 \times$	gram
centi	$0.01 \times$	centigram
milli	$0.001 \times$	milligram
micro	$1 \times 10^{-6} \times$	microgram
nano	$1 \times 10^{-9} \times$	nanogram
pico	$1 \times 10^{-12} \times$	picogram
femto	$1 \times 10^{-15} \times$	femtogram
atto	$1 \times 10^{-18} \times$	attogram

(23)

2. **(C)** In this example, consider 1 μg as equaling 1,000 ng, thus 100 μg = 100,000 ng. Since 1 mg equals 1,000 μg, 100 μg equals 0.1 mg. If 1 mg equals 0.001 g, 0.1 mg or 100 μg equals 0.0001 g. It may be clearer if one solves this conversion using dimensional analysis

$$100 \text{ μg} \times \frac{1 \text{ mg}}{1,000 \text{ μg}} \times \frac{1 \text{ g}}{1,000 \text{ mg}} = 0.00001 \text{ g.} \quad \textit{(1; 23)}$$

3. **(C)** 2.4 megaunits is 2.4 million units or a total of 2,400,000 units. The final dilution will have a volume of 14 mL.

$$\frac{2,400,000 \text{ units}}{14 \text{ mL}} =$$

171,400 units/mL or 170,000 units/mL. *(1; 23)*

4. **(C)** An increasing number of laboratory test values and drug doses are being reported in terms of millimoles (mM). Weight quantities expressed in molar amounts allow a more realistic evaluation of the actual number of drug molecules present, for example, when comparing salts of a drug. In this problem, the mM/L concentration is converted by recognizing that 1 mol of cholesterol weighs 386 g and 4 mmol equals 0.004 mol.

$$386 \times 0.004 \text{ mol} = 1.544 \text{ g or } 1,540 \text{ mg/L}$$
$$1,540 \text{ mg/L} = 154 \text{ mg/dL} \quad \textit{(1; 23)}$$

5. **(B)** The minimum weight that can be measured on any balance can be determined if the balance's sensitivity requirement (SR) and the acceptable percentage of error have been established. The equation is

$$SR = (\text{minimum weighable amount}) \times (\text{acceptable error}).$$

In this problem, the SR was given as 6 mg and an accuracy of at least 95% or an error of not more than 5% is permissible.

$$6 \text{ mg} = (x \text{ mg}) (5\%)$$
$$6 \text{ mg} = (x \text{ mg}) (0.05)$$
$$x = 120 \text{ mg} \quad \textit{(1; 23)}$$

6. **(B)** 6 mg equals 6,000 μg.

$$6{,}000 \div 250 \ \mu g = 24\times$$

7. **(D)** Use of a child's BSA will usually result in more accurate dosing than the other methods mentioned in the question. *(1; 23)*

8. **(B)** 1 kg = 2.2 lb.

$$140 \ lb \times \frac{1 \ kg}{2.2 \ lb} = 64 \ kg$$

$$64 \ kg \times 2 \ mg \ dose = 128 \ mg \qquad (23)$$

9. **(A)** Neonates have an age span from birth to 1 month of age. Infants are 1 month to 1 year, early childhood is 1 to 5 years, and late childhood is 6 to 12 years. *(23)*

10. **(C)**

$$60 \ lb \times \frac{1 \ kg}{2.2 \ lb} \times \frac{1.2 \ mg}{kg} = 32 \ mg \qquad (23)$$

11. **(D)** Patient weight of 175 lb × 1 kg/2.2 lb = 79.5 kg

$$79.5 \ kg \times 0.5 \ mg/kg = 40 \ mg$$

$$\frac{20 \ mg}{1 \ mg} = \frac{40 \ mg}{x \ mL} \qquad (23)$$

$$x = 2 \ mL$$

12. **(B)** 1 mol of tobramycin = 470 g/L *(23)*

1 mmol/L = 0.470 g or 470 mg or 470,000 μg

1 μmol/L = 470 μg

2 μg/mL = 2,000 μg/L

$$\frac{1 \ mmol}{470 \ mg/L} = \frac{x \ mmol}{2{,}000 \ mg/L} \qquad (1; 23)$$

$$x = 4.25 \ mmol/L$$

13. **(A)** 20 mL × 2% = 0.4 g of pure dye *(23)*

$$\frac{0.4 \ g}{20 \ mL + 250 \ mL} \times 100\% = 0.148 \ or \ 0.15\%$$

$$(1; 23)$$

14. **(D)** There are two factors that may lead to a final concentration slightly lower than the targeted concentration. When aseptically transferring the 20 mL of concentrated dye solution, the technician should inject the dye solution and then draw up 20 mL of the normal saline solution to rinse the syringe of dye solution. Also one must realize that LVPs of 250, 500, and 1,000 mL have volumes greater than the labeled claim. For example, the 250 mL bag of normal saline is likely to have between 260 and 270 mL. Both factors will reduce the final concentration of dye by a small amount. *(1; 13; 23)*

15. **(E)** Because the volume of a standard teaspoon is considered to be 5 mL, the patient in this prescription is receiving four daily doses for a total of 20 mL.

$$\frac{200 \ mg \ codeine}{120 \ mL \ of \ Rx} = \frac{x \ mg \ codeine}{20 \ mL \ of \ Rx}$$

$$x = 33 \ mg \qquad (23)$$

16. **(A)** The weight of codeine phosphate present in each dose is

$$\frac{200 \ mg}{120 \ ml} = \frac{x \ mg}{5 \ mL}$$

$$x = 8.3 \ mg \ per \ teaspoon$$

The relationship between codeine and codeine phosphate is easily seen when viewed as a chemical reaction:

$$\begin{array}{ccc} x \ mg & & (8.3 \ mg) \\ cod. + phosphoric \ acid & \rightarrow & cod. \ phosphate \\ (mol. \ wt. = 299) & & (mol. \ wt. = 406) \end{array}$$

$$x = 6 \ mg \ codeine \ base \qquad (1; 23)$$

17. **(B)** Young's rule relates a child's dose to the child's age.

$$Child's \ dose = \frac{age \ (year)}{(age[year] + 12)} \times adult \ dose$$

$$Child's \ dose = \frac{6}{(6 + 12)} \times 250 \ mg$$

$$Dose = 83.3 \ or \ 85 \ mg$$

Although well intended, rules such as Young's (child's age), Cowling's (age at next birthday divided by 24), and Clark's [weight divided by average weight of an adult (150 lb)] are only rough estimates. Pharmacists should check the literature for individual drug dosing for children. In some instances, the child's dose will be similar to that for the adult. *(1; 23)*

18. **(D)** The nomogram in the USP consists of three parallel vertical lines. The left line is calibrated with height measurements in both centimeters and inches, whereas the right line lists weights in kilograms and pounds. Using data based on the patient's measurements, a line is drawn between the two outside parallel lines. The intercept on the middle line, which is calibrated in square meters of BSA, allows the estimation of the patient's BSA. *(23)*

19. **(D)** In this problem one of two methods could be used, Young's rule or a BSA calculation. Since the BSA is usually more accurate, it is the preferred method. The average adult BSA is estimated to be 1.73 m². A child's dose can be estimated by

$$\frac{\text{BSA (child)}}{\text{BSA (adult)}} \times \text{adult dose} = \text{child's dose}$$

In this question,

$$\frac{0.6 \text{ m}^2}{1.73 \text{ m}^2} \times 200 \text{ mg} = 69 \text{ or } 70 \text{ mg} \quad (1; 23)$$

20. **(E)** Many drugs, especially chemotherapeutic agents, have their dosage expressed as mg/m² of BSA. One simply has to multiply the dose by the specific patient's BSA to obtain the dose.

$$135 \text{ mg/m}^2 \times 1.5 \text{ m}^2 = 202 \text{ mg} \quad (23)$$

Answer (B) of 120 or 117 is incorrect since it involved the use of the surface area equation, which was not needed.

Answer (A) of 110 or 108 is incorrect since it attempted to correct the dose based on the patient's body weight.

21. **(C)** To avoid decimal point errors, one should always include a "leading zero" before decimal points, that is, 0.5 not .5. The correct term of weight measurement is gram, which is abbreviated as g not gm, Gm, or gr. The abbreviation "gr" should be discouraged since one may mistake it for the grain, an outdated apothecary weight. The designation "q.s." is acceptable as the Latin abbreviation for "a sufficient quantity to make." *(1; 23)*

22. **(D)** The median value in a series of numbers is that value in the middle (ie, the number of values lower than the median value is equal to the number of values higher than the median value). The median may not be the same as the average or mean value, which is obtained by adding all of the values together and dividing by the number of values. *(23)*

23. **(A)** The mean value of a series of numbers is obtained by adding all of the values and then dividing by the actual number of values. In this example, the diastolic readings were 70 + 84 + 88 + 90 + 70 = 402 divided by 5 = 80.4. *(23)*

24. **(D)** A SD is calculated mathematically for experimental data. It shows the dispersion of numbers around the mean (average value). One SD will include approximately 67% to 70% of all values, whereas two SDs will include approximately 97% to 98%. *(1; 23)*

25. **(C)** The sensitivity of a test is determined by its ability to detect the presence of the disease. The sensitivity expressed as a percentage is determined by dividing the number of subjects with the detected disease (positive) by the total number of subjects that actually has the disease (positive + false negative). In this example,

80 divided by (80 + 10) = 0.89 or 90%. *(1; 23)*

26. **(B)** The prevalence of a disease is determined by dividing the total number of subjects with the disease—(both those testing positive plus those testing negative but with the disease) by the total population tested. In this example,

(80 + 10) divided by 910 = 0.099 or 10%. *(1; 23)*

27. **(A)** The original dilution would be

$$\frac{100 \text{ units}}{1 \text{ mL}} = \frac{1,000 \text{ units}}{x \text{ mL}}$$

$x = 10$ mL (final volume, of which 1 mL is the volume occupied by the dissolved powder)

If a 120 unit/mL concentration is requested, the new volume will be

$$\frac{120 \text{ units}}{1 \text{ mL}} = \frac{1,000 \text{ units}}{x \text{ mL}}$$

$$x = 8.3 \text{ mL}$$

Since 1 mL is dissolved powder, the remaining 7.3 mL is diluent. *(1; 23)*

28. **(E)** The final volume obtained by using 10 mL of diluent instead of 9 mL is as follows:

10 mL + 1 mL (powder volume in solution) = 11 mL   *(1; 23)*

$$x = 1.3 \text{ mL}$$

29. **(D)** Since alcohol USP contains 95% v/v ethanol.

Alcohol 200 mL × 95% = 190 mL ethanol

Mouthwash 800 mL × 12% = 96 mL ethanol

Total ethanol = 286 mL

286 mL ÷ 1,000 mL = 28.6% v/v

Note: There is a minor error in calculating the final percentage of alcohol since minor volume shrinkage of alcohol will occur due to hydrogen bonding. *(1; 23)*

30. **(C)** The patient is placing one drop in each eye three times a day, thus a total of six drops. This equates to 0.3 mL, since the dropper calibration was 20 drops per milliliter.

$$\frac{20 \text{ drops}}{1 \text{ mL}} = \frac{6 \text{ drops}}{x \text{ mL}}$$

$$x = 0.3 \text{ mL}$$

Since a 4% Pilocar solution contains 4,000 mg of drug per 100 mL.

$$\frac{4,000 \text{ mg}}{100 \text{ mL}} = \frac{x \text{ mg}}{0.3 \text{ mL}} \qquad (23)$$

$$x = 12 \text{ mg}$$

31. **(E)** The body weight will be

$$16 \text{ lb} \times \frac{1 \text{ kg}}{2.2 \text{ lb}} = 7.27 \text{ kg}$$

$$\frac{0.08 \text{ mg}}{\text{kg}} \times 7.27 \text{ kg} = 0.58 \text{ mg/h} \times 12 \text{ h}$$

$$= 7 \text{ mg in } 12 \text{ h}$$

The low dosing of theophylline is correct because the metabolic pathway of theophylline in young babies has yet to develop sufficiently. *(19; 23)*

32. **(D)** First, convert the weight in pounds to kilograms

$$180 \text{ lb} \times \frac{1 \text{ kg}}{2.2 \text{ lb}} = 82 \text{ kg}$$

Second, determine the total daily dose

82 kg × 2 mg × 6 doses = 980 mg   *(23)*

33. **(D)** One hundred milliliters of Clorox will contain 5.25 g of sodium hypochlorite. The final dilution will be 1 qt, which is 946 mL. The ratio strength will be

$$\frac{5.25 \text{ g}}{946 \text{ mL}} = \frac{1}{x}$$

$$x = 180 \text{ or } 1{:}180 \text{ w/v of}$$
$$\text{sodium hypochlorite}$$

In actual practice, Clorox is recommended as a disinfectant for HIV-contaminated equipment when used in a 1:10 dilution. However, this designation refers to 1 mL of Clorox in every 10 mL of final dilution. *(23)*

34. **(E)** Four milliliters of a 4% cocaine HCl solution will contain 0.16 g, or 160 mg, of cocaine HCl (4 mL × 4%), or, by proportions

$$\frac{4,000 \text{ mg}}{100 \text{ mL}} = \frac{x \text{ mg}}{4 \text{ mL}} \quad x = 160 \text{ mg} \qquad (23)$$

35. (D) Use the equation of

$$Q_1 \times C_1 = Q_2 \times C_2$$

$$4 \text{ mL} \times \frac{1}{2{,}000} = x \text{ mL} \times \frac{1}{1{,}000} \quad (20; 23)$$

$$\frac{4}{2{,}000} = \frac{x}{1{,}000}$$

$$x = 2 \text{ mL}$$

36. (B) The dosing regimen for this patient consists of 400 mg of cefazolin every 6 hours. When the pharmacist reconstitutes the 1,000-mg vials, the strength will be 1,000 mg/3 mL of solution.

$$\frac{1{,}000 \text{ mg}}{3 \text{ mL}} = \frac{1{,}600 \text{ mg}}{x \text{ mL}} \quad (23)$$

$$x = 4.8 \text{ mL}$$

37. (E) The original order requested that the solution be infused over a 20-minute time span. Therefore, 100 mL divided by 20 minutes equals 5 mL/min. *(23)*

38. (B) Determine the total time for the infusion by using the relationship of

$$\frac{40 \text{ mEq}}{x \text{ min}} = \frac{0.5 \text{ mEq}}{1 \text{ min}}$$

$$0.5x = 40 \text{ min} \quad (4; 23)$$

$$x = 80 \text{ min}$$

39. (A) First determine the mL/h flow rate to obtain 2 mEq/h.

$$\frac{2 \text{ mEq}}{x \text{ mL}} = \frac{40 \text{ mEq}}{1{,}000 \text{ mL}}$$

$$x = 50 \text{ mL/h}$$

Now determine the equivalent flow per minute

$$\frac{50 \text{ mL}}{60 \text{ min}} = \frac{x \text{ mL}}{1 \text{ min}} \quad (23)$$

$$x = 0.83 \text{ mL/min}$$

40. (B) This calculation may be done by several methods

$$Q_1 \times C_1 = Q_2 \times C_2$$

$$1 \text{ mL} \times \frac{1}{1{,}000} = x \text{ mL} \times \frac{1}{2{,}500}$$

$$\frac{1}{1{,}000} = \frac{x}{2{,}500} \quad x = 2.5 \text{ mL} \quad (23)$$

2.5 mL − 1 mL (original volume) = 1.5 mL

41. (D) Two hundred milligrams dopamine in 500 mL = 0.4 mg/mL. Because 1 mg = 1,000 μg, 0.4 mg = 400 μg; therefore, the final concentration of dopamine will be 400 μg/mL. *(23)*

42. (C)

$$155 \text{ lb} \times \frac{1 \text{ kg}}{2.2 \text{ lb}} \times \frac{5 \text{ mg}}{\text{kg}/1 \text{ min}} = 352 \text{ μg/min}$$

Because the solution concentration is 400 μg/mL, divide the dosage rate by the concentration

$$\frac{352 \text{ μg/min}}{400 \text{ μg/mL}} = 0.88 \text{ mL/min} \quad (23)$$

43. (B)

$$50 \text{ mL} \times 100 \text{ U/mL} = 5{,}000 \text{ U total}$$

$$\frac{10{,}000 \text{ U}}{1 \text{ mL}} = \frac{5{,}000 \text{ U}}{x \text{ mL}} \quad (23)$$

$$x = 0.5 \text{ mL}$$

44. (C)

$$Q_1 \times C_1 = Q_2 \times C_2$$

$$(15 \text{ g})(0.05\%) = (x \text{ g})(0.02\%)$$

$$0.02x = 0.75$$

$$x = 37.5 \text{ g (final weight)}$$

Therefore, 37.5 g − 15 g = 22.5 g *(23)*

45. (B)

$$\frac{500 \text{ mg}}{x \text{ mL}} = \frac{25 \text{ mg}}{1 \text{ mL}} \quad (23)$$

$$x = 20 \text{ mL}$$

46. (A)

$$\frac{0.05 \text{ mg}}{x \text{ mL}} = \frac{500 \text{ mg}}{100 \text{ mL}} \quad (23)$$

$$x = 0.01 \text{ mL/min}$$

47. (B) The maximum volume used per hour will be

$$0.01 \text{ mL/min} \times 60 \text{ min} = 0.6 \text{ mL}$$

plus bolus dosing of 2 mg (0.4 mL) = 1 mL total

Since the total volume in the PCA is 100 mL, it should last at least 100 hours or 4.2 days. *(23)*

48. **(C)**

$$\frac{5 \text{ g salicylic acid}}{100 \text{ mL of lotion}} = \frac{x \text{ g}}{473 \text{ mL of lotion}} \qquad (23)$$

$$x = 23.7 \text{ g}$$

49. **(B)** When concentrations of alcohol are listed on labels, the % v/v is based on absolute alcohol (100% ethanol), although this form of alcohol is seldom used during manufacturing or compounding. Alcohol USP was specified for the formula. Its strength is 95% v/v

$$20 \text{ mL} \times 95\% = 19 \text{ mL}$$

$$\frac{19 \text{ mL}}{120 \text{ mL}} = 15.8\% \text{ v/v} \qquad (23)$$

50. **(B)** Eighty Proof Vodka consists of 40% pure ethanol without additional ingredients, therefore, $Q_1 \times C_1 = Q_2 \times C_2$

$$[x \text{ mL}] [40\% \text{ v/v}] = [20 \text{ mL}]$$
$$[95\% \text{ v/v}]$$

$$x = 47.5 \text{ mL}$$

The other two choices are incorrect, not because of the math but because of their composition. SDA alcohol (specially denatured alcohol) is grain alcohol to which has been added additional ingredients to render it unsuitable for drinking. It could only be used with the permission of the prescriber after the additives have been identified since there are a number of SDA formulas. Isopropyl alcohol is an entirely different chemical and could only be used with the prescriber's permission. *(1; 23)*

51. **(B)**

$$\frac{0.25 \text{ g}}{120 \text{ mL}} = \frac{x \text{ g}}{240 \text{ mL}}$$

$$x = 500 \text{ mg pure triamcinolone}$$

$$\frac{40 \text{ mg}}{1 \text{ mL}} = \frac{500 \text{ mg}}{x \text{ mL}} \qquad (23)$$

$$x = 12.5 \text{ mL of the injection solution}$$

52. **(D)** The mL in 1 lb of propylene glycol can be calculated as

$$SG = \frac{W}{V}$$

$$1.04 = \frac{454 \text{ g}}{x \text{ mL}}$$

$$x = 436 \text{ mL of propylene glycol in 1 lb}$$

$$\frac{\$24.00}{436 \text{ mL}} = \frac{\$x}{100 \text{ mL}}$$

$$x = \$5.50 \qquad (1; 23)$$

53. **(B)** Total amount of pure tobramycin will be as follows:

in ophthalmic solution 4 mL $\times$ 0.3% = 0.012 g
in injection 2 mL $\times$ 40 mg/mL = 0.08 g
Total amount in 6 mL = 0.092 g

$$\frac{0.092 \text{ g}}{6 \text{ mL}} = 0.0153 \text{ g/mL} \qquad (4)$$

54. **(A)** One avoirdupois pound contains 454 g. The total number of bacitracin units required is

$$454 \text{ g} = 200 \text{ U/g} = 90{,}800 \text{ U}$$

$$\frac{500 \text{ U}}{1 \text{ g}} = \frac{90{,}800 \text{ U}}{x \text{ g}} \qquad x = 182 \text{ g} \quad (23)$$

55. **(B)** Five hundred milliliters of $D_{30}W$ will contain 150 g of dextrose while $D_{50}W$ contains 50 g of dextrose per 100 mL.

$$\frac{50 \text{ g dextrose}}{100 \text{ mL of solution}} = \frac{150 \text{ g dextrose}}{x \text{ mL of solution}}$$

$$x = 300 \text{ mL} \qquad (23)$$

Or, this problem may be solved by using the following equation:

$$Q_1 \times C_1 = Q_2 \times C_2$$

$$(x \text{ mL}) (50\%) = (500 \text{ mL}) (30\%)$$

$$x = 300 \text{ mL} \qquad (23)$$

56. **(D)** This problem can be solved by the alligation alternate or simple parts method

1%		0.3 parts
	0.8%	
0.5%		0.2 parts

Thus, the final solution will contain 0.2 parts of the 0.5% HC cream for every 0.3 parts of 1%

HC cream for a total of 0.5 parts. (One may refer to the above parts as 2 parts to every 3 parts for a total of 5 parts.)

$$1\% \text{ HC cream} = \frac{0.3 \text{ parts}}{0.5 \text{ parts}} \times 60 \text{ g} = 36 \text{ g}$$

$$0.5\% \text{ HC cream} = \frac{0.2 \text{ parts}}{0.5 \text{ parts}} \times 60 \text{ g} = 24 \text{ g} \text{ (23)}$$

57. **(B)** Because the amount of 0.5% HC cream is exactly 60 g, the final weight of the cream will be greater when HC powder is added. Therefore, the problem may be solved by the alligation alternate method or by simple algebra

100% HC		1.5 parts
	2%	
0.5% HC		98 parts

$$\frac{60 \text{ g of } 0.5\%}{98 \text{ parts}} = \frac{x \text{ g of } 100\%}{1.5 \text{ parts}}$$

$$x = 0.92 \text{ g}$$

Or, by algebra, let x = weight of 100% HC powder, then

$$(x \text{ g}) (100\%) + (60 \text{ g}) (0.5\%) = (60 \text{ g} + x \text{ g}) (2\%)$$

$$x + 0.3 = 1.2 + 0.02\, x$$

$$x = 0.92 \text{ g} \qquad (23)$$

58. **(C)** Step 1—Determine the amount of sodium thiosulfate in the Rx

$$100 \text{ mL} \times 1.2\% = 1.2 \text{ g or } 1{,}200 \text{ mg}$$

Step 2—Multiply the amount of chemical by its "E" value

$$1{,}200 \text{ mg} \times 0.31 = 372 \text{ mg}$$

(equivalent amount of NaCl)

Step 3—Determine the amount of NaCl needed as if no other chemical was present

$$100 \text{ mL} \times 0.9\% = 900 \text{ mg}$$

Step 4—Subtract contribution by chemical (Step 2) from amount of NaCl (Step 3)

$$900 \text{ mg} - 372 \text{ mg} = 528 \text{ mg}$$

(The amount of NaCl needed to render the solution isotonic.) *(1)*

59. **(B)** Since the 5 mL of Atrovent inhalation solution is already isotonic, the pharmacist has to render the remaining volume of solution (diluent) isotonic.

$$30 \text{ mL} - 5 \text{ mL} = 25 \text{ mL}$$

$$25 \text{ mL} \times 0.9\% \text{ sodium chloride} = 225 \text{ mg}$$
$$(1; 23)$$

60. **(D)** The dissociation factor or constant is usually referred to as the "i" value. It may be determined as

$$i = \frac{\text{number of solute particles in solution after dissociation}}{\text{number of particles before dissociation}}$$

$$CaCl_2 \rightarrow Ca \text{ ion} + 2 Cl \text{ ions}$$

If only 70% ionization occurs

100 molecules $\rightarrow$ 70 Ca ions + 70% (100 $\times$ 2) Cl ions + 30 molecules $CaCl_2$

for a total of 240

$$i = \frac{240}{100} = 2.4 \qquad (12; 23)$$

When describing colligative properties of solutions, the concept of dissociation factor is similar to the van's Hoff "i" values.

61. **(B)** One liter of normal saline contains 0.9% NaCl or 9 g. To calculate the milliosmolarity of the solution, we have the following steps:

Step 1—Determine the moles present.

$$\frac{\text{wt. of chemical}}{\text{mol. wt.}} = \frac{0.9 \text{ g}}{58.5 \text{ g/mol}}$$

$$= 0.154 \text{ mol or } 154 \text{ mmol}$$

Step 2—Multiply the millimoles by the "i" value. The i value is the theoretical number of ions or particles formed by one molecule of chemical assuming complete ionization.

$$154 \text{ mmol} \times 2 = 308 \text{ mOsm/L} \quad (1; 23)$$

62. **(D)** Three chemicals are contributing to the osmolarity.

Potassium chloride 2 g ÷ 74.5 = 0.0268 mol or 26.8 mM

26.8 mM × i value of 2 = 53.6 mOsm

Dextrose 50 g ÷ 198 = 0.253 mol or 253 mM

253 mM × i value of 1 = 253 mOsm

Sodium chloride 1,000 mL × 0.45% = 4.5 g

4.5 g ÷ 58.5 = 0.0769 mol or 76.9 mM

76.9 mM × i value of 2 = 153.8 mOsm

Total in 1 L = 53.6 + 253 + 153.8 = 460 mOsm/L $(1; 23)$

63. **(E)** The final mixture consists of three solutions each contributing to its osmolarity.

(1) 240 mL of supplement formula with osmolarity of 400 mOsm/L.

$$\frac{400 \text{ mOsm}}{1,000 \text{ mL}} = \frac{x \text{ mOsm}}{240 \text{ mL}} \quad x = 96 \text{ mOsm}$$

(2) 250 mL $D_{10}W$ = 25 g dextrose

$$\frac{25 \text{ g}}{180 \text{ g/mol}} = 0.14 \text{ mol or } 140 \text{ mmol}$$

140 mmol × i value of 1 = 140 mOsm

(3) $\frac{5 \text{ g CaCl}_2}{111 \text{ g/mol}}$ = 0.045 mol or 45 mmol

45 mmol × i value of 3 = 135 mOsm

Total mOsm of 96 + 140 + 135 = 371 mOsm in a volume of 690 mL; therefore,

$$\frac{371}{690 \text{ mL}} = \frac{x}{1,000 \text{ mL}} \quad x = 538 \text{ mOsm/L } (1; 23)$$

64. **(C)** One of the most convenient methods of solving this problem is using the following equation:

$$Q_1 \times C_1 = Q_2 \times C_2$$

(500 mL) (520 mOsm/L) = (x mL) (300 mOsm/L)

300x = 260,000

x = 867 mL of final product

Therefore, the amount of water diluent needed = 867 mL − 500 mL = 367 mL. $(1; 23)$

65. **(C)** One equivalent weight of KCl = 74.6 g, therefore,

$$1 \text{ mEq} = 74.6 \text{ mg}$$

$$\frac{1 \text{ mEq}}{74.6 \text{ mg}} = \frac{x \text{ mEq}}{5,860 \text{ mg}}$$

$$x = 78.5 \text{ mEq}$$

Or, the problem may be solved by using the following equation:

$$\text{mg of chemical} = \frac{(\text{mEq})(\text{mol. wt.})}{\text{valence}}$$

$$5,860 \text{ mg} = \frac{(x)(74.6)}{1} \quad (23)$$

$$x = 78.5 \text{ mg}$$

66. **(B)** The formula weight of ferrous sulfate is 278. The amount of iron present in 300 mg of the chemical will be

$$\frac{\text{Atomic wt. Fe}}{\text{Formula wt. salt}} = \frac{55.9}{278} = \frac{x \text{ mg}}{300 \text{ mg}}$$

$$x = 60.4 \text{ mg} \quad (23)$$

Choices (A) or (D) would be obtained if the correct answer was either doubled or halved to reflect the + 2 valence of iron. The valence of iron has no significance in this type of problem because only one atom of iron is present in each molecule of ferrous sulfate.

Choice C assumes that the ferrous sulfate is anhydrous with a molecular weight of 152. This is incorrect, because the 300-mg weight is based on a chemical formula containing seven waters of hydration.

Choice E is the amount of anhydrous ferrous sulfate present in each 300 mg. The question asks for iron (Fe) only.

67. **(B)**

$$\text{mg} = \frac{[\text{mEq}][\text{formula wt.}]}{\text{valence}}$$

$$300 \text{ mg} = \frac{[x \text{ mEq}][278]}{2}$$

$$x = 2.2 \text{ mEq} \quad (4; 23)$$

68. **(D)** One equivalent of calcium chloride = 147 (mol. wt.) divided by 2 (valence of calcium) = 73.5 g and 1 mEq = 73.5 mg. Therefore, 40 mEq is 40 × 73.5 mg = 2,940 mg, which is 2.94 g.

Or, the problem can be solved by the following equation:

$$\text{mg of chemical} = \frac{(\text{mEq})\,(\text{mol. wt.})}{\text{valence}}$$

$$x \text{ mg} = \frac{(40 \text{ mEq})\,(147)}{2}$$

$$x = 2{,}940 \text{ mg or } 2.94 \text{ g}$$

It must be remembered that 40 mEq of calcium combines with 40 mEq of chloride to form 40 mEq of calcium chloride. *(1; 23)*

(A, incorrect)—This answer is obtained if one multiplies the 40 mEq desired by the atomic weight of calcium and then divides by the valence of 2. The use of the atomic weight of calcium is incorrect because the official hydrated calcium chloride is being weighed to obtain the correct amount of calcium. The right answer can be obtained by adding the following step:

$$\frac{0.80 \text{ g (Ca)}}{40 \text{ (atomic wt. Ca)}}$$

$$= \frac{x \text{ g (hydrated calcium chloride)}}{147 \text{ (formula wt. of hydrated salt)}}$$

$$x = 2.94 \text{ hydrated calcium chloride}$$

(C, incorrect)—The answer of 2.22 g is incorrect because it assumes that anhydrous calcium chloride (mol. wt. = 111) was used. However, the problem specified that the official form, which contains two waters of hydration, was available.

(E, incorrect)—The answer of 5.88 g is obtained if one ignores the + 2 valence of calcium. *(23)*

69. **(B)** Magnesium carbonate has the structure of $MgCO_3$ therefore,

$$\frac{\text{magnesium}}{MgCO_3} = \frac{24.3}{84.3} \times 15 \text{ g} = 4.32 \text{ g} \quad (4)$$

70. **(C)** Since the written formula is based on a total volume of 350 mL, reduce the amounts for a percentage formula based on 100%.

$$\frac{27.4 \text{ g (anhydrous citric acid)}}{350 \text{ mL}}$$

$$= \frac{x \text{ g anhydrous citric acid}}{100 \text{ mL}}$$

$$x = 7.83 \text{ g anhydrous citric acid}$$

Since the hydrated form of citric acid contains 10% impurities (water!), an adjustment may be made by

$$Q_1 \times C_1 = Q_2 \times C_2$$

$$[7.83 \text{ g anhydrous citric acid}]\,[100\%]$$

$$= [x \text{ g hydrous}]\,[90\%]$$

$$x = 8.7 \text{ g of hydrated citric acid} \quad (1; 4; 23)$$

71. **(B)** Since the concentration expression parts per million is usually based on 1 g of chemical in 1,000,000 mL of solution, conversion of 2 mg/L will involve

$$\frac{2 \text{ mg}}{\text{L}} = \frac{0.002 \text{ g}}{1{,}000 \text{ mL}} = \frac{x \text{ g}}{1{,}000{,}000 \text{ mL}}$$

$$1{,}000\,x = 2{,}000 \quad x = 2 \text{ ppm} \quad (23)$$

72. **(B)** Mercury is a solid chemical. Thus, the 5-ppm concentration indicates 5 g of mercury per 1,000,000 mL of solution. Therefore, the grams present in 100 mL will be

$$\frac{5 \text{ g mercury}}{1{,}000{,}000 \text{ mL}} = \frac{x \text{ g}}{100 \text{ mL}}$$

$$1{,}000{,}000x = 500 \quad (23)$$

$$x = 0.0005\%$$

73. **(A)** Step 1—Determine the drug concentration present in every milliliter

$$\frac{20{,}000 \text{ U}}{250 \text{ mL}} = \frac{x \text{ U}}{1 \text{ mL}} \quad x = 80 \text{ U/mL}$$

Step 2—Determine the milliliter needed to obtain the concentration requested

$$\frac{80 \text{ U}}{1 \text{ mL}} = \frac{20 \text{ U}}{x \text{ mL}} \quad x = 0.25 \text{ mL}$$

Step 3—Calculate the number of drops needed, based on the administration set being used, to obtain the required volume

$$\frac{60 \text{ drops}}{1 \text{ mL}} = \frac{x \text{ drops}}{0.25 \text{ mL}} \quad x = 15 \text{ drops} \quad (23)$$

74. **(D)** 200 mg = 200,000 µg

$$\frac{200,000 \text{ µg}}{500 \text{ mL}} = \frac{x \text{ µg}}{1 \text{ mL}}$$

$$x = 400 \text{ µg/mL} \quad (1; 23)$$

75. **(B)** One gallon contains 3,785 mL; thus 3,785 mL × 0.25% = 9.46 or 9.5 g.

Because the volume contributed by the acetic acid is insignificant when compared to 3,785 mL, it does not enter into the calculation of the final volume. *(1; 23)*

76. **(D)** Two pounds would contain 454 × 2 = 908 g of ointment. The final preparation would contain 908 g × 2% = 18.18 g of pure HC. Because the available hydrocortisone ointment is 5% strength, one would need

$$\frac{5 \text{ g}}{100 \text{ g}} = \frac{18.6 \text{ g}}{x \text{ g}}$$

$$x = 363.2 \text{ g of the 5\% ointment}$$

Or, using the equation

$$Q_1 \times C_1 = Q_2 \times C_2$$

$$(908 \text{ g}) (2\% \text{ w/w}) = (x \text{ g}) (5\% \text{ w/w})$$

$$x = 363.2 \text{ g} \quad (23)$$

77. **(B)** The total content of the vial will be 20 mL (4 mg/mL) = 80 mg.

The total amount of morphine prescribed per day = 3 mg × 4 (every 6 hours around the clock) = 12 mg. 80 mg ÷ 12 mg = 6.67 days. The nearest answer is 6 whole days.

78. **(A)** First-order half-lives relate to kinetic constant rate values by the following equation:

$$t_{0.5} = \frac{0.693}{k}$$

$$14.3 \text{ days} = \frac{0.693}{k}$$

$$k = 0.048 \text{ per day or } 4.8\% \text{ per day} \quad (23)$$

79. **(B)** Because the time interval between preparation and administration is 6 hours, and the half-life of the radiopharmaceutical is 6 hours, approximately one-half of the original strength has decayed. Therefore, 1 mL of the solution, which now assays at 20 mCi/mL, is needed. *(23)*

80. **(E)** The loss in first-order kinetics is a constant fraction of the immediate past concentration. In this example, the half-life of 6 hours allows a quick comparison of the amount of radioactivity remaining.

Original activity	40 mCi/mL
After 6 h	20 mCi/mL
After 12 h	10 mCi/mL
After 18 h	5 mCi/mL
After 24 h	2.5 mCi/mL *(13; 23)*

81. **(B)** A decomposition expressed in amount per unit of time indicates zero-order kinetics. Thus the half-life time interval will occur when the original concentration of 2,000 units is reduced to 1,000 units. This loss of 1,000 units divided by 50 units/month = 20 months. *(1; 24)*

82. **(B)** The product will be considered expired when the drug level has decreased by 10% from the original 4,000 units. Since 4,000 units times 10% = 400 units, the stability limit is 4,000 minus 400 or 3,600 units. Since 50 units are lost every month, 400 units divided by 50 units/month = 8 months. *(1; 24)*

83. **(C)** Since 1,000 µg = 1 mg and 100 mL = 1 dL, 40 µg/mL = 0.04 mg/mL or 4 mg/dL. This problem may be solved by dimensional analysis: When dimensional analysis is used, all of the units cancel except those appropriate for the final answer.

$$\frac{40 \text{ mg}}{1 \text{ mL}} \times \frac{1 \text{ mg}}{1,000 \text{ mg}} \times \frac{100 \text{ mL}}{1 \text{ dL}} = 4 \text{ mg/dL}$$

$$(13; 23)$$

CHAPTER 3

Pharmacy

When one peruses the definitions of pharmacy as presented by various state boards of pharmacy, one notices an expansion from the traditional definition of "the art of preparing and dispensing drugs" to "the art or practice of preparing, preserving, compounding, and dispensing drugs plus administering drugs and discovering new drugs through research." With the expanding role of the pharmacist in health care, many states include wording allowing the pharmacist to diagnose and prescribe, usually under set protocols.

Today, pharmacy encompasses all aspects of drug preparation and dispensing, as well as evaluation of therapeutic effects in patients. The term "pharmaceutical care" is being used to stress the duty of the pharmacist to ensure that drug therapy produces maximum beneficial outcomes. This chapter includes basic material with which the practicing pharmacist should be familiar in order to dispense drug products successfully and to serve as the resource person to other health professionals and the general public. This includes knowledge of the manufacture and characteristics of the dosage form, trade names and generic names, drug strengths and commercial dosage forms, packaging, dispensing advice, recognition of significant drug interactions, and the selection of over-the-counter (OTC) products including dietary supplements and herbal products. Actually, this chapter is intended to include topics and information not specifically designated in the other books. Subsequent book chapters stress the pharmacokinetics and therapeutic actions of drugs in the body, the selection of specific drugs to treat various diseases, and the evaluation of therapeutic outcomes.

Questions

DIRECTIONS (Questions 1 through 338): Each of the numbered items or incomplete statements in this section is followed by answers or completions of the statement. Select the one lettered answer or completion that is most correct in each case.

1. Where are official standards for individual drugs and chemicals formulated into dosage forms published?

   (A) *United States Pharmacopeia/National Formulary (USP/NF)*
   (B) *USP DI* Volume I
   (C) *USP DI* Volume II
   (D) *USP DI* Volume III
   (E) *PDR*

2. Which agency in the United States is responsible for selecting appropriate nonproprietary names for drugs?

   (A) AMA
   (B) APhA
   (C) FDA
   (D) United States Adopted Names (USAN)
   (E) USP

3. Where may descriptions of the Federal Controlled Substances Act, Approved Drug Products with Therapeutic Equivalence Evaluations, and USP/NF dispensing requirements be found?

   (A) *USP DI* Volume I
   (B) *USP DI* Volume II
   (C) *USP DI* Volume III
   (D) *Facts and Comparisons*
   (E) *PDR*

4. Where may prescription drug descriptions expressed in layperson's terms, useful as handouts for patients, be found?

   (A) *USP DI* Volume I
   (B) *USP DI* Volume II
   (C) *USP DI* Volume III
   (D) *Facts and Comparisons*
   (E) *Remington's Pharmaceutical Sciences*

5. Which of the following is (are) methods used to reduce the cost of medical therapy?

   I. CAM
   II. biosimilar drugs
   III. use of single-source drugs

   (A) I only
   (B) III only
   (C) I and II only
   (D) II and III only
   (E) I, II, and III

6. Which one of the following practices would NOT be classified as "alternative medicine" in the United States?

   (A) allopathy
   (B) chiropractic
   (C) naturopathy
   (D) nutraceutical
   (E) reflexology

7. What is alternative medical practice that stresses the use of extremely small doses of drugs known as?

   (A) folk medicine
   (B) holistic medicine
   (C) homeopathic medicine
   (D) orthomolecular medicine
   (E) faith healing

8. Which one of the following series correctly reflects the rates of disintegration for most commercial tablets?

   (A) coated tablets > sublingual tablets > uncoated tablets
   (B) coated tablets > uncoated tablets > sublingual tablets
   (C) sublingual tablets > coated tablets > uncoated tablets
   (D) sublingual tablets > uncoated tablets > coated tablets
   (E) uncoated tablets > coated tablets > sublingual tablets

9. Which of the following types of tablet coatings is (are) employed to mask the bitter taste of drugs?

   I. enteric
   II. film
   III. sugar

   (A) I only
   (B) III only
   (C) I and II only
   (D) II and III only
   (E) I, II, and III

10. Which of the following is NOT used primarily as a diluent in tablet formulations?

   (A) magnesium stearate
   (B) dicalcium phosphate
   (C) lactose
   (D) mannitol
   (E) starch

11. Which of the following is NOT a function of the lubricant in a tablet formulation?

   (A) improving flow properties of granules
   (B) reducing powder adhesion onto the dies and punches
   (C) improving tablet wetting in the stomach
   (D) reducing punch and die wear
   (E) facilitating tablet ejection from the die

12. Which of the following trademarked dosage forms is enteric coated?
   (A) Kapseal
   (B) Enseal
   (C) Extentab
   (D) Filmtab
   (E) Spansule

13. Which of the following is a sweetener that is widely employed in chewable tablet formulations?
   (A) aspartame
   (B) glucose
   (C) lactose
   (D) mannitol
   (E) sucrose

14. What is starch in tablet formulations used as?

   I. binder
   II. disintegrant
   III. lubricant

   (A) I only
   (B) III only
   (C) I and II only
   (D) II and III only
   (E) I, II, and III

15. The Commission E Monographs are mainly related to which of the following?

   (A) dietary supplements
   (B) herbs
   (C) homeopathic drugs
   (D) nonprescription drugs
   (E) safety of drugs during pregnancy

16. A specific drug is available in both oral tablet and liquid dosage forms. Which of the following statements is (are) most likely to be correct?

    I. The liquid product will have better stability.

    II. The liquid product is more economical to manufacture.

    III. The liquid product is likely to be absorbed faster.

    (A) I only
    (B) III only
    (C) I and II only
    (D) II and III only
    (E) I, II, and III

17. Which one of the following general characteristics is NOT true for alkaloids?

    (A) contain nitrogen in the molecule
    (B) have good alcohol solubility
    (C) have pK_as less than 7
    (D) often exhibit stereoisomerism
    (E) have poor water solubility

18. Which of the following drugs would exhibit good water solubility?

    I. morphine HCl
    II. cocaine
    III. atropine

    (A) I only
    (B) III only
    (C) I and II only
    (D) II and III only
    (E) I, II, and III

19. Which of the following forms of the basic drug haloperidol will have good water solubility?

    I. hydrochloride
    II. lactate
    III. decanoate

    (A) I only
    (B) III only
    (C) I and II only

    (D) II and III only
    (E) I, II, and III

20. Which one of the following dosage forms is most frequently dispensed in the United States?

    (A) oral capsule
    (B) oral solution
    (C) parenteral solution
    (D) oral tablet
    (E) topical ointment or cream

21. Which one of the following chemicals may be included in a drug solution as a chelating agent?

    (A) ascorbic acid
    (B) hydroquinone
    (C) edetate
    (D) sodium bisulfite
    (E) fluorescein sodium

22. Which of the following ions may be effectively chelated?

    I. sodium
    II. lithium
    III. lead

    (A) I only
    (B) III only
    (C) I and II only
    (D) II and III only
    (E) I, II, and III

23. Which one of the following organizations is responsible for Medline?

    (A) USP
    (B) APhA
    (C) ASHP
    (D) FDA
    (E) US National Library of Medicine

24. Although most drugs in pharmaceutical dosage forms decompose following first-order kinetics, exceptions are drugs formulated in which of the following?

(A) capsules

(B) oral solutions

(C) oral suspensions

(D) tablets

(E) suppositories

25. The presence of the following is an early sign of a decomposing epinephrine solution?

(A) brown precipitate

(B) pink color

(C) white precipitate

(D) crystal

(E) red color

26. A pharmacist is assigned the task of evaluating new drug products with respect to pharmacoeconomics, including efficacy and relative cost when compared to other drugs in the same category. Which one of the following reference sources is likely to be most useful for gathering this information?

(A) Drug Facts and Comparisons

(B) Merck Index

(C) Medical Letter

(D) Merck Manual

(E) USP/NF

27. What type of substance does the term "impalpable" refer?

(A) bad tasting

(B) not perceptible to the touch

(C) greasy

(D) nongreasy

(E) tasteless

28. Tartrazine may be included in drug products as which of the following?

(A) antimicrobial agent

(B) coloring agent

(C) sweetener

(D) solubilizer

(E) antioxidant

29. To what aspect of a drug is the term "chiral" related?

(A) chelating ability

(B) eutectic properties

(C) stereoisomerism

(D) partition coefficient

(E) complexation

30. What are advantages of developing chiral forms of a drug?

I. more specific drug action

II. decreased toxicity

III. more economical product

(A) I only

(B) III only

(C) I and III

(D) II and III

(E) I, II, and III

31. Which of the following outcomes are different in crystalline forms (polymorphs) of the same drug?

I. metabolism rates

II. melting points

III. solubilities

(A) I only

(B) III only

(C) I and II only

(D) II and III only

(E) I, II, and III

32. Which of the following is an example of a nonionic surfactant?

(A) ammonium laurate

(B) cetylpyridinium chloride

(C) docusate sodium

(D) sorbitan monopalmitate

(E) triethanolamine stearate

33. The literature lists albuterol with two pK_as of 9.3 and 10.3. Which one of the following descriptions is most appropriate for this drug?

    (A) a weak acid
    (B) a weak base
    (C) a strong acid
    (D) almost 100% in unionized form at a pH of 9.3
    (E) almost 100% ionization at pH of 10.3

34. Patients following low-sodium diets may resort to the use of sodium-free salt substitutes such as NoSalt. What is the major ingredient in these products?

    (A) ammonium chloride
    (B) calcium chloride
    (C) potassium chloride
    (D) potassium iodide
    (E) none of these

35. Potassium supplements are administered in all of the following manners except which of the following?

    (A) IV infusion
    (B) IV bolus
    (C) elixirs, po
    (D) effervescent tablets
    (E) slow-release tablets, po

36. Which of the following statements concerning fluorouracil is not true?

    (A) Its chemical structure is a modified pyrimidine similar to uracil and idoxuridine.
    (B) It is effective only when administered by injection.
    (C) Anorexia and nausea and vomiting are very common side effects.
    (D) The drug interferes with the synthesis of ribonucleic acid.
    (E) Leukopenia is a major clinical toxic effect.

37. A pharmacist associates a "black box warning" with which of the following?

    (A) drug company disclaimers concerning a product
    (B) drug product inserts
    (C) medical devices
    (D) off-label claims
    (E) TV advertising of drugs

38. Which one of the following sequences lists the three types of cautions found in drug product inserts in the order of least serious to most serious?

    (A) contraindication, precaution, warning
    (B) precaution, warning, contraindication
    (C) warning, contraindication, precaution
    (D) warning, precaution, contraindication
    (E) contraindication, warning, precaution

39. Where can a comparison of individual amino acids present in commercial amino acids injection solutions be found?

    I. *Facts and Comparisons*
    II. *Trissel's Handbook on Injectable Drugs*
    III. *Remington's Pharmaceutical Sciences*

    (A) I only
    (B) III only
    (C) I and II only
    (D) II and III only
    (E) I, II, and III

40. The containers used to package drugs may consist of several components and/or be composed of several materials. Which term describes the release of an ingredient from packaging components into the actual product?

    (A) absorption
    (B) adsorption
    (C) leaching
    (D) permeation
    (E) porosity

41. What do gauge numbers used to size hypodermic needles reflect?

    (A) bevel size
    (B) external diameter of the cannula
    (C) internal diameter of the cannula
    (D) length of the needle
    (E) size of the lumen opening

42. The designation, "winged" needles, is most closely associated with which type of injection?

    (A) intradermal
    (B) intramuscular
    (C) intrathecal
    (D) intravenous
    (E) subcutaneous

43. Which of the following dosage forms is (are) are suitable for IV injections?

    I.   sterile solutions
    II. sterile suspensions
    III. sterile vegetable oils

    (A) I only
    (B) III only
    (C) I and II only
    (D) II and III only
    (E) I, II, and III

44. Which one of the following needles is most suited for the administration of insulin solutions?

    (A) 16G 5/8"
    (B) 21G 1/2"
    (C) 21G 5/8"
    (D) 25G 5/8"
    (E) 25G 1"

45. With what is the term "venoclysis" is most closely associated?

    (A) intravenous injections
    (B) intrathecal injections
    (C) intravenous infusions
    (D) intrapleural withdrawals
    (E) peritoneal dialysis

46. With what does the designation "minibottles" refer?

    (A) partially filled parenteral bottles with 50- to 150-mL volumes
    (B) any parenteral bottle with a capacity of less than 1 L

    (C) 10–30 mL glass vials
    (D) prescription bottles with capacities of 4 oz or less
    (E) vials with a capacity of less than 10 mL

47. With what is the term "piggyback" most commonly associated?

    (A) intermittent therapy
    (B) intrathecal injections
    (C) intravenous bolus
    (D) slow intravenous infusions
    (E) total parenteral nutrition

48. Which of the following acronyms refer(s) to parenteral nutrition?

    I.   TPN
    II. TNA
    III. PMN

    (A) I only
    (B) III only
    (C) I and II only
    (D) II and III only
    (E) I, II, and III

49. What is the approximate maximum volume of fluid that should be administered daily by intravenous infusion to a stabilized patient?

    (A) 1 L
    (B) 4 L
    (C) 8 L
    (D) 12 L
    (E) 16 L

50. Although isotonicity is desirable for almost all parenterals, it is particularly critical for which injections?

    (A) intra-articular
    (B) intradermal
    (C) intramuscular
    (D) intravenous
    (E) subcutaneous

51. A suspension is not a suitable dosage form for what type of injection?

    (A) intra-articular
    (B) intradermal
    (C) intramuscular
    (D) intravenous
    (E) subcutaneous

52. Which one of the following designations is most appropriate for a medical order requiring an intravenous bolus injection?

    (A) per IV
    (B) IVP
    (C) IVPB
    (D) po
    (E) KVO

53. When can even distribution of a drug into the blood after an IV bolus injection be expected?

    (A) instantaneously
    (B) within 4 minutes
    (C) in 5–10 minutes
    (D) within 30 minutes
    (E) only after a few hours

54. The quantities of all ingredients present in parenteral solutions must be specified on the label EXCEPT for which of the following?

    I. antimicrobial preservatives
    II. isotonicity adjustors
    III. pH adjustors

    (A) I only
    (B) III only
    (C) I and II only
    (D) II and III only
    (E) I, II, and III

55. What is the usual expiration dating that should be placed on a parenteral admixture prepared in a hospital pharmacy?

    (A) 1 hour
    (B) 24 hours
    (C) 48 hours
    (D) 72 hours
    (E) 1 week

56. Parenteral solutions that are isotonic with human RBCs have an osmolality of approximately how many mOsm/L?

    (A) 20
    (B) 40
    (C) 50
    (D) 150
    (E) 300

57. Which of the following injectables is (are) isotonic with human RBCs?

    I. D_5W
    II. $D_{2.5}W/0.45NS$
    III. D_5W/NS

    (A) I only
    (B) III only
    (C) I and II
    (D) II and III
    (E) I, II, and III

58. The osmotic pressure of a 0.1-mol dextrose solution will be approximately how many times that of a 0.1-mol sodium chloride solution?

    (A) 0.5
    (B) 1
    (C) 2
    (D) 3
    (E) 4

59. Which one of the following parenteral solutions is considered to most closely approximate the extracellular fluid of the human body?

    (A) Dextrose 2.5% and Sodium Chloride 0.45% injection
    (B) Lactated Ringer's injection
    (C) Ringer's injection
    (D) Sodium Chloride injection
    (E) Sodium Lactate injection

60. Which of the following types of injection routes should be limited to volumes 1 mL or less?

I. intramuscular into gluteus maximus

II. intramuscular into deltoid

III. subcutaneous

(A) I only

(B) III only

(C) I and III

(D) II and III

(E) I, II, and III

61. Which one of the following parenterals antibiotics is least suitable for surgical prophylaxis?

(A) cefazolin 1 g IV at induction of anesthesia and q 8 h for up to 24 hours

(B) cefuroxime 1.5 g q 8–12 h up to 24 hours

(C) clindamycin if patient is allergic to penicillin

(D) tetracycline

(E) vancomycin 1 g IV

62. Which is an IM injection site suitable for a small child (<3 years of age)?

(A) gluteus maximus

(B) gluteus minimal

(C) gluteus ultima

(D) ventrogluteal

(E) vastus lateralis

63. Which of the following parenteral routes of administration is (are) considered suitable for heparin sodium injection USP?

I. continuous IV infusion

II. subcutaneous

III. intramuscular

(A) I only

(B) III only

(C) I and II only

(D) II and III only

(E) I, II, and III

64. Which of the following parenteral routes of administration is (are) commonly employed for the administration of insulin USP?

I. continuous IV infusion

II. subcutaneous

III. intramuscular

(A) I only

(B) III only

(C) I and III only

(D) II and III only

(E) I, II, and III

65. Which of the following facts concerning regular insulin is (are) true?

I. Degradation occurs only in the liver.

II. Product is available without a prescription.

III. Drug has a short plasma half-life.

(A) I only

(B) III only

(C) I and III only

(D) II and III only

(E) I, II, and III

66. How is the parenteral system known as "ADD-Vantage" best described?

(A) disposable needle and syringe

(B) premixed minibag of drug solution

(C) two-compartment container

(D) vial attached to a minibag of diluent

(E) burette type of administration set

67. How is the IVAC's controlled-release infusion system (CRIS) best described?

(A) a plastic disposable adaptor

(B) a minipump

(C) a volumetric burette

(D) an implantable catheter

(E) a magnetically controlled infusion device

68. What is an example of an implantable catheter for the administration of parenteral solutions?

(A) Hickman

(B) Foley

(C) Broviac

(D) Port-A-Cath

(E) Port-In-Fuse

69. Which of the descriptions of Pharmacy Bulk Packages is (are) true?

    I. units intended for preparation of sterile parenterals
    II. do not have an antimicrobial preservative
    III. may be used for direct infusion of drugs into patients

    (A) I only
    (B) III only
    (C) I and II only
    (D) II and III only
    (E) I, II, and III

70. How must parenteral containers of potassium chloride concentrate be packaged?

    (A) as single-dose units only
    (B) in vials not greater than 20 mL capacity
    (C) in vials with a capacity of 10 mL or less
    (D) with a black flip-off button
    (E) with a red flip-off button

71. What is the usual maximum volume allowed as a parenteral package for Bacteriostatic Water for Injection?

    (A) 10 mL
    (B) 20 mL
    (C) 30 mL
    (D) 50 mL
    (E) 60 mL

72. In which of the following populations is the antimicrobial agent, benzyl alcohol, of specific danger?

    (A) alcoholics
    (B) neonates
    (C) geriatrics
    (D) pediatrics
    (E) HIV patients

73. Which of the following vitamins possesses antioxidant properties?

    I. ascorbic acid
    II. ergocalciferol
    III. pantothenic acid

    (A) I only
    (B) III only
    (C) I and III only
    (D) II and III only
    (E) I, II, and III

74. Which one of the following parenteral antibiotics is the most stable in an aqueous solution?

    (A) gentamicin sulfate
    (B) amoxicillin sodium
    (C) oxacillin sodium
    (D) tetracycline hydrochloride
    (E) vancomycin hydrochloride

75. Biologicals can be used to obtain either active or passive immunity. Which one of the following pairs is not correct?

    (A) antiserum, passive immunity
    (B) antitoxin, passive immunity
    (C) human immune serum, active immunity
    (D) toxoid, active immunity
    (E) vaccine, active immunity

76. For which population is the vaccine Gardasil recommended?

    (A) females older than 20 years
    (B) females older than 55 years
    (C) females between the ages of 9 and 26
    (D) both sexes older than 20 years
    (E) both sexes younger than 8 years

77. What is the route of administration for tuberculin USP?

    (A) intradermal
    (B) subcutaneous
    (C) intramuscular
    (D) intra-arterial
    (E) interarticular

78. Which of the following is correct about tuberculin syringes?

    I. They are only suitable for administration of TB vaccine.
    II. They are prefilled syringes.

III. They are 1 mL units with 0.05 mL accuracy.

(A) I only
(B) III only
(C) I and III
(D) II and III
(F) I, II, and III

79. All of the following vaccines are intended for administration to children except which of the following?

(A) herpes
(B) MMR
(C) pneumococcal conjugate
(D) rotavirus
(E) varicella

80. Immune serum globulin (gamma globulin) is usually administered by what type of injection?

(A) intradermal
(B) intramuscular
(C) intravenous
(D) subcutaneous
(E) any of the usual methods of injection

81. Pediarix is a combination vaccine for protection against all of the following except?

(A) diphtheria
(B) hepatitis B
(C) hepatitis C
(D) pertussis
(E) polio

82. Which of the vaccines should not be administered to pregnant women?

I. measles
II. mumps
III. rubella

(A) I only
(B) III only
(C) I and III only
(D) II and III only
(E) I, II, and III

83. Which of the following preparations will induce passive rather than active immunity?

(A) tetanus toxoid
(B) botulism antitoxin
(C) typhoid vaccine
(D) mumps virus vaccine, attenuated
(E) cholera vaccine

84. Which description of toxoids is incorrect?

(A) detoxified toxins
(B) antigens
(C) produce permanent immunity
(D) are often available in a precipitated or adsorbed form
(E) produce artificial active immunity

85. The DTP series of injections is intended for administration to which type of patient?

(A) infants
(B) children
(C) children 6 years and older
(D) children and adults
(E) only after puberty

86. Both Adacel and Boostix are examples of the newer Tdap vaccines. How does Adacel differ from Boostix?

(A) It is for children younger than 2 years.
(B) It is administered orally.
(C) It may be used in an older population.
(D) It is intended for a one-time injection only.
(E) There are no differences.

87. Which of the following populations are good candidates for the pneumonia vaccine?

I. geriatrics
II. young adults
III. infants

(A) I only
(B) III only
(C) I and II only
(D) II and III only
(E) I, II, and III

88. What is the usual storage condition specified for biologicals?

    (A) below 2°C
    (B) 2–8°C
    (C) a cool place
    (D) 8–15°C
    (E) room temperature

89. All of the following are viral infections except which of the following?

    (A) influenza
    (B) measles
    (C) mumps
    (D) hepatitis
    (E) typhoid fever

90. Techniques used in the development of "biotechnological drugs" include?

    I. gene splicing
    II. preparation of monoclonal antibodies
    III. lyophilization

    (A) I only
    (B) III only
    (C) I and II only
    (D) II and III only
    (E) I, II, and III

91. Which of the following are used to prepare "targeted drug delivery systems"?

    I. liposomes
    II. nanoparticles
    III. transdermal patches

    (A) I only
    (B) III only
    (C) I and II only
    (D) II and III only
    (E) I, II, and III

92. Most of the recently developed biotechnological drugs are formulated into which dosage form?

    (A) inhalation solutions
    (B) parenteral
    (C) capsules
    (D) tablets
    (E) topicals

93. Which of the following home diagnostic tests incorporates monoclonal antibodies into the testing procedure?

    I. fecal occult blood
    II. ovulation prediction
    III. pregnancy determination

    (A) I only
    (B) III only
    (C) I and II only
    (D) II and III only
    (E) I, II, and III

94. What acronym has been given to describe tablets that quickly dissolve in the mouth with the intent of being swallowed for GI tract absorption?

    (A) ET
    (B) RDT
    (C) SC
    (D) s.l.
    (E) TTS

95. By which mechanism do OraSolv compressed tablets disintegrate?

    (A) acid/base reaction
    (B) effervescence
    (C) inclusion of methyl cellulose
    (D) surfactant activity
    (E) use of a starch disintegrant

96. Which one of the following descriptions best fits units such as Baxter's Intermates?

    (A) elastomeric balloons
    (B) minibags containing preset amounts of a drug
    (C) disposable prefilled plastic syringes
    (D) patient-controlled analgesias (PCAs)
    (E) multidose vials

97. Which of the following is (are) true concerning PCA devices?

    I. Unit is intended to be used only with analgesics.

    II. Patient may be ambulatory when using the unit.

    III. Bolus dosing is possible with the unit.

    (A) I only
    (B) III only
    (C) I and II only
    (D) II and III only
    (E) I, II, and III

98. A hospital pharmacist has reviewed several clinical papers concerning irritable bowel syndrome and is preparing a summary comparing the findings for publication. What term is used to describe this type of review?

    (A) dimensional analysis
    (B) double blind study
    (C) meta-analysis
    (D) peer review
    (E) crossover design

99. A client in a retail pharmacy asks the pharmacist where she might find the new lotion product that contains ecamsule. To which section of the pharmacy should the pharmacist direct her?

    (A) antiaging lotions
    (B) antiacne agents
    (C) insect bite remedies
    (D) sunscreening products
    (E) teeth brighteners

100. The medical intern wishes to initiate iron therapy on a patient who has been undergoing hemodialysis. Which of the following products may be administered by intramuscular injection?

    I. INFeD (iron dextran) injection

    II. Ferrlecit (sodium ferric gluconate) injection

    III. Venofer (iron sucrose) injection

    (A) I only
    (B) III only
    (C) I and II only
    (D) II and III only
    (E) I, II, and III

101. Which of the following parenteral iron products have a black box warning concerning risks of fatal anaphylactic-type reactions?

    I. INFeD (iron dextran) injection

    II. Ferrlecit (sodium ferric gluconate) injection

    III. Venofer (iron sucrose) injection

    (A) I only
    (B) III only
    (C) I and II only
    (D) II and III only
    (E) I, II, and III

102. Which of the following statements concerning iron sucrose injection is (are) accurate?

    I. Indications are similar to those for iron dextran injection.

    II. It may be administered using Z-track injection techniques.

    III. It is indicated for treatment of iron deficiency anemia in hemodialysis patients.

    (A) I only
    (B) III only
    (C) I and II only
    (D) II and III only
    (E) I, II, and III

103. Which one of the following chemicals is an effective and safe drug in the treatment of either diarrhea or constipation?

    (A) activated charcoal
    (B) bismuth salts
    (C) kaolin
    (D) attapulgite
    (E) polycarbophil

104. Simethicone is most likely to be included in what type of OTC product?

    (A) antacid
    (B) cough product
    (C) decongestant
    (D) laxative
    (E) weight control

105. Which one of the following ingredients has been substituted in many OTC antidiarrheal products as a replacement for the adsorbent attapulgite?

    (A) bismuth subsalicylate
    (B) kaolin
    (C) loperamide
    (D) polycarbophil
    (E) methyl cellulose

106. What is the suggested dosing regimen for loperamide 2 mg tablets for diarrhea?

    (A) one tablet every 4–6 hours
    (B) two tablets immediately then one tablet after each loose stool
    (C) one or two tablets every 6–8 hours
    (D) two tablets immediately then one tablet every 6 hours
    (E) one tablet immediately then two tablets every 2 hours

107. What is a common building block for liposomes?

    (A) anionic surfactants plus mineral oil
    (B) nonionic surfactants plus mineral oil
    (C) phospholipids
    (D) polyethylene glycols (PEGs)
    (E) straight chain hydrocarbons combined with phosphoric acid

108. Liposomal dosage forms can be administered by which route(s) of administration?

    I. parenteral
    II. topical
    III. oral

    (A) I only
    (B) III only
    (C) I and II only
    (D) II and III only
    (E) I, II, and III

109. Which of the following parenteral product(s) have been formulated into liposomal dosage forms?

    I. amphotericin
    II. daunorubicin
    III. vancomycin

    (A) I only
    (B) III only
    (C) I and II only
    (D) II and III only
    (E) I, II, and III

110. Which one of the following descriptions is given to Doxorubicin HCl (Doxil) liposomal formula?

    (A) depo
    (B) gelated
    (C) pegylated
    (D) emulsified
    (E) stealth

111. Which one of the following OTC internal analgesics contains magnesium salicylate?

    (A) Bromo-Seltzer
    (B) Doan's Original
    (C) Ecotrin
    (D) Pamprin
    (E) Sinarest

112. Which one of the following is not a characteristic of dextromethorphan as a cough suppressant?

    (A) as effective as codeine on a wt/wt basis
    (B) does not cause respiratory depression
    (C) is nonaddicting
    (D) doses of 10–15 mg suppress coughing for at least 4 hours
    (E) maximum daily adult dose is 30 mg

113. Which one of the following is NOT true of calcium carbonate as an antacid?

   (A) some patients may develop hypercalcemia
   (B) capacity for acid neutralization is poor
   (C) may cause constipation
   (D) may induce gastric hypersecretion
   (E) prolonged use may induce renal calculi and decreased renal function

114. Which of the following products contain calcium carbonate as the active ingredient?

   I. Basaljel capsules
   II. Rolaids chewable tablets
   III. Titralac chewable tablets

   (A) I only
   (B) III only
   (C) I and II only
   (D) II and III only
   (E) I, II, and III

115. Which one of the following antacid products is a chemical combination of aluminum and magnesium hydroxides?

   (A) Gelusil
   (B) Maalox
   (C) Mylanta
   (D) Riopan
   (E) Tums

116. Which of the following drugs have label warnings against their use during pregnancy, especially during the last trimester?

   I. acetaminophen
   II. aspirin
   III. ibuprofen

   (A) I only
   (B) III only
   (C) I and II only
   (D) II and III only
   (E) I, II, and III

117. Which one of the following statements concerning bisacodyl is not true?

   (A) Laxative action occurs within 6 hours after oral administration.
   (B) Action of the suppositories occurs within 1 hour of insertion.
   (C) Suppositories may cause rectal irritation with continued administration.
   (D) Tablets should be swallowed whole.
   (E) Tablets should be administered with milk to avoid gastric irritation.

118. Which one of the following OTC products does not contain bisacodyl as the active ingredient?

   (A) Correctol
   (B) ExLax, Regular Strength
   (C) ExLax, Ultra
   (D) Carter's Laxative
   (E) Fleet Stimulant Laxative

119. Which one of the following statements concerning tablet dissolution is not true?

   (A) Disintegration precedes dissolution.
   (B) In vivo disintegration is usually a good predictor of dissolution.
   (C) Changing a drug's crystalline state may change dissolution rates.
   (D) Increasing tablet compression will increase dissolution rates.
   (E) Micronization of drug powder will decrease dissolution times.

120. A product label indicates storage in a refrigerator. Which of the following condition is most appropriate for the product?

   (A) a location held between 0°C and 4°C
   (B) a cold place held between 2°C and 8°C
   (C) any place with temperature between 0°C and 32°F
   (D) an air-conditioned room with temperature below 32°C
   (E) a freezer

121. A patient requests a container of Abreva. In which section of a pharmacy would this product most likely be stocked?

    (A) cold sore remedies
    (B) cough products
    (C) with the prescription drugs
    (D) in the refrigerator of the prescription department
    (E) vitamins

122. Aspartame is included in some drug products as a (an)

    (A) nutrient
    (B) vitamin
    (C) solubilizer
    (D) sweetener
    (E) stimulant

123. The term "circadian rhythm" refers to which of the following?

    (A) irregular heart beats
    (B) biological events that occur in 1-month intervals
    (C) normal consequential heart beat
    (D) cycles of approximately 24 hours
    (E) breathing patterns

124. Which antihypertensive drug product is based on circadian rhythm?

    (A) Catapres (clonidine)
    (B) Covera-HS (verapamil)
    (C) Aldomet (methyldopa)
    (D) Monopril (fosinopril)
    (E) Vasotec (enalapril)

125. Which of the following properties is desirable in a pharmaceutical suspension?

    I. caking
    II. pseudoplastic flow
    III. thixotropy

    (A) I only
    (B) III only

    (C) I and II only
    (D) II and III only
    (E) I, II, and III

126. Which of the following are characteristics of inhalation aerosol dosage forms?

    I. avoid first-pass effect
    II. rapid onset of action
    III. can administer large amounts of drug to intended site

    (A) I only
    (B) III only
    (C) I and II only
    (D) II and III only
    (E) I, II, and III

127. Which of the following internal analgesic products contain ketoprofen?

    I. Actron
    II. Aleve
    III. Nuprin

    (A) I only
    (B) III only
    (C) I and II only
    (D) II and III only
    (E) I, II, and III

128. Burns are classified according to relative severity. What are characteristics of a first-degree burn?

    (A) erythema, pain, no blistering
    (B) erythema, pain, blistering
    (C) blisters, pain, skin will regenerate
    (D) no blisters, leathery appearance of skin, skin grafting necessary
    (E) blackened skin, danger of deep infection

129. Which one of the following statements concerning dextranomer (Debrisan by Johnson & Johnson) is not correct?

    (A) aids in the removal of wound exudates
    (B) can be used to treat decubitus ulcers
    (C) consists of spherical hydrophilic beads

(D) is effective in the healing of both secreting and nonsecreting wounds

(E) must be physically removed after treatment

130. Which of the following local anesthetics should not be suggested by the pharmacist to remedy sunburns?

    I. benzocaine

    II. lidocaine

    III. phenol

(A) I only

(B) III only

(C) I and II only

(D) II and III only

(E) I, II, and III

131. For effectiveness as a local anesthetic, the level of benzocaine in a topical preparation should be at least of what percentage?

(A) 0.1

(B) 1.0

(C) 2.0

(D) 5.0

(E) 25

Questions 132 through 134
Alcohol has many pharmaceutical uses and is available in several concentrations. MATCH the lettered concentration (%V/V) with the associated numbered official product.

(A) 49%

(B) 70%

(C) 92%

(D) 95%

(E) 100%

132. Alcohol USP

133. Diluted alcohol

134. Rubbing alcohol

135. Which one of the following statements concerning allergic reactions to insect bites and stings is NOT true?

(A) Cross-sensitization to bites of different insects (ants, wasps, bees, etc) can be expected.

(B) Death may occur due to anaphylactic reaction.

(C) The initial systemic reaction will usually occur within 20 minutes of the time of the bite.

(D) The toxicity of the venom is the prime cause of the severe reaction or death.

(E) Subsequent sting episodes usually cause more severe reactions than the earlier stings.

136. Which one of the following is not included in emergency insect sting and bite kits?

(A) antiseptic pads

(B) antihistamines

(C) epinephrine HCl injection

(D) tourniquet

(E) tweezers

137. Lotions with high SPFs are intended to prevent which one of the following conditions?

(A) hidrosis

(B) melanogenesis

(C) pruritus

(D) Sjogren syndrome

(E) skin cell damage

138. Which one of the following chemicals is used as a sunscreening agent?

(A) aloe

(B) ecamsule

(C) liquid petrolatum

(D) milk thistle

(E) white petrolatum

139. Pamabrom is present in certain OTC products as a (an)?

(A) analgesic

(B) diuretic

(C) antirheumatic

(D) sedative

(E) mild stimulant

140. Which one of the following procedures or ingredients has been recognized by the FDA for the removal of ear cerumen?

    (A) carbamide peroxide
    (B) diluted acetic acid
    (C) cotton tips wetted with warm water
    (D) cotton tips wetted with alcohol
    (E) vinegar

141. Which one of the following procedures would NOT improve the absorption of a drug into the skin?

    (A) applying the ointment and covering the area with an occlusive bandage or Saran wrap
    (B) incorporating an oil-soluble drug in PEG ointment rather than white ointment
    (C) applying the medicated ointment on the back of the hand rather than on the palms
    (D) increasing the concentration of the active drug in the ointment bases
    (E) using an ointment base in which the active drug has excellent solubility

142. Melatonin is available in some products as a (an)?

    (A) amino acid supplement
    (B) sleep aid
    (C) digestant
    (D) noncaloric sweetener
    (E) coloring agent

143. Which of the following is the most appropriate procedure for using Melatonin to prevent jet lag?

    (A) Take the drug for 1 week before flying.
    (B) Take the drug daily for 3 days before flying.
    (C) Take the drug daily for 3 days before and 3 days after flying.
    (D) Take a large dose of the drug the morning of the flight.
    (E) Start taking the drug after arriving at the new time zone.

144. What do the most commercial vaginal suppositories use as a base?

    (A) beeswax
    (B) cocoa butter
    (C) glycerin
    (D) glycerinated gelatin
    (E) PEGs

145. Which one of the following diluents is usually used for compressed vaginal tablet formulation?

    (A) lactose
    (B) starch
    (C) sucrose
    (D) talc
    (E) glucose

146. Which one of the following is not a characteristic of rectal drug administration?

    (A) neutral pH of colon fluids lessens possible drug inactivation by stomach acidity
    (B) drugs may avoid first-pass hepatic inactivation
    (C) drugs intended for systemic activity can be administered
    (D) the release and absorption of drugs is predictable
    (E) irritating drugs have less effect on the rectum than on the stomach

147. Which of the following vaginal suppository products have contraceptive properties?

    I. Norforms
    II. Terazol
    III. Semicid

    (A) I only
    (B) III only
    (C) I and II only
    (D) II and III only
    (E) I, II, and III

148. Carbomers may be included in a topical product as?

    (A) antimicrobial preservatives
    (B) buffers

(C) penetration enhancers

(D) sweeteners

(E) thickening agents

149. Colligative properties are useful in determining?

(A) tonicity

(B) pH

(C) solubility

(D) sterility

(E) stability

150. The colligative properties of a solution are related to?

(A) total number of solute particles

(B) pH

(C) number of ions

(D) number of unionized molecules

(E) the ratio of the number of ions to the number of molecules

151. Which one of the following values must be similar for a solution to be considered isotonic with blood?

(A) total salt content

(B) pH

(C) fluid pressure

(D) osmotic pressure

(E) level of sodium chloride present

152. What may mixing a hypertonic solution with RBCs cause to happen to the RBCs?

(A) bursting

(B) chelating

(C) crenation

(D) hemolysis

(E) hydrolysis

153. Sodium chloride equivalents are used to estimate the amount of sodium chloride needed to render a solution isotonic. The sodium chloride equivalent or "E" value may be defined as which of the following?

(A) amount of sodium chloride that is theoretically equivalent to 1 g of a specified chemical

(B) amount of a specified chemical theoretically equivalent to 1 g of sodium chloride

(C) milliequivalents of sodium chloride needed to render a solution isotonic

(D) weight of a specified chemical that will render a solution isotonic

(E) percent sodium chloride needed to make a solution isotonic

154. Which one of the following reference sources has the most extensive listings of sodium chloride equivalents and freezing point depression values?

(A) *Merck Manual*

(B) *Merck Index*

(C) *Remington*

(D) *USP/NF*

(E) *USP DI*

155. What is a second method commonly used for adjusting solutions to isotonicity?

(A) boiling point elevation

(B) blood coagulation time

(C) freezing point depression

(D) milliequivalent calculation

(E) refractive index

156. Evaluate the following two statements: (1) All aqueous solutions that freeze at $-0.52°C$ are isotonic with RBCs. (2) They are also iso-osmotic with each other. Which of the following is correct about these statements?

(A) Both statements are true.

(B) Both statements are false.

(C) The first statement is true but the second is false.

(D) The second statement is true but the first is false.

(E) There is no correlation between freezing points and osmotic pressures of solutions.

157. What is the approximate capacity of the human eye for instilled ophthalmic drops?

    (A) 0.01–0.05 mL
    (B) 0.1 mL
    (C) 0.5 mL
    (D) 1.0 mL
    (E) 2.0 mL

158. Which one of the following has not been included in ophthalmic solutions as viscosity builders?

    (A) hydroxypropylmethylcellulose
    (B) polyvinyl alcohol
    (C) polyvinylpyrrolidone
    (D) methylcellulose
    (E) Veegum

159. What is the main reason for including methylcellulose and similar agents in ophthalmic solutions?

    (A) increase drop size
    (B) increase ocular contact time
    (C) reduce inflammation of the eye
    (D) reduce tearing during instillation of the drops
    (E) reduce drop size

160. In which ophthalmic solution would the presence of *Pseudomonas aeruginosa* be particularly dangerous?

    (A) atropine sulfate
    (B) fluorescein sodium
    (C) pilocarpine hydrochloride
    (D) silver nitrate
    (E) zinc sulfate

161. Which microorganism has resulted in ophthalmic infections in patients using contact lens solutions?

    (A) *Acanthamoeba*
    (B) *Aspergillus*
    (C) *Escherichia*
    (D) *Helicobacter*
    (E) *Trichophyton*

162. Which combination of preservatives appears to be most effective for ophthalmic use?

    (A) benzalkonium chloride and edetate
    (B) benzalkonium chloride and chlorobutanol
    (C) chlorobutanol and EDTA
    (D) methyl and propyl paraben
    (E) phenylmercuric nitrate and phenylethyl alcohol

163. Which of the following ingredients may be present in soft contact lens cleaning products to remove protein buildup?

    I. benzalkonium chloride
    II. subtilisin
    III. papain

    (A) I only
    (B) III only
    (C) I and II only
    (D) II and III only
    (E) I, II, and III

164. What does the presence of sodium bisulfite in a drug solution imply about the drug?

    (A) it has poor water solubility
    (B) it is heat labile
    (C) it is susceptible to oxidation
    (D) alkaline media is required
    (E) it will sustain growth of microorganisms

165. Which one of the following side effects occurs in some individuals who are sensitive to bisulfites?

    (A) difficulty in breathing
    (B) a dry cough
    (C) diarrhea
    (D) dizziness
    (E) upset stomach

166. Which of the following descriptions is (are) correct concerning the sterilization by membrane filtration of an extemporaneously prepared solution?

    I. suitable for heat labile drug solutions
    II. convenient for sterilizing small volumes

III. greater assurance of sterility than using autoclaving

(A) I only
(B) III only
(C) I and II only
(D) II and III only
(E) I, II, and III

167. Which of the following methods is (are) suitable for an eye clinic to sterilize 15 mL of a heat stable solution packaged in glass bottles?

I. exposure to ethylene oxide gas
II. steam autoclaving
III. membrane filtration

(A) I only
(B) III only
(C) I and II only
(D) II and III only
(E) I, II, and III

168. What is the prime reason why pharmaceutical companies will utilize a lyophilized powder in a parenteral vial?

(A) enhance the solubility of the active drug
(B) increase the rate of dissolution of the active drug
(C) increase the stability of the drug
(D) improve the bioavailability of the drug
(E) reduce the production cost

169. Which one of the following ingredients may be included in lyophilized products as a bulking agent?

(A) benzalkonium chloride
(B) mannitol
(C) magnesium oxide
(D) aspartame
(E) zinc chloride

170. What purpose does benzyl alcohol serve in some parenteral solutions?

(A) antimicrobial preservative
(B) antioxidant
(C) chelating agent

(D) buffering agent
(E) tonicity adjuster

171. Which one of the following is true about pH mathematically?

(A) the log of the hydroxyl ion concentration
(B) the negative log of the hydroxyl ion concentration
(C) the log of the hydronium ion concentration
(D) the negative log of the hydronium ion concentration
(E) none of the above

172. Data required to determine the pH of a buffer system include which of the following?

I. molar concentration of the weak acid present
II. the pK_a of the weak acid
III. the volume of solution present

(A) I only
(B) III only
(C) I and II only
(D) II and III only
(E) I, II, and III

173. pH is equal to pK_a at which of the following?

(A) pH 1
(B) pH 7
(C) the neutralization point
(D) the end point
(E) the half-neutralization point

Answer questions 174 through 177 by referring to the following table as necessary.

TABLE OF pK_a VALUES FOR ACIDS

Acid	pK_a
Acetic	4.76
Acetylsalicylic	3.49
Boric	9.24
Lactic	3.86
Salicylic	2.97

174. Which one of the following acids would have the greatest degree of ionization in water?

(A) acetic
(B) boric
(C) hydrochloric
(D) lactic
(E) salicylic

175. Which one of the following acids would be considered the weakest (with the least amount of ionization) in water?

(A) acetic
(B) acetylsalicylic
(C) boric
(D) lactic
(E) salicylic

176. To prepare a buffer system with the greatest buffer capacity at a pH of 4.0, one would use which one of the following acids?

(A) acetic
(B) acetylsalicylic
(C) boric
(D) lactic
(E) salicylic

177. A pharmacist prepares a buffer system by mixing 1 dL of 0.005 mol boric acid with 1 dL of 0.05 mol sodium borate in sufficient water to make 1 L. What will be the approximate pH of this solution?

(A) 8.24
(B) 9.24
(C) 10.24
(D) <8.0
(E) >10.5

178. Ibuprofen has a pK_a of 5.5. If the pH of a patient's urine is 7.5, what would be the ratio of disassociated to undisassociated drug?

(A) 2:1
(B) 100:1
(C) 20:1

(D) 1:2
(E) 1:100

179. A patient has consumed a large number of aspirin tablets. The pH of her urine is 4.5. What percentage of aspirin is present in the unionized form if the pK_a of aspirin is 3.5?

(A) 10
(B) 20
(C) 50
(D) 90
(E) 100

180. Which of the following are characteristics of drugs intended for formulation into sustained-release dosage forms?

  I. usually given in doses of 500 mg t.i.d.
 II. intended for treatment of chronic conditions
III. have a high therapeutic index

(A) I only
(B) III only
(C) I and II only
(D) II and III only
(E) I, II, and III

181. Drugs with which one of the following half-lives are the best candidates for oral sustained-release formulations?

(A) <1 hour
(B) 1–2 hours
(C) 4–8 hours
(D) 12–16 hours
(E) >16 hours

182. Which of the following trademarked sustained-release systems are based on encapsulated drug particles that will dissolve at various rates?

  I. Sequels
 II. Spansules
III. Extentabs

(A) I only
(B) III only

(C) I and II only

(D) II and III only

(E) I, II, and III

183. The USP has established requirements for the amount of active ingredient in dosage forms. Unless otherwise specified in the monograph what is the extreme lowest limit below labeled claim allowed for an active ingredient in capsules?

(A) 5%

(B) 10%

(C) 15%

(D) 20%

(E) 30%

184. Drug products that utilize the osmotic pressure controlled drug delivery system include?

I. Procardia XL

II. Glucotrol XL

III. Contac

(A) I only

(B) III only

(C) I and II only

(D) II and III only

(E) I, II, and III

185. Which of the following drug products is (are) suitable for sprinkling the contents of the opened capsule onto applesauce before consuming?

I. Depakote

II. Effexor XR

III. Ditropan XL

(A) I only

(B) III only

(C) I and II only

(D) II and III only

(E) I, II, and III

186. According to the USP, the instruction "protect from light" in a monograph indicates storage should be in a (an)

(A) dark place

(B) amber glass bottle

(C) light-resistant container

(D) hermetic container

(E) tight glass container

187. The label for trazodone tablets indicates the presence of yellow ferric oxide. For which one of the following reasons is this ingredient most likely to be present?

(A) prevent oxidation of the active drug

(B) keep the drug in the oxidized state

(C) increase the rate of absorption

(D) give color to the tablet

(E) provide a daily dose of iron

188. The expiration date on a pharmaceutical container states "Expires July 2014." This statement means that by that expiration date, what may the product have lost?

(A) up to 5% of its activity

(B) up to 10% of its activity

(C) at least 10% of its activity

(D) at least 50% of its activity

(E) sufficient activity to be outside USP monograph requirements

189. A pharmacist has reconstituted a powder dosage form to form a solution. Which of the following statement(s) concerning a beyond-use date is (are) appropriate when determining an expiration date for this product?

I. The beyond-use date is identical to the manufacturer's expiration date.

II. The beyond-use date is never more than 10 days for reconstituted products.

III. The beyond-use date for nonsolid dosage forms shall not be greater than 1 year from the date of dispensing.

(A) I only

(B) III only

(C) I and II only

(D) II and III only

(E) I, II, and III

190. A reconstituted drug solution assays at 1.5 mg/mL after 24 hours. What is the first-order reaction rate if the original solution concentration was 2.0 mg/mL?

    (A) 0.2/day
    (B) 0.25/day
    (C) 0.3/day
    (D) 0.33/day
    (E) 0.5/day

191. By storing the above-reconstituted drug solution in the refrigerator, its half-life is extended to 4 days. What will be the concentration of the drug solution (mg/mL) after 12 days?

    (A) 0.25
    (B) 0.5
    (C) 1.0
    (D) 1.2
    (E) 1.5

192. When reconstituted, an experimental biotech drug follows first-order kinetics and has a half-life of 24 hours. If the original solution has a concentration of 10,000 units/mL, how many milliliters should be injected into a rabbit 3 days after the solution was reconstituted if a dose of 2,000 units is desired?

    (A) 1.0
    (B) 1.6
    (C) 2.0
    (D) 3.2
    (E) 5.8

193. For which one of the following categories of chemicals is denaturation a major stability problem?

    (A) amino acids
    (B) benzodiazepines
    (C) catecholamines
    (D) cephalosporins
    (E) proteins

194. Which one of the following chemicals is not suitable for use as an antioxidant?

    (A) ascorbyl palmitate
    (B) ascorbic acid
    (C) butylated hydroxytoluene
    (D) chlorobutanol
    (E) vitamin E

195. What do units expressing radioisotope decay include?

    I. Rad
    II. Curie
    III. Becquerel

    (A) I only
    (B) III only
    (C) I and II only
    (D) II and III only
    (E) I, II, and III

196. How does the decay of radioactive atoms occur?

    (A) at a constant rate
    (B) as a first-order reaction
    (C) as a zero-order reaction
    (D) as a second-order reaction
    (E) at constantly increasing rates

197. Which one of the following forms of radiation has the greatest penetrating power?

    (A) alpha radiation
    (B) beta radiation
    (C) gamma radiation
    (D) x-rays
    (E) ultraviolet radiation

198. Which of the following widely used radioisotopes is considered to be an almost ideal isotope for medical applications and is commercially available as a radioisotope generator?

    (A) ^{131}I (iodine)
    (B) ^{99m}Tc (technetium)
    (C) ^{32}P (phosphorus)
    (D) ^{59}Fe (iron)
    (E) ^{198}Au (gold)

199. What is a radioisotope generator?

(A) pharmaceutical product labeled with a radioactive substance

(B) ion-exchange column on which a nuclide has been adsorbed

(C) ionization chamber

(D) high-energy-yielding radioactive isotope that produces one or more isotopes, emitting low-energy radiation

(E) apparatus in which radioactive isotopes are incorporated into biological molecules

200. A cough syrup is labeled as containing 20% alcohol by volume. Which of the following statements is (are) true?

I. Each 100 mL of syrup contains exactly 20 mL Alcohol USP.

II. There is an equivalent of 20 mL of absolute alcohol present in every 100 mL of syrup.

III. The strength of this product may be expressed as 40 proof.

(A) I only

(B) III only

(C) I and II only

(D) II and III only

(E) I, II, and III

201. Which of the following chemicals is (are) included in topical formulas as sunscreens?

I. benzophenones

II. cinnamates

III. methyl salicylate

(A) I only

(B) III only

(C) I and II only

(D) II and III only

(E) I, II, and III

202. A fair-skinned client claims that he normally begins to sunburn in approximately 30 minutes when exposed to the midday sun. What maximum length of protection could he expect using a sun lotion with a sun protection factor (SPF) of 12?

(A) 1 hour

(B) 2–3 hours

(C) 4–6 hours

(D) 10–12 hours

(E) 24 hours

203. Vehicles for nasal medications should not possess which of the following properties?

(A) an acid pH

(B) isotonicity

(C) high buffer capacity

(D) ability to resist growth of microorganisms

(E) all of the above are important properties; no exceptions

DIRECTIONS (Questions 204 through 208): For each of the following drug trade names, select the dosage strength(s) that is (are) commercially available for oral administration. Use the following response key:

(A) I only

(B) III only

(C) I and II only

(D) II and III only

(E) I, II, and III

204. Singulair

I. 10 mg

II. 20 mg

III. 40 mg

205. Coumadin

I. 5 mg

II. 10 mg

III. 20 mg

206. Prozac

I. 5 mg

II. 10 mg

III. 40 mg

207. Januvia

I. 50 mg

II. 100 mg

III. 250 mg

208. Tricor

    I. 48 mg

    II. 96 mg

    III. 200 mg

209. Which of the following products is (are) combinations of two active ingredients?

    I. Augmentin

    II. Ziac

    III. Zithromax

    (A) I only

    (B) III only

    (C) I and II only

    (D) II and III only

    (E) I, II, and III only

210. What of the following are active ingredients in Percodan include?

    I. aspirin

    II. hydrocodone

    III. acetaminophen

    (A) I only

    (B) III only

    (C) I and II only

    (D) II and III only

    (E) I, II, and III

Questions 211 and 212

MATCH the lettered brand name of anesthetic with the numbered nonproprietary name most closely related to it.

    (A) Marcaine

    (B) Carbocaine

    (C) Novocaine

    (D) Xylocaine

    (E) Tronothane

211. Lidocaine

212. Procaine

DIRECTIONS (Questions 213 through 217): SELECT the brand-name product(s) that may be substituted for the numbered brand-name product when filling a hospital medication order. Assume that a formulary system that allows same drug substitution is in effect.

    (A) I only

    (B) III only

    (C) I and II only

    (D) II and III only

    (E) I, II, and III

213. Avinza

    I. Percodan

    II. Endocet

    III. Kadian

214. Synthroid

    I. Levo-T

    II. Levoxyl

    III. Eltroxin

215. Cardizem CD 120-mg capsule

    I. Dilacor XR

    II. Tiazac

    III. Verelan

216. Coumadin

    I. Hytrin

    II. Sofarin

    III. Panwarfin

217. Vicodin

    I. Oxycontin

    II. Tylox

    III. Zydone

DIRECTIONS (Questions 218 through 303): Each group of items in this section consists of lettered answers followed by numbered questions. Select the lettered answer that is most closely associated with each question. A lettered answer may be selected once, more than once, or not at all.

Questions 218 through 224

MATCH the lettered manufacturer with the associated numbered trademarked dosage form.

(A) Abbott

(B) GlaxoSmithKline

(C) Lilly

(D) Teva

(E) Alza

(F) Pfizer

(G) Schering

218. Filmtab

219. Pulvule

220. Diskus

221. Gradumet

222. Reditab

223. Repetab

224. Oros

Questions 225 through 230

MATCH the lettered biotechnology technique that best applies to the numbered drug.

(A) antisense drug

(B) colony-stimulating factor (CSF)

(C) erythropoietin (EPO)

(D) interleukin (IL)

(E) monoclonal antibodies

225. Humira (adalimumab)

226. Sustiva (efavirenz)

227. Neupogen (filgrastim)

228. Remicade (infliximab)

229. Neumega (oprelvekin)

230. Procrit

231. Recombinant alteplase (Activase) is best described as which of the following?

(A) antisense drug

(B) CSF

(C) proteolytic enzyme

(D) IL

(E) tissue plasminogen activator

Questions 232 through 235

MATCH the lettered dosage strength with its most closely corresponding numbered drug brand name.

(A) 10 mg

(B) 20 mg

(C) 50 mg

(D) 100 mg

(E) 250 mg

232. Zetia

233. Ultram

234. Strattera

235. Ambien

Questions 236 through 240

MATCH the lettered dosage strength with its most closely corresponding numbered drug brand name.

(A) 1 mg

(B) 10 mg

(C) 50 mg

(D) 60 mg

(E) 80 mg

236. Paxil

237. Prilosec

238. Allegra

239. Claritin

240. Zyrtec

Questions 241 through 249
MATCH the lettered generic name most closely corresponding to the numbered drug brand name.

    (A) latanoprost

    (B) atomoxetine

    (C) paroxetine

    (D) pantoprazole

    (E) aripiprazole

    (F) clopidogrel

    (G) esomeprazole

    (H) olanzapine

    (I) valsartan

    (J) zaleplon

241. Xalatan

242. Strattera

243. Abilify

244. Paxil

245. Nexium

246. Plavix

247. Diovan

248. Zyprexa

249. Sonata

Questions 250 through 253
MATCH the lettered trade name most closely corresponding to the numbered generic name.

    (A) Altace

    (B) Avandia

    (C) Plavix

    (D) Diovan

    (E) Novasc

250. Amlodipine

251. Clopidogrel

252. Ramipril

253. Valsartan

Questions 254 through 258
MATCH the lettered antacid ingredients with the corresponding numbered commercial antacid product.

    (A) aluminum hydroxide

    (B) mixture of aluminum and magnesium hydroxides

    (C) mixture of aluminum hydroxide, magnesium trisilicate, and sodium bicarbonate

    (D) calcium carbonate

    (E) sodium bicarbonate

254. Amphojel suspension

255. Alka Selzer tablets

256. Tums

257. Maalox suspension

258. ALternaGEL liquid

Questions 259 through 262
MATCH the lettered drug brand name having the same active therapeutic ingredient as the numbered drug brand name.

    (A) Pentasa

    (B) Calan

    (C) Flovent

    (D) Levoxyl

    (E) Dilacor

259. Asacor

260. Synthroid

261. Flonase

262. Covera HS

Questions 263 through 265
MATCH the lettered generic name with the associated numbered trade name.

    (A) celecoxib

    (B) citalopram

    (C) clonazepam

(D) divalproex

(E) fosphenytoin

263. Celebrex

264. Cerebyx

265. Celexa

Questions 266 through 268
MATCH the lettered trade name of each of the following topical decongestant products with the related numbered nonproprietary name.

(A) Benzedrex

(B) Afrin

(C) Privine

(D) Neo-Synephrine Extra

(E) Otrivin

266. Phenylephrine

267. Xylometazoline

268. Oxymetazoline

Questions 269 through 272
MATCH the lettered vitamin B numbers with the correct nonproprietary name.

(A) vitamin B_1

(B) vitamin B_2

(C) vitamin B_6

(D) vitamin B_{10}

(E) vitamin B_{12}

269. Cyanocobalamin

270. Pyridoxine

271. Riboflavin

272. Thiamine

273. A patient presents a prescription for vitamin B_{12} 1 mg/mL, Dispense 1 vial with the directions: "0.5 mL IM when needed." Which of the following information should the pharmacist communicate to the patient?

I. The vial must be stored in the refrigerator.

II. Discard the vial if the color of the solution appears to be pink or red.

III. Please clarify with the prescriber as to the frequency of administration.

(A) I only

(B) III only

(C) I and II only

(D) II and III only

(E) I, II, and III

274. Which one of the following oils has not been utilized as solvents for parenteral dosage forms?

(A) castor

(B) cottonseed

(C) mineral

(D) peanut

(E) sesame

Questions 275 through 278
MATCH the lettered manufacturer with the associated numbered parenteral syringe system that it markets.

(A) Novo Nordisk

(B) Pfizer

(C) Roche

(D) GlaxoSmithKline

(E) Hospira

275. FlexPEN

276. Isoject

277. Carpuject

278. STATdose

279. A customer questions the purpose of stevia as an ingredient in a cough product.
The pharmacist should explain that its main purpose is as a (an)

(A) antimicrobial preservative

(B) antioxidant

(C) solvent enhancer

(D) sweetener

(E) thickening agent

Questions 280 through 281
MATCH the lettered manufacturer with the associated numbered parenteral container system that it manufactures.

(A) Abbott
(B) Baxter
(C) Lilly
(D) McGaw
(E) Wyeth-Ayerst

280. Lifecare

281. Viaflex

Questions 282 through 285
MATCH the lettered term concerning hypodermic needles with the associated numbered description.

(A) bevel
(B) cannula
(C) hub
(D) heel of bevel
(E) lumen

282. Extension of needle that fits onto the syringe

283. Portion of needle that is ground for sharpness

284. Shaft portion of the needle

285. The hole in the needle

Questions 286 through 289
As a pharmacist you may be asked for advice in selecting a suitable product for a skin condition. MATCH the lettered OTC ointment with the most appropriate numbered request.

(A) calamine 10%
(B) hydrogen peroxide 2%
(C) coal tar 2%
(D) ichthammol 10%
(E) salicylic acid 17%

286. To treat inflammation and boils

287. An astringent/protective

288. To treat a wart on the finger

289. To treat a mild case of psoriasis

DIRECTIONS (Questions 290 through 293): It is often desirable to formulate a dosage form so that its pH approximates that of the area to which it is administered. MATCH the lettered pH value that is nearest to the pH usually found in the numbered body areas. Answers may be used once, more than once, or not at all.

(A) 4.0–4.5
(B) 5.5
(C) 6.4
(D) 7.0
(E) 7.4

290. blood

291. eye

292. skin

293. vagina

Questions 294 through 298
MATCH the lettered formulation design that best describes the mechanism of release for each of the following delayed, extended, or sustained-release drug products.

(A) enteric-coated granules in a capsule
(B) drug microencapsulated with celluloses
(C) coated pellets in a capsule with an immediate release followed by slower release
(D) drug impregnated in an inert, porous, plastic matrix
(E) osmotic pump system

294. Compazine Spansule

295. Desoxyn Gradumet

296. Allegra-D

297. K-Dur

298. Prilosec Delayed-Release

Questions 299 through 303
MATCH the numbered herb with its most appropriate lettered therapeutic use.

(A) mild sedative

(B) improve memory

(C) reduce severity of a cold or virus infection

(D) improve urinary flow

(E) reduce GI spasms

299. Echinacea

300. Ginkgo biloba

301. St. John's wort

302. Saw palmetto

303. Valerian

304. Advantages of transdermal drug delivery systems include

  I. avoids first-pass effect

  II. improves patient compliance

  III. suitable for drugs with relatively short half-lives

(A) I only

(B) III only

(C) I and II only

(D) II and III only

(E) I, II, and III

305. All of the following drugs are available as transdermal drug dosage forms EXCEPT

(A) scopolamine

(B) estradiol

(C) bupropion

(D) fentanyl

(E) testosterone

306. Which one of the following ranges of pH is most suitable for an extemporaneously prepared nasal solution?

(A) <4.0

(B) 4.0–5.5

(C) 5.5–7.5

(D) 7.5–8.0

(E) >8.0

Questions 307 through 312
A community pharmacist is presenting a talk at a senior citizens center. How would she answer each of the following questions from the audience?

307. Why has my physician suggested that I take daily doses of Coenzyme Q10?

(A) as a blood thinner

(B) prevent or treat congestive heart failure

(C) improve short-term memory

(D) help prevent respiratory infections

(E) aid in digestion

308. What would you suggest to reduce my recurring tendency for urinary tract infections (UTIs)?

  I. daily dose of 500 mg TMZ

  II. daily dosing with penicillin VK 500 mg

  III. drinking 10 oz cranberry juice daily

(A) I only

(B) III only

(C) I and II only

(D) II and III only

(E) I, II, and III

309. What are the possible advantages of taking garlic on a daily basis?

  I. counteract hyperlipidemia

  II. for relieving hypertension

  III. prevention of colds due to its antioxidant properties

(A) I only

(B) III only

(C) I and II only

(D) II and III only

(E) I, II, and III

310. An elderly gentleman has been taking the expensive drug, Proscar, and has heard that there is an herb with similar activity. To which of the following drugs is he likely referring?

    (A) cranberry juice
    (B) garlic
    (C) ginseng
    (D) gingko
    (E) saw palmetto

311. A nursing home resident complains of chronic constipation, which is only occasionally relieved by a mail-order herbal mixture. What should the pharmacist suggest?

    (A) increase the dose of the present product
    (B) switch to a bulk-forming laxative
    (C) switch to a senna product such as Senokot
    (D) switch to biscodyl tablets
    (E) use a tablespoonful of mineral oil each day

312. Another older woman is confused about the meaning of the "C" impressed on her Zyrtec tablet. This letter represents which of the following?

    (A) Tablet contains codeine.
    (B) Tablet is chewable.
    (C) Active ingredient is cetirizine.
    (D) Product is intended for children.
    (E) Strength of active ingredient is 100 mg.

313. Potential advantage(s) of valerian as a sleep aid include which of the following?

    I.   no residual morning effects
    II. safe during pregnancy
    III. may be safely combined with prescription sedatives such as Ambien or Sonata

    (A) I only
    (B) III only
    (C) I and II only
    (D) II and III only
    (E) I, II, and III

314. Ginger root has been shown to be effective in?

    (A) the treatment of nausea or motion sickness
    (B) reducing bronchial spasms
    (C) treating constipation
    (D) treating diarrhea
    (E) reducing blood pressure

315. Which one of the following herbals is classified as an adaptogen?

    (A) cassia
    (B) eleuthero
    (C) hawthorn
    (D) ginger
    (E) milk thistle

316. Which one of the following herbals is believed to possess hepatoprotective effects?

    (A) garlic
    (B) ginger
    (C) milk thistle
    (D) ginkgo biloba
    (E) peppermint

317. Which one of the following herbals exhibits the LEAST effect on blood coagulation?

    (A) echinacea
    (B) garlic
    (C) ginseng
    (D) ginkgo
    (E) St. John's wort

318. Which of the following are standard methods for extracting active ingredients from crude herbals?

    I.   maceration
    II. percolation
    III. reverse osmosis

    (A) I only
    (B) III only
    (C) I and II only
    (D) II and III only
    (E) I, II, and III

319. A customer purchasing a nonprescription drug combination containing glucosamine is probably using the product to prevent/treat which of the following?

(A) joint pain
(B) malnutrition
(C) mild hypertension
(D) obesity
(E) high cholesterol values

320. Which one of the following herbals is most likely to interfere with the activity of oral birth control tablets?

(A) garlic
(B) ginger
(C) ginseng
(D) ginkgo biloba
(E) St. John's wort

321. Which one of the following herbal products may be useful for a 60-year-old who is experiencing hot flashes?

(A) black cohosh
(B) feverfew
(C) ginseng
(D) milk thistle
(E) valerian

322. A client is purchasing a bottle of feverfew extract. What is the most likely use for this herb?

(A) adaptogen
(B) analgesic
(C) for fever reduction
(D) prevent migraines
(E) mild sedative

323. A customer is seeking the highest concentration of topical hydrocortisone available without a prescription. The pharmacist could suggest which one of the following products?

(A) Aveeno Anti-itch Cream
(B) Cortaid, J & J

(C) Cortizone Maximum Strength
(D) Cortizone-10
(E) any of the above

324. SAMe has been advocated for which one of the following?

(A) antidepressant
(B) antihypertensive
(C) cardioprotective
(D) sedative
(E) vitamin

325. Which of the following herbal products is (are) intended for topical use?

  I. aloe vera
 II. tea tree oil
III. milk thistle

(A) I only
(B) III only
(C) I and II only
(D) II and III only
(E) I, II, and III

326. Which one of the following nonprescription drug products may be useful for weight reduction?

(A) Alli
(B) Aloe
(C) Aspartame
(D) Senokot
(E) Doxylamine

327. An OTC product that may relieve a child's sour and upset stomach is Children's Pepto. What is the active ingredient in this product?

(A) aluminum hydroxide
(B) calcium carbonate
(C) bismuth subcarbonate
(D) bismuth subnitrate
(E) magnesium hydroxide

328. How may a pharmacist explain to a consumer the difference between Senokot-S and Senokot?

(A) Senokot-S has double the amount of senna.

(B) Senokot-S is less irritating.

(C) Senokot-S contains biscodyl instead of senna.

(D) Senokot-S contains docusate plus senna.

(E) Senokot does not require a prescription.

Questions 329 through 331

A hospital pharmacy intern receives the following three orders on a medication sheet. Indicate for each what action should be taken.

(A) Ask the prescriber to clarify desired strength.

(B) Fill the order as written.

(C) Question the order based on route of administration.

(D) Question the order based on product availability in indicated strength.

(E) Consult with prescriber concerning directions for use.

329. Hep Lock Flush Solution. Use as directed.

330. Synthroid 0.15 mg. Take one after breakfast.

331. ASA 325 mg every AM followed by niacin 500 mg po after 30 minutes.

Questions 332 through 334

The Stevens family has a limited annual income of approximately $28,000 and must discontinue the use of their expensive prescriptions. Mrs. Stevens asks the pharmacist if there are any economical products available that may be used in place of each of the following drug products that they no longer can afford.

MATCH the lettered OTC product that may have similar therapeutic action as the corresponding numbered drug.

(A) Coenzyme Q10

(B) Omega-3 fish oil

(C) Pepcid AC

(D) Tylenol PM

(E) Ginseng

332. Ambien

333. Lovaza

334. Nexium

335. Mrs. Stevens has been consuming Lipitor for 3 years. Which one of the following vitamins may also help to control her cholesterol levels?

(A) Vitamin A

(B) Vitamin B_1

(C) Vitamin B_2

(D) Vitamin B_3

(E) Vitamin B_6

336. Which one of the following transdermal patches may be cut in half to reduce therapeutic action and/or reduce cost to the patient?

(A) Climara

(B) Estraderm

(C) Lidoderm

(D) Nitroglycerin

(E) Emsam

337. Pharmaceutical products with the designation of "HFA" included in their names are administered in which dosage form?

(A) aerosols

(B) oral tablets

(C) oral capsules

(D) sustained-release products

(E) injections

338. To which of the following herbs is eleutherococcus most closely related?

(A) feverfew

(B) ginseng

(C) hawthorn

(D) St. John's wort

(E) valerian

Answers and Explanations

Numbers within parentheses at the end of the answers refer to the numbered references that are listed in the front matter.

1. **(A)** Official standards in the form of drug monographs are presented in the USP/NF. These monographs may describe the rapeutically active drugs or other ingredients, known as excipients, which one essential for formulating a stable drug product. However, the book does not provide information concerning therapeutic activity. *(24)*

2. **(D)** The USAN Council establishes nonproprietary drug names. The Council is jointly sponsored by the AMA, United States Pharmacopoeial Convention, and the APhA. Because the USAN is not an official government agency, the chosen names are not formally recognized until they are published in the Federal Register. *(24)*

3. **(C)** Federal drug laws and regulations are described in the USP Dispensing Information (DI), Volume III, which also contains listings of therapeutic equivalent drugs and drugs that are biologically inequivalent. The latter information is from the FDA's Orange Book. *(18c section:VI)*

4. **(B)** Volume II of the USP DI contains drug monographs written for the layperson. Pharmacists have the permission to photocopy individual drug descriptions for distribution to the patient when dispensing the drug. Volume I of the USP DI contains drug information for health professionals. It includes more detailed and more scientific information than Volume II. *(18a; 18b)*

5. **(C)** CAM is an acronym for "complementary alternative medicine." The FDA includes in this definition herbals, dietary supplements, and other addiction treatments. Many of these have costs lower than traditional drug products. The term, biosimilar drug, usually refers to a biotech drug that is similar to a brand-name product but not identical mainly because the drugs are so molecularly complex that current science does not allow exact duplication. However, similar therapeutic activity is expected. A single-source drug product is one that is available from only one company. These are usually more expensive than a generic product. *(1; 5)*

6. **(A)** Allopathy is the treatment of disease by using remedies that produce effects on the body that differ from those produced by the disease. This new set of conditions is incompatible with or antagonistic to the original symptoms of the disease. The term is now used when referring to standard or orthodox medical practice. *(1; 14)*

    (C—incorrect) Naturopathy indicates healing by the exclusive use of natural remedies (heat, light, vegetables, fruits, etc) but no surgery or drugs.

    (D) Nutraceutical practice is one in which foods are used to promote healing and health.

7. **(C)** Homeopathy involves the use of substances that produce symptoms similar to the symptoms of the disease (the law of similarity). The drugs used, mainly herbals, are administered as very high dilutions, that is, in extremely low doses. *(1; 27)*

8. **(D)** The speed at which tablets disintegrate usually correlates with the drug dissolution rate and speed at which drug action will occur. Sublingual tablets are intended to provide fairly fast activity that is accelerated by fast disintegration and dissolution under the tongue. While tablet compression is an important factor, uncoated compressed tablets usually disintegrate faster than coated tablets. *(1; 17)*

9. **(D)** Both film and sugar coats are water soluble and most will readily disintegrate in the stomach. However, the smooth tablet surface makes the tablet easier to dissolve with less chance of bitter drug powder remaining in the mouth or throat. Enteric coats are intended to prevent the disintegration of the tablet until it reaches the small intestine. *(1; 24)*

10. **(A)** Magnesium stearate (as well as other stearates) is included in tablet formulations as a lubricant. *(1; 24)*

11. **(C)** Tablet lubricants are characterized by lubricity, as they are usually water insoluble and difficult to wet. The waterproofing property might retard disintegration and dissolution. *(1)*

12. **(B)** Products such as Potassium Chloride Enseals are enteric coated to protect the stomach from irritating substances or to prevent drug decomposition in the stomach. *(1; 10)*

    (A—incorrect) Kapseal is a hermetically sealed capsule. An example is Dilantin Kapseal.

    (C—incorrect) Extentabs are prolonged-action tablets (eg, Dimetapp Extentabs).

    (D—incorrect) Filmtabs are tablets coated with a transparent protective coating (eg, K-Tab Filmtabs).

13. **(D)** Mannitol possesses characteristics that make it an almost ideal sweetener for chewable tablets. Although not as sweet as sucrose, it has good body, leaves a cool taste in the mouth, and is not hygroscopic. Mannitol is also easily compressed by wet granulation. *(24)*

14. **(C)** When moistened, starch will swell, thus aiding in the disintegration of a tablet. Corn starch in the form of a paste will bind powders during the formation of granules suitable for compression into tablets. *(1)*

15. **(B)** The German Commission E Monographs are publications that describe in detail information collected worldwide concerning herbs and herbal products. Included are common names, chemistry, therapeutic uses, contraindications, side effects, and dosing. *(1; 2)*

16. **(B)** The liquid product bypasses the disintegration and dissolution steps in the GI tract; therefore, the drug molecules are available for absorption in a shorter period of time. However, the molecules in solution are more susceptible to decomposition in the dosage form because of greater mobility when compared to solid forms, thus, less stability. For the manufacturer, tablets are the faster dosage form to manufacture in large quantities, and should be the most economical. *(24)*

17. **(C)** Most alkaloids have a pK_a above 7; therefore, they are weak bases that will form salts with an acid (eg, pilocarpine hydrochloride, morphine sulfate). *(1)*

    (D—incorrect) Stereoisomerism is common in alkaloid structures; large differences in therapeutic activity can be expected among isomers.

18. **(A)** Naturally occurring alkaloids that are weak organic bases have relatively poor water solubility but are soluble in alcohol. Most pharmaceutical products use the alkaloid salts such as morphine HCl, cocaine HCl, and atropine sulfate to increase the drugs' water solubility. *(1)*

19. **(C)** Haloperidol is a butyrophenone derivative and the base form has very poor water solubility (1 g in more than 10,000 mL). The hydrochloride salt is water soluble, as is the lactate salt, which is utilized in preparing the aqueous injection of haloperidol. Haloperidol decanoate is the ester form that is dissolved in an oil vehicle. This injection product

is injected intramuscularly and has a half-life of approximately 3 weeks. *(1)*

20. **(D)** The compressed tablet is the most commonly manufactured dosage form for several reasons. It is the most economical product for a manufacturer to produce, package, and ship. The tablet is easy for the pharmacist to dispense, and it is very convenient for most patients to consume. *(1; 24)*

21. **(C)** A chelating agent forms a compound by the combination of an electron donor with a metal ion to form a ring structure. The molecule that forms the ring structure is called a ligand or chelating agent. The metals that may be chelated must have valences of two or more. A major pharmaceutical use for chelating agents is to bind trace metals such as iron and copper that would otherwise catalyze oxidation of active drugs. Edetate (ethylenediamine tetraacetic acid) is commonly used in parenteral solutions. *(24)*

22. **(B)** Edetate calcium disodium (Versenate) is usually administered by intramuscular parenteral injection to reduce blood levels and depot stores of lead in acute and chronic lead poisoning and lead encephalopathy. The chelate formed with lead is stable, water soluble, and readily excreted by the kidneys. The other choices, lithium and sodium, are monovalent ions and will not complex with EDTA. *(1)*

23. **(E)** Medline is an online computerized system that contains up-to-date information on drugs. *(1)*

24. **(C)** Drugs in suspensions are likely to follow zero-order kinetics because the limiting factor is the amount of drug actually in solution. The classic example is aspirin suspension. *(12)*

25. **(B)** Epinephrine, a catecholamine, is very sensitive to oxidation, which results in biologically inactive products. The first indication of oxidation is the development of a pink color that darkens to form a brown precipitate. *(1; 24)*

26. **(C)** The Medical Letter is a biweekly newsletter that mainly describes newly marketed drugs with information concerning pharmacokinetics, clinical studies, adverse effects, and dosage. Comparisons to other drug products in the same therapeutic category with respect to efficacy and cost of therapy are also included. *(30)*

27. **(B)** Powders that are either directly applied to the skin or are incorporated into topical products should be extremely fine or impalpable. Trituration is often needed to reduce particles to an extremely fine size so that the patient will not discern individual particles when the product is rubbed on the skin. Usually a particle size of 50 μm or smaller is desired. *(1; 4; 24)*

28. **(B)** Tartrazine (F D & C Yellow 5) is a popular coloring agent in both oral tablets and solutions. There are reported cases of individuals being sensitive to this dye. *(1; 14)*

29. **(C)** Chiral relates to the optical activity of a molecule. Stereoisomers of a specific drug may exhibit distinctly different degrees of therapeutic activity. For some drugs, the activity or major side effects may be due to only one of the isomers present. *(1)*

30. **(C)** A specific stereoisomer may possess greater desired activity than its mixture. If the more active form is isolated and used exclusively in a dosage form, there will usually be less toxicity and side effects. The actual synthesis, formulation, and manufacturing of the purified isomer into a commercial dosage form will not significantly result in a more economical drug than by using a mixture. *(1)*

31. **(D)** Polymorphs differ in their melting points, x-ray diffractions, infrared spectra, and dissolution rates. For example, riboflavin has three polymorphs, each with significantly different solubilities. Theobroma oil (cocoa butter) can exist in four forms, each differing in melting point. Gentle heating of cocoa butter will favor the formation of the stable beta polymorph. This crystalline form is desired because it melts at 34.5°C, which is close to, but lower than, body temperature. Metabolic

rates of a drug's polymorphs will not vary because once the drug has dissolved, the polymorphs no longer exist. *(1)*

32. **(D)** Sorbitan monopalmitate is a sorbitan fatty acid ester, commercially available as Span 40. It is classified as nonionic because the molecules do not have the tendency to migrate to either pole in an electric field. *(1)*

   (A, C, E—incorrect) These compounds are anionic surfactants. This designation implies that the large active portion of the surfactant molecule bears a negative charge and, therefore, migrates to the anode in an electric field. For example, the stearate portion of triethanolamine stearate is considered the active ion.

   (B—incorrect) Cetylpyridinium chloride is a cationic surfactant. The active surfactant portion, cetylpyridinium, has a positive charge and migrates to the cathode.

33. **(B)** Since the salt form of albuterol is the sulfate, the drug itself most likely is a weak base. The presences of two pK_as indicate two active sites for combining, but complete ionization will not occur until the pH of the solution is well below a pH of 9.3. *(20)*

34. **(C)** Potassium chloride is an obvious substitute for sodium chloride because it has a similar salty taste, is crystalline, and is an electrolyte already present in the body. However, the use of this salt substitute is contraindicated in patients with severe kidney disease or oliguria. Symptoms such as weakness, nausea, and muscle cramps indicate excessive sodium depletion. Increased sodium intake is warranted. *(10)*

35. **(B)** IV injection of high concentrations of potassium may cause cardiac arrest. Intravenous administration must be by slow infusion to allow dilution of the potassium to occur. When plasma potassium levels are above 2.5 mEq/L, rates up to 10 mEq/h (total of 100–200 mEq/d) may be set. In more serious conditions, with plasma levels below 2 mEq/L, rates of 40 mEq/h (total of 400 mEq/d) have been employed. Available injection forms contain 10 to 80 mEq per vial. IV admixtures are prepared by diluting these solutions to 250 to 1,000 mL. Oral dosage forms include Kay Ciel elixir, Kaon tablets, K-Lor, and K-Lyte packets. Slow-K tablets have a wax matrix from which the KCl slowly dissolves in the GI tract. *(1)*

36. **(B)** Topical dosage forms are used. For example, both creams and solutions are available under the trade names of Efudex and Fluoroplex. In fact, however, fluorouracil is usually administered by IV injection. It is not given orally because of irregular absorption from the GI tract. *(3; 6)*

37. **(B)** The product inserts for many drug products contain various categories of statements including drug description, pharmacokinetics, warnings, precautions, indications for use, dosage, and administration. Both the prescriber and the pharmacist carefully review any black box warnings since these are of extreme importance. The boxed material is usually located at the beginning of the product insert so that it is readily visible. *(1; 24)*

38. **(B)** A precaution is intended to advise the physician of possible problems that may occur with the use of a drug. For example, the use of tetracycline may result in overgrowth of non-susceptible microorganisms. A warning signifies a more serious problem with greater potential for harm to a patient. For example, renal impairment may require reduction in the drug dose. A contraindication is the most restrictive limitation because it refers to an absolute prohibition against the use of a drug under certain conditions. For example, the use of penicillin derivatives is prohibited in patients known to be sensitive to penicillin. *(24)*

39. **(C)** Both *Facts and Comparisons* and the *Handbook on Injectable Drugs* present tables comparing the commercial amino acid injections. *(21; 10)*

40. **(C)** The term leaching is used specifically to designate the release of a container ingredient into the product itself. For example, zinc and

accelerators may be leached from rubber closures into a parenteral vial. *(24)*

(A—incorrect) Adsorption would refer to the binding of a substance onto the surface of the container wall.

(B—incorrect) Diffusion is the passage of a substance through a second substance. For example, volatile oil or dye may diffuse from a solution through the walls of a plastic container.

(D—incorrect) Permeation would denote the solution of a substance in the cell wall followed by passage through the wall.

(E—incorrect) Porosity indicates small holes or passages through which a substance could pass.

41. **(B)** Hypodermic needle sizes are expressed by a gauge system based on the external diameter of the cannula: the larger the number, the smaller the diameter of the needle. For example, the 21-gauge needle is smaller in diameter than the 19-gauge needle. Generally, the length of the cannula is also specified. This measurement, expressed in inches, represents the distance from the needle tip to the junction with the hub. *(13)*

42. **(D)** The winged (scalp–vein, scalp, or butterfly) needle consists of a stainless steel needle with two flexible plastic winglike projections. The wings serve two purposes: they ease manipulation of the needle during insertion into the vein and then allow the needle to be anchored with tape to the skin. *(13)*

43. **(A)** The physical form of drugs given intravenously is the solution. Other systems such as suspensions or vegetable oil solvents may block small veins. Also, a suspended drug will quickly dissolve in the large volume of blood in the body thus resulting in an overdose in many situations. *(1; 24)*

44. **(D)** Insulin solutions have low viscosities, and only small volumes are injected. Therefore, small-bore needles (25 gauge up to 30 gauge) may be used. Short-length (3/8–5/8 in.) needles are usually adequate for the usual subcutaneous route of insulin administration. *(13)*

45. **(C)** The term venoclysis is synonymous with intravenous infusion. *(13)*

46. **(A)** Partially filled glass containers (minibottles) usually consist of 250-mL bottles containing 50, 100, or 150 mL of either D_5W or NS. To these bottles one can easily add drug solutions, taking advantage of the vacuum present in the minibottle. Plastic bags are also employed for preparing parenteral admixtures. The plastic units do not have a vacuum but are flexible enough to accommodate additional liquids. *(1)*

47. **(A)** Intermittent therapy refers to administration of parenteral drugs at spaced intervals. One of the most convenient methods of administration for the pharmacist is to prepare a minibottle containing active drug solution such as an antibiotic added to a diluent. This unit is attached to the tubing of a large-volume parenteral (LVP) bottle already hanging on the patient. This piggyback concept saves the patient from multiple injections and assures high blood levels of the additive drug because the minibottle solution is infused in a short period of time. *(1; 13)*

48. **(C)** TPN (total parenteral nutrition) and TNA (total nutritional admixture) refer to solutions administered parenterally to provide calories, amino acids, and other nutrients by parenteral infusion. PMN is an abbreviation sometimes used for phenylmercuric nitrate, an antimicrobial preservative. *(4)*

49. **(B)** Although the maximum volume will vary depending on the condition of the patient, the normal daily water requirement is approximately 25 to 40 mL/kg of body weight. Daily volumes greater than 3 to 4 L in normal (nondehydrated) patients may cause a fluid overload. A dehydrated patient will require larger quantities. Water replacement therapy (hydration therapy) in an adult may be 70 mL/kg. Thus, a 50-kg patient will need 3,500 mL (replacement) plus 2,400 mL (maintenance). *(24)*

50. **(E)** A subcutaneous injection will come into contact with a large number of nerve endings

and may remain at the injection site for a long period of time. Pain will be experienced if the solution is not isotonic. The potential effects of hypotonic or hypertonic intravenous solutions are offset by their dilution in the large volume of blood into which they are injected, provided the volume injected is not excessive and the rate of injection is slow. *(1; 24)*

51. **(D)** There is the potential danger of suspension particles blocking blood vessels. Also, relatively insoluble particles of suspension may dissolve faster than desired if injected intravenously into a relatively large volume of patient's blood, thus giving immediate therapeutic activity, when a sustained-release activity was desired. For example, only insulin solution is administered by the IV route while the various suspension dosage forms are intended for subcutaneous injection. *(1; 24)*

52. **(B)** The abbreviation of IVP represents intravenous push (bolus) administration indicating fast injection (usually <1 minute) of the parenteral solution. IVPB requires a minibottle or minibag setup known as the piggyback arrangement. These bottles are usually infused over a time span of 20 minutes to 1 hour. KVO means to keep the vein open, by setting up an LVP of 5% dextrose or 0.9% sodium chloride injection for very slow infusion. The intent is to allow the quick hookup of additional drug solutions without having to enter the vein several times. *(13)*

53. **(B)** Factors affecting the distribution of a drug in the blood after an IV bolus include the blood volume, heart rate, and injection rate. Assuming that even distribution occurs within 4 minutes, drug sampling may be initiated after that time. *(1)*

54. **(D)** The pH of solutions is often adjusted during the manufacturing procedure by the addition of either acid (hydrochloric acid) or alkali (sodium hydroxide). The amount needed may vary from batch to batch. Therefore, the label cannot specify an exact quantity. Also, isotonicity adjusters may be listed by name only with a statement as to their purpose. *(18c)*

55. **(B)** Although many of the parenteral admixtures are chemically stable for long periods of time, potential contamination of the products during preparation by the pharmacist is of prime concern. Usually no significant microbial growth will occur until after 24 to 36 hours. Therefore, an expiration date of 24 hours is safest unless the solution is known to be less stable chemically. Some hospitals use a 28-hour expiration date. Refrigeration also helps to retard microbial growth. *(13)*

56. **(E)** Osmolarity, expressed as mOsm/L, is included on the labels of LVPs. Those injections with a value of approximately 300 mOsm/L will be iso-osmotic and presumably isotonic with the blood. For example, 5% dextrose injection has a value of 280 mOsm/L, whereas 0.9% sodium chloride injection has a value of 308 mOsm/L. One calculates the osmolarity of a solution by first determining the millimoles of chemical present, then multiplying by the number of ions formed from one molecule. One liter of 0.9% sodium chloride solution contains 9 g of sodium chloride (mol. wt. = 58.4). The millimole concentration will be

$$9 \text{ g}/58.4 = 0.154 \text{ mol or } 154 \text{ mM.}$$

The milliosmole (mOsm) concentration will be

$$154 \text{ mM} \times 2 \text{ (ions present in NaCl)} = 308 \text{ mOsm/L. } (1)$$

57. **(C)** Dextrose 5% injection (D_5W) has an osmolarity of approximately 300 mOsm/L, as does 0.9% sodium chloride injection (NS). If 1 L of solution contains both 5% dextrose and 0.9% sodium chloride, its osmolarity will be approximately 600 mOsm/L and will be hypertonic. Fortunately, infusing hypertonic solutions such as D_5W/NS is not dangerous, since the solution is rapidly diluted by the blood with no significant damage to the RBCs. One formula often used for infusion is $D_{2.5}W$/0.45NS, which is isotonic. *(1; 23)*

58. **(A)** The osmotic pressure of the dextrose solution will be approximately one-half that of an equimolar sodium chloride solution. The osmotic pressure of a substance in solution is

an example of a colligative property. Equimolar concentrations of nonelectrolytes will have similar osmotic pressures. However, electrolytes ionize to form particles that quantitatively increase the magnitude of the colligative property. Because sodium chloride ionizes into two particles, a 0.1-mol solution has twice the osmotic pressure of a 0.1-mol solution of a nonelectrolyte such as dextrose. Deviations from this simple theory arise from interionic attractions, solvation, and other factors. *(1)*

59. **(B)** Except for the lactate concentration and the absence of sodium bicarbonate, lactated Ringer's (Hartmann's) solution closely approximates the extracellular fluid. Although the injection has a pH of 6 to 7.5, it has an alkalinizing effect because the lactate is metabolized to bicarbonate. *(1)*

60. **(B)** To avoid pain at the injection site, solutions injected into subcutaneous sites should be limited to not more than 1 mL. The usual limit suggested for deltoid IM injections is up to 2 mL, while IM injections into the gluteal medial muscle may be up to 5 mL. *(4)*

61. **(D)** Presurgical prophylactic administration of an antibiotic is routine in most hospitals. The choice of antibiotic is subjective to several parameters including causative microbes in a given area and the experience of the surgical staff. Either cefazolin 1 g IV at induction of anesthesia and every 8 hours for up to 24 hours or cefuroxime 1.5 g every 8 to 12 hours up to 24 hours are commonly used. Clindamycin may be used if a patient is allergic to penicillin. Vancomycin 1 g infused over an hour with a second dose in 12 hours is effective but many hospitals prefer to reserve vancomycin for serious cases. Tetracycline is seldom used. *(1; 14)*

62. **(E)** The vastus lateralis is the largest developed muscle in young children and is free of major nerves and veins. The volume limitation should be 1 mL. *(4)*

63. **(C)** Heparin sodium is given by both IV bolus and infusion as well as by subcutaneous injection. The IM route is not used since it may be painful and also cause a localized hematoma. *(1)*

64. **(C)** Self-administration of insulin is most readily accomplished by subcutaneous injection into the abdomen or thigh. Intravenous infusion is used in institutional settings and, in emergencies, IV bolus doses may be given. The development of portable infusion pumps and other devices is expanding the methods for insulin administration. *(1; 13)*

65. **(D)** There are two main sites of degradation for insulin—the liver and the kidneys. Insulin is filtered through the glomeruli and reabsorbed by the tubules, where some degradation occurs. When injected by the IV route, the half-life is estimated to be 5 to 6 minutes. Approximately 50% of the insulin that reaches the liver through the portal vein is destroyed. U-100 insulin is available OTC. *(10)*

66. **(D)** The ADD-Vantage system consists of a vial usually containing a powder which is already attached to a minibag. The health professional simply has to engage the vial into the bag thus allowing reconstitution of the powder and subsequent mixing with the main body of diluent. *(1; 24)*

67. **(A)** The CRIS unit is a plastic disposable adaptor that allows the quick transfer of a drug solution into an infusion container. A vial is hooked to the adaptor, the valve device is turned, and the vial contents will enter the infusion line mixing with the infusion solution flowing into the patient. The unit avoids the need to initially mix the additive with the primary infusion solution. *(1)*

68. **(D)** Pharmacia's Port-A-Cath is a stainless steel unit with a self-sealing septum through which drug solutions may be injected over 100 times. The unit is implanted under the skin in a location allowing the patient to self-administer solutions. A similar unit is Infusaid's Infuse-A-Port. Answers A and C are incorrect. These two catheters are classified as central catheters and are mainly

used for infusing hypertonic TPN solutions. *(1; 13; 22)*

69. **(C)** Pharmacy bulk packages are intended to provide the compounding pharmacist with a unit, the contents of which may be aseptically subdivided into several parenteral admixtures. The package is pierced only once, and used within a short period of time; therefore it does not contain an antimicrobial preservative. Bulk packages are ideal when reconstituting an antibiotic powder for transfer into several minibottles or bags. *(4; 13)*

70. **(D)** Potassium chloride concentrate solutions are potentially very dangerous if infused undiluted. Because of numerous fatalities in hospitals, the FDA specifies that it is the only product that must be packaged in vials with black flip-off buttons. There is no color code for other parenteral solutions that are packaged in vials. *(18c)*

71. **(C)** The inclusion of an antimicrobial preservative in parenteral solutions is intended only for multidose containers from which fairly small volumes of solution are used at one time. When large volumes of solution are infused, the presence of an antimicrobial preservative may increase potential toxicity of the product. *(24)*

72. **(B)** Benzyl alcohol is an effective antimicrobial preservative. However, it is contraindicated in solutions being administered to neonates. These very young babies have not developed the liver enzyme to detoxify benzyl alcohol, and a clinical condition known as the gasping syndrome will develop. The USP requires labels to state "Not for Use in Neonates." *(24)*

73. **(A)** Although vitamin C's main attribute is in the prevention and cure of scurvy, it has been advocated for the prevention and alleviation of symptoms of the common cold, to facilitate absorption of iron by maintaining iron in the ferrous state, and as an antioxidant in both pharmaceuticals and foods. The fat-soluble vitamin E also possesses antioxidant proper-

ties and is sometimes employed as a preservative in lipid pharmaceutical and cosmetic products. *(1)*

Ergocalciferol (Vitamin D_2) prevents or treats rickets and is used in the management of hypoparathyroidism and hypocalcemia. *(1)*

Pantothenic acid is biologically important as a component in coenzyme A (CoA). *(1)*

74. **(A)** Gentamicin sulfate (Garamycin) is stable for 2 years at room temperature. Of the five antibiotics listed, it is the only one marketed as an aqueous solution, ready for injection. The others are packaged as powders for reconstitution. *(21)*

75. **(C)** Human immune serum is obtained from human blood. It contains specific antibodies reflecting the diseases contracted by the donor. The immunity is passive because the recipient's body does not actively develop either antibodies or sensitized lymphocytes in response to a foreign antigen. Passive immunity does not last long; usually not more than 2 or 3 weeks of protection are achieved. Active immunity implies that the recipient of the biological resource will develop specific immunity due to an active response to the introduction of antigenic substances. *(24)*

76. **(C)** The Human Papillomavirus Quadrivalent vaccine, Recombinant is available under the brand names of Gardasil and Cervarix. The original intent was protection for females in the age bracket of 9 to 26 years against infections from four types of papillomavirus (HPV 6, 11, 16, and 18). HPV types 16 and 18 are responsible for most cervical cancers while HPV types 6 and 11 cause about 90% of genital warts. However, inoculation of males may also decrease the incidence of genital warts. An IM injection of 0.5 mL suspension is administered followed by 2 and 6 months with additional injections. A second product, Cervarix, main indication is for prevention of HPV types 16 and 18 infections. *(10; 30:52,37,2010)*

77. **(A)** Tuberculin is a solution of soluble products of tubercle bacillus. The solution is used as a diagnostic aid for exposure to the bacillus. It is administered intradermally. *(24)*

78. **(B)** Tuberculin syringes are made of either plastic or glass with a total capacity of 1 mL. Despite their name, they are suitable for measuring small volumes of any liquid. *(13)*

79. **(A)** Herpes vaccine is a live virus vaccine intended for the prevention of herpes zoster in adults. It will also prevent postherpetic neuralgia and reduce both acute and chronic shingles-associated pain in adults. The vaccine, Zostavax, is administered as a single subcutaneous injection.

MMR (measles, mumps, rubella vaccine) is a live attenuated vaccine usually given in two doses at 12 to 15 months and 4 to 6 years of age.

Pneumococcal Conjugate Vaccine (Prevnar) will reduce the incidence of bacterial meningitis in children.

Rotavirus vaccine (RotaTeq) is a live oral pentavalent vaccine for infants to protect against rotavirus gastroenteritis. Varicella vaccine is a live attenuated vaccine recommended for healthy individuals at least 12 months old for protection against chickenpox caused by the *Varicella zoster*. *(1; 24)*

80. **(B)** The immune gamma globulin is used to prevent or modify several diseases, including measles, infectious hepatitis, German measles, and chickenpox. The immunity is passive, lasting for 1 to 2 months. There are also special forms for individuals exposed to mumps, pertussis, tetanus, vaccinia, and rabies. *(1; 24)*

81. **(C)** Pediarix is a vaccine offering protection against diphtheria, tetanus, acellular pertussis, hepatitis B, and poliovirus. However, it does not protect against hepatitis C. *(3; 25)*

82. **(E)** There may be some danger to both mother and fetus if live attenuated vaccines are administered. Although the evidence is not conclusive, neither the individual nor combination MMR (measles, mumps, and rubella vaccine) should be administered during pregnancy or during the previous 3 months for women considering pregnancy. *(24)*

83. **(B)** Passive immunizations are usually accomplished by the administration of purified and concentrated antibody solutions (antitoxins) derived from humans or animals that have been actively immunized against a live antigen. Active immunizations are usually accomplished by the administration of one of the following: (1) toxoids (eg, A—incorrect), (2) inactivated (killed) vaccines (eg, choices C and E—incorrect), (3) live attenuated vaccines (eg, choice D—incorrect). *(1; 24)*

84. **(C)** Booster doses of the common toxoids are required to sustain immunity. For example, a 0.5 mL dose of tetanus toxoid should be administered as a routine booster about every 10 years, or, as a booster in the management of minor clean wounds, not more frequently than every 6 years. *(1)*

85. **(A)** Diphtheria, tetanus toxoid, and pertussis vaccine (DTP) is administered as a series of four injections starting when the baby is 6 weeks to 2 months of age. Two additional injections are given at 6-week intervals, with a final dose given 1 year later. If needed, a booster injection can be given when the child is 4 to 6 years old. DTP must never be given to children older than 6 years because of serious reactions that may occur. *(1; 24)*

86. **(C)** Both vaccines protect against tetanus (T), diphtheria (d), acellular pertussis (ap) and are intended as booster shots following the normal immunization schedule for infants and young children. Adacel may be administered to individuals aged between 11 and 64 while the intended target group for Boostrix is individuals with ages between 10 and 18. Once administered, booster injections should be scheduled for every 10 years. *(1; 10; 25)*

87. **(C)** All people over the age of 2 are appropriate candidates for pneumonia vaccinations. There are several products on the market such as Merck's Pneumovax and Wyeth's Pnu-Imune. The vaccine is given by either intramuscular or subcutaneous injection and provides active immunization. *(24)*

88. **(B)** The labeling on biologicals is required to specify the recommended storage temperature.

With few exceptions, biologicals are stored in a refrigerator at 2°C to 8°C. *(24)*

89.   (E) Typhoid fever is a bacterial infection. *(1)*

90.   (C) Monoclonal antibodies (MAb) are antibodies derived from single hybrid cells. The resulting product has enhanced selectivity, making it invaluable as a specific diagnostic agent or drug. Gene splicing refers to those procedures resulting in alterations of the DNA make-up of a microorganism. Using recombinant DNA technology, specific antibodies useful for medical and agricultural applications can be developed. *(1; 24)*

91.   (C) Liposomes consist of phospholipids that when dispersed in water form multilamellar vesicles. These liposomes can be utilized as drug carriers delivering drugs to specific body sites. Nanoparticles refer to a dispersed drug consisting of colloidal size particles with diameters between 200 and 500 nm. After IV injection, the nanoparticles are taken up by the reticuloendothelial system and localized in the liver. Transdermal delivery systems allow diffusion of a drug through the skin into the general circulation. They do not target specific sites for drug delivery. *(1; 24)*

92.   (B) Most biotechnological drugs consist of amino acid sequences. Because these proteins have relatively poor stability in the GI tract and have erratic absorption, most of the drugs are intended for parenteral administration. *(13; 24)*

93.   (D) The increased sensitivity of both types of tests is due to the use of MAb, which allow earlier determination of the specific hormones involved. Ovulation prediction tests detect surges in luteinizing hormone (LH), which indicate that ovulation is about to occur. Pregnancy determination tests detect an increased level of human chorionic gonadotropin hormone that occurs when the egg is fertilized. The fecal occult blood tests are based on the colorimetric detection of hemoglobin. Various chemicals, such as guaiac and tetramethylbenzidine, are used to elicit a characteristic color. The occult blood tests are not very selective or sensitive. *(2)*

94.   (B) Rapidly dissolving tablets (RDTs) are tablets that will quickly dissolve in the mouth without the patient having to take any water. This makes convenient dosing in many situations especially for children and the elderly. The formulation principles vary. Zydis is Cardinal Health's system in which water is removed from a powder mix by freeze drying, then the tablets are compressed. Products such as Zyprexa, Zofran ODT, Risperdal M-Tab, Claritin Reditabs use the above technique.

Another system is the WOWTAB that utilizes physically modified polysaccharides for high compressibility yet fast disintegration. An example is Benadryl Fastmelt. A second acronym used for the above phenomenon is ODT representing orally disintegrating tablet.

ET refers to an enteric-coated tablet. SC is a sugar-coated tablet. Sublingual (s.l.) tablets also dissolve quickly in the mouth but the drug is absorbed directly from under the tongue. TTS represents transdermal therapeutic systems. *(10; 24)*

95.   (B) OraSolv allows the direct compression of drugs combined with effervescent excipients. When exposed to water, the tablet will quickly disintegrate due to effervescence caused by the production of carbon dioxide. Drug products using this principle include Zomig-ZMT (zolmitriptan for migraine), Remeron SolTab (mirtazapine for depression), and Alavert (loratadine for allergy). *(10; 24)*

96.   (A) Intermates are transparent plastic units containing an elastic balloon that may be aseptically filled with sterile solutions. The unusual characteristic of the balloon is that it collapses at a constant rate when the administration set is opened, thus giving a constant flow rate. For example, the Intermate 100 will deliver 100 mL in a 1-hour period. The pharmacist may control the amount of drug received by the patient by either changing the fill volume or the concentration of drug present.

However, the flow rate is preset and cannot be changed. A similar unit is provided by Block Medical as the Homepump. *(22)*

97. **(D)** PCA devices such as Pharmacia's CADD models allow the slow infusion of drug solutions into the patient. Not only can small volumes be infused, the units may be programmed to vary flow at different intervals and also provide bolus doses when desired. There is also a lockout device that prevents too frequent bolus doses. The PCA units are not only very convenient for delivery of analgesics but also may be used for other drug solutions. *(22)*

98. **(C)** The term meta-analysis is used to describe the statistical analysis of collection of data from numerous papers. By analyzing and evaluating the data one may compare similarities and differences in the results and conclusions from the studies. *(1)*

99. **(D)** In 2006, the FDA approved the marketing of the sunscreen agent, ecamsule. This chemical, long available in Canada and Europe, has good blocking properties against UVB and UVA. Although most currently available sunscreens concentrate on blocking UVB, there is evidence that UVA may increase the incidence of basal and squamous cell cancers and melanomas. One product, Anthelios SX, contains ecamsule plus the standard sunscreening agents avobenzone and octocrylene. *(10)*

100. **(A)** Of all the injectable forms of iron, only iron dextran (INFeD) is intended for intramuscular injection. The nurse should use the Z-Track technique for a deep IM injection to reduce potential discoloration of the skin surface. This involves sliding the upper layer of the muscle to one side, injecting, then allowing the muscle to return to normal position while removing the needle. The objective is that none of the solution should reach the skin surface. INFeD and DexFerrum are colloidal solutions of ferric hydroxide complexed with partially hydrolyzed dextran. However, DexFerrum, as well as Ferrlecit, Venofer, and Feraheme (Ferumoxytol) are

indicated only for intravenous administration. *(1; 3)*

101. **(A)** Test doses of INFeD should be administered prior to starting therapy. The other agents have lower incidences of severe hypersensitivity and are now preferred for treating iron deficiency anemias. Both DexFerrum and InFeD are parenteral products containing iron dextran. Because of incidences of fatal anaphylactic-type reactions, their use should be limited to the treatment of confirmed cases of iron-deficiency anemia, particularly among those patients who cannot tolerate or fail to respond to oral administration of iron. *(1; 3)*

102. **(B)** Iron sucrose injections are available under the trade name of Venofer. It is intended for treating iron-deficiency anemia in patients undergoing chromin hemodialysis and are receiving EPO therapy. The solution is administered only intravenously into the dialysis line. The Z-track technique used to prevent skin discoloration that may occur when administering IM iron dextran is not used for iron sucrose since this drug solution is given IV. *(1; 3)*

103. **(E)** Polycarbophil absorbs large quantities of water, allowing the formation of stools. There does not appear to be any effect on the action of digestive enzymes or nutrients. The drug itself is not absorbed systemically. Polycarbophil is present in Mitrolan and FiberCon. *(1; 2)*

(A—incorrect) Activated charcoal possesses good adsorption properties but is seldom used as an antidiarrheal.

(C, D—incorrect) Kaolin and attapulgite are typical examples of adsorbent clays. Attapulgite is a colloidal hydrated magnesium aluminum silicate clay. Studies have indicated that it is an effective adsorbent for alkaloids, toxins, bacteria, and strains of human enteroviruses. However, attapulgite and kaolin are not selective and will also adsorb nutrients and digestive enzymes. Probably their greatest efficacy is in the treatment of mild functional diarrhea. *(2; 11)*

104. **(A)** Simethicone is a mixture of inert silicon polymers that may be used as a defoaming agent to relieve GI tract gas. This antiflatulent ingredient is present in Mylicon drops and Phazyme tablets. Simethicone is included in a number of combination antacid products (Mylanta, Riopan, and Gelusil). A newer antiflatulent agent is alpha-galactosidase, an enzyme that breaks down oligosaccharides before they form intestinal gas. A commercial product containing this compound is Beano. *(2)*

105. **(A)** For a long time, the adsorbent clay, attapulgite, was a popular absorbent, but many antidiarrheal products have replaced the clay with bismuth subsalicylate. Insoluble bismuth salts are effective adsorbents and also possess useful astringent and protective properties. Pepto-Bismol and many other antidiarrheal products contain bismuth subsalicylate. The subsalicylate salt is the preferred insoluble form because the subnitrate may form the nitrite ion in the gut. Absorption of this ion could cause hypotension and possibly methemoglobinemia. Bismuth salicylate is safe when taken orally but should not be consumed by patients sensitive to aspirin. Patients should be counseled that black-stained stools, which may occur with bismuth intake, are harmless. *(2; 11)*

106. **(B)** Loperamide is an effective drug for the relief of diarrhea. It slows intestinal motility and may stimulate GI mu receptors to decrease GI secretion.

   The recommended dosing is two tablets (4 mg) immediately, then one tablet (2 mg) after each loose stool until the diarrhea subsides. The maximum daily dose should not exceed 16 mg per day. *(2)*

107. **(C)** Liposomes are small vesicles of a bilayer of phospholipid encapsulating an aqueous compartment. Since phospholipids have both hydrophilic and hydrophobic portions, either lipophilic or hydrophilic drugs may be incorporated into the structure. Liposomes may vary in shape, usually with sizes between 0.5 and 100 μm. *(17; 24)*

108. **(E)** Liposomal dosage forms may be developed for any route of administration, but their parenteral use is exciting. Liposomal forms of amphotericin B have activity-targeted fungi localized in tissue, thus allowing lower doses and fewer side effects. The chemotherapeutic agent, doxorubicin, has been formulated into parenteral liposomes with reduced cardiotoxicity when compared to the conventional product. *(17; 24)*

109. **(C)** Amphotericin is available as AmBisome and Abelcet for antifungal activity. Daunorubicin as DaunoXome is used for treating Kaposi sarcoma. To avoid medication errors, pharmacists must be cognizant that regular solutions of these two drugs are still being used. *(24; 25)*

110. **(E)** Doxorubicin HCl liposome injection has the drug encapsulated in Stealth liposomes. The liposomes are protected by surface-bound methoxy PEG from detection by the phagocyte system, thus increasing blood circulation time. *(24)*

111. **(B)** Magnesium salicylate is similar to sodium salicylate in its analgesic activity, but there is the danger of systemic magnesium toxicity, especially in the renal-impaired patient. *(2)*

112. **(E)** The usual adult dose of dextromethorphan is 30 mg every 8 hours, with a maximum daily dose of 120 mg. Individual doses of 30 mg or higher do not appreciably increase antitussive activity. *(2; 11)*

113. **(B)** Calcium carbonate is a rapid, prolonged, potent neutralizer of gastric acid. Some scientists and consumer groups have advocated its use because of its high effectiveness and low cost. However, the listed side effects should warrant curtailment of its use, particularly for chronic therapy. *(2)*

   (A—incorrect) Some of the insoluble calcium carbonate is converted to soluble calcium chloride, which is absorbed. Significant amounts of calcium may be absorbed after a few days of antacid therapy.

   (D—incorrect) Gastric hypersecretion is believed to be caused by the local effect of calcium on the gastrin-producing cells.

114. (D) Calcium carbonate appears to be the antacid of choice when formulating chewable tablets. Although both the Titralac and Rolaids products contain calcium carbonate, Rolaids chewable tablets also contain magnesium hydroxide. Basaljel capsules contain only aluminum hydroxide. Other antacids containing only aluminum hydroxide include Amphojel and ALternaGEL. *(2; 11)*

115. (D) The generic name for Riopan is magaldrate. The product is a chemical rather than a physical combination of aluminum and magnesium hydroxides. Although this chemical form has a lower neutralizing capacity, it is still considered to be an effective antacid with a low sodium level and does not cause electrolyte imbalance in the body. *(1; 2)*

116. (D) Of the three analgesics, acetaminophen appears the safest for use during pregnancy. Aspirin, as well as all other salicylates, is especially dangerous during the last trimester and when breastfeeding mainly due to increased fetal and maternal morbidity. Ibuprofen may also cause postpartum bleeding and prolonged labor. *(2; 11)*

117. (E) The tablets are enteric coated to avoid gastric irritation. They should not be taken within 1 hour of ingestion of milk or antacids because the enteric coating may be dissolved prematurely. *(4)*

118. (B) Since companies have a degree of latitude in changing their OTC formulas, it is difficult for health professionals and laypersons to be certain of specific active ingredients in a specific product. The best procedure is to read recent labels. All of the products mentioned in the question contain 5 mg of biscodyl per tablet except Regular Strength ExLax, which contains 15 mg of sennosides. There is also an ExLax Maximum Strength which contains 25 mg of sennosides per tablet. Another active ingredient, docusate, is present in Correctol Gentle Laxative. *(2)*

119. (D) Excessive tablet compression may hinder tablet disintegration into aggregates, thus slowing the dissolution process. Other factors that affect dissolution include drug solubility, particle size, and crystalline structure; though these factors may not influence the disintegration rate. However, there is usually a fairly good correlation between tablet disintegration characteristics and dissolution, and disintegration times are a convenient in-house manufacturing control. Increasing drug particle surface area by micronization of drugs such as griseofulvin, chloramphenicol, and sulfadiazine have increased their dissolution rates (decreased dissolution times) and improved absorption. *(1)*

120. (B) The USP/NF has established official storage conditions that the pharmacist should follow for all pharmaceutical products. Temperatures within a refrigerator are described as being between 2°C and 8°C. *(1; 24)*

121. (A) Abreva is a nonprescription topical preparation intended to be placed on cold sores to speed healing time. Present in the formula are moisturizers that relieve dryness and prevent painful cracking, thus reducing pain, burning, and itching of the sore. *(2; 3)*

122. (D) Aspartame is a dipeptide that is approximately 200 times sweeter than sucrose. Because it provides less than 1 calorie per dose and does not impart the bitter aftertaste experienced by some people after consuming saccharin, it is a popular sweetening agent in drug products and foods. Its tendency to disintegrate on heating limits potential uses. Patients with phenylketonuria should avoid aspartame because one breakdown ingredient is phenylalanine. *(2)*

123. (D) Circadian refers to rhythmic cycles that recur in approximately 24-hour intervals. *(1; 14)*

124. (B) Searle's Covera-HS is formulated into a COFR-24 delivery system. The 180 or 240 mg tablets are intended for bedtime dosing to insure maximum plasma levels in the early morning. This time factor design is intended to take advantage of the body's circadian rhythm because blood pressures tend to be higher when the patient arises in the morning. *(10)*

125. **(D)** Thickening a suspension will slow its sedimentation, but it is still necessary to get the product out of the bottle. A pseudoplastic flow is desirable because it is characterized by a greater flow rate after the system has been agitated. Thixotropy refers to a reversible sol-gel system; it is characterized by a gel that forms a flowable sol when shaken. On standing, the reformation of the gel will slow particle settling. Caking is undesirable because settling particles form a dense pack at the bottom of the container. It is very difficult to break this cake and reconstitute the original suspension. *(1)*

126. **(C)** Inhalation aerosol products may be intended for either localized activity (bronchodilators for asthma) or systemic action (ergotamine for migraine). In either situation, the onset of action will be rapid. When the drug is absorbed through the alveolar-capillary membrane, the first-pass metabolism in the liver is avoided. Because of the limited capacity of aerosol units, especially in the small-chamber metered valves only a limited amount of drug can be administered. *(1)*

127. **(A)** Actron contains 12.5 mg of ketoprofen. Aleve contains 225 mg naproxyn sodium, and Nuprin has 200 mg ibuprofen. *(2; 3)*

128. **(A)** The first-degree burn is the mildest injury because only the epidermis is affected.

    (C—incorrect) These are characteristics of a second-degree burn, which affects the epidermis and portions of the dermis.

    (D—incorrect) A third-degree burn penetrates through the entire skin. Damage may be permanent.

    (E—incorrect) These are characteristics of the fourth-degree or char burn. Both the skin and underlying tissues are affected. *(2)*

129. **(D)** Debrisan is not useful in the treatment of nonsecreting wounds. Its action appears to be absorption of fluids and particles that impede tissue repair. The product is available as 0.1- to 0.3-mm spherical beads (4 g packets) that are sprinkled onto secreting wounds. The hydrophilic nature of the beads creates a strong suction force; each gram absorbs about 4 mL of fluid. The beads become grayish yellow when they are saturated with fluid; they should then be washed away by irrigating with sterile water or saline. *(1; 24)*

130. **(B)** Although phenol (carbolic acid) possesses both antiseptic and local anesthetic effects, there is the possibility that it may accentuate tissue damage because of its caustic properties. *(1; 2)*

    Benzocaine is widely used for surface anesthesia of the skin and mucous membranes. It remains on the skin for a long period of time because of its poor water solubility and slow absorption. Systemic toxicity is rare. Although the possibility of local sensitization should be considered, the incidence is low considering the frequent use of benzocaine. Although the incidence of hypersensitivity to lidocaine is lower than that of benzocaine, prolonged administration of lidocaine to a large skin area may result in systemic side effects. Lidocaine is present in Medi-Quik Aerosol, Bactine, and Unguentine Plus. *(1)*

131. **(D)** A topical preparation should contain a minimum of 5% benzocaine. Some studies have indicated that 10% to 20% of the drug is needed. *(2; 11)*

132. **(D)** Alcohol USP, sometimes known as grain alcohol, contains 94.9% v/v or 92.3% w/w of ethanol (C_2H_5OH). The remaining portion is water. It may be used as a solvent and as a source of alcohol for oral dosage forms. *(1; 24)*

133. **(A)** Diluted alcohol is prepared by mixing equal volumes of Alcohol USP and purified water with the final strength being 49%. Some volume shrinkage occurs because of hydrogen bonding. This attractive force between hydrogen atoms and electronegative atoms such as oxygen, fluorine, and nitrogen results in the miscibility of certain solvents and increases the solubility of certain chemicals. The

shrinkage phenomenon that occurs when mixing equal volumes of Alcohol USP (95%) and purified water results in approximately 3% shrinkage from the theoretical volume. If one wishes to prepare 100 mL of diluted Alcohol USP, a solution that contains 49% v/v ethanol plus purified water, equal volumes of each are used. However, one must also remember to use an excess of at least 3% of both liquids to ensure obtaining the required volume. *(1; 12)*

134. **(B)** Rubbing alcohol is a form of denatured alcohol containing approximately 70% of absolute alcohol. This product is used as a germicide and as an external rubefacient. *(1; 24)*

135. **(D)** Although the venoms of some insects are potent, the amounts injected are too small to be toxic. The severity of the sting reaction in some individuals is due to their hypersensitivity to certain proteins in the venom. This results in the anaphylactic shock. *(2; 11)*

136. **(D)** Persons who experience severe anaphylactic reactions to insect sting or bites should carry emergency kits. These kits usually contain antiseptic pads (to clean and disinfect the area), both an antihistamine and epinephrine injection (to counteract the anaphylactic reaction), and tweezers (to remove the stingers). A tourniquet would be of little value because the amount of venom is very small. Self-injectable units of epinephrine, such as EpiPen, are also available for individuals known to be susceptible to stings. *(3; 10)*

137. **(E)** Products used to reduce the potential of skin cell damage due to excessive sun exposure have designated SPF's numbers on their labeling. The higher the number the greater the extent of protection. *(27)*

Incorrect answers include: **(A)** Hidrosis refers to the production and excretion of sweat. **(B)** Melanogenesis refers to the formation of melanin in the skin layers with subsequent migration to the surface thus resulting in tanning. **(C)** Pruritus refers to itching. **(D)** One of the major symptoms of Sjogren syndrome is dryness of mucous membranes.

138. **(B)** Ecamsule (Mexoryl) is one of the newer topical sunscreening agents often used in combination with avobenzone and octocrylene. Commercial products containing ecamsule include Anthelios and Helioplex. Ecamsule blocks some dangerous UV-A wavelengths as well as UV-B wavelengths.

139. **(B)** Pamabrom, a xanthine derivative, is present in several OTC products for the prevention of premenstrual syndrome (PMS), specifically bloating. Its diuretic activity is obtained with a dose of 25 to 50 mg four times a day. Examples of products containing pamabrom include Midol PMS and Pamprin. *(2; 11)*

140. **(A)** The carbamide peroxide will effervesce, thereby softening the waxy material. An example of an OTC product is Debrox that also contains glycerin and propylene glycol that act as solvents. *(2; 11)*

141. **(E)** Diffusion of a drug from a vehicle into the skin is often related to the solubility of the drug in the vehicle relative to the solubility in the skin, that is, the partition coefficient. Drugs that are very soluble in a vehicle will tend to remain in the vehicle and will penetrate more slowly than drugs with poorer solubility in the vehicle. *(1)*

(A—incorrect) Covering the area to which a topical drug product has been applied will often enhance the rate of drug absorption. Sweat accumulation at the skin—vehicle interface induces hydration of the skin, a condition that facilitates penetration of drugs.

(B—incorrect) Poorer solubility of the drug in PEG ointment than in white ointment may lead to faster diffusion. This is the converse of choice E.

(C—incorrect) The thicker epidermis of the palms results in slower drug penetration than that which occurs on the backs of the hands.

(D—incorrect) Higher drug concentrations will increase the rate of diffusion and penetration. *(1; 24)*

142. **(B)** Melatonin is an endogenous hormone produced by the human pineal gland. It appears to shift the circadian rhythm and may

serve as a sleep aid when taken 1 to 2 hours before bedtime. *(2)*

143. (E) A major use for melatonin is to reduce jet lag caused by crossing several time zones; the best course of action is probably to start taking melatonin after arrival at the new location. One wants to readjust his/her circadian sleep pattern to the new location. While dosing may vary, 2 to 5 mg on the day of arrival and continuing for 2 to 5 days will suffice. *(2)*

144. (E) Selected combinations of the PEGs can be formulated into water-miscible suppositories with a range of consistency. They are easy to insert and do not require refrigeration. *(24)*

145. (A) Lactose is a readily compressible and water-soluble inert ingredient. It also encourages the growth of Doderlein's bacilli, a microorganism present in the healthy vagina. *(24)*

146. (D) The extent of drug release and absorption will vary depending upon the properties of the drug, the suppository base, and the condition of the colon. Oil-soluble drugs will be poorly released from a cocoa-butter base because of their high lipid/water solubility. *(24)*

(A—incorrect) The rectal fluid pH is essentially neutral and has a low buffer capacity. Therefore, drugs that can be destroyed by the acidity of the stomach may be successfully administered rectally.

(B—incorrect) Drugs that are absorbed through the colon pass into the lower hemorrhoidal veins and into the general systemic circulation. Avoidance of first-pass exposure to the liver may enhance the effect of those drugs inactivated by the liver. Drugs that are absorbed from the upper intestinal tract pass directly through the portal vein into the liver, where metabolism may occur.

(E—incorrect) The lesser dose frequency and lower propensity for irritation are the reasons certain drugs can be administered rectally but not orally.

147. (B) Semicid inserts contain 100 mg of the spermicide nonoxynol-9. The active ingre-

dient in Norforms vaginal suppositories is the quaternary ammonium germicide, benzethonium chloride, which decreases odor-producing microorganisms. Terazole contains terconazole for the treatment of moniliasis. *(2; 24)*

148. (E) Carbomers (Goodrich's Carbopols) are polymers with a number of carboxy groups present. When the pH of a solution containing the carbomer is increased, there will be a significant increase in viscosity. *(1)*

149. (A) Solutions with equal osmotic pressure are iso-osmotic; they also will be isotonic if separated by a membrane permeable to the solvent but impermeable to the solute. Any of the colligative properties can be used to determine tonicity of solutions. Freezing-point depression values are used most frequently. The freezing point of a 0.9% sodium chloride aqueous solution is $-0.52°C$, the same as that of human blood and tears. Saline solutions of this concentration are isotonic with these body fluids. More concentrated solutions are hypertonic, while less concentrated are hypotonic. *(1)*

150. (A) Properties of a solution that depend on the number of particles of the solute and are independent of the chemical nature of the solute are termed colligative properties. The magnitude of vapor pressure, freezing-point reduction, boiling-point elevation, and osmotic pressure are all related to the number of particles in solution. *(1)*

151. (D) Solutions with the same osmotic pressure as blood are usually isotonic with blood. Solutions that have a higher osmotic pressure (ie., hypertonic) will cause water to pass out of the RBCs. Solutions that have a lower osmotic pressure (ie, hypotonic) will allow water to pass into the cells. This causes them to swell and rupture with a release of hemoglobin (hemolysis). *(1; 24)*

152. (C) A hypertonic solution will draw water from within the cell until an equilibrium is reached with equal pressure on each side of the cell membrane. Because of the loss of volume, the cell will shrink and take on a wrinkled appearance (crenation). *(1; 24)*

153. **(A)** A sodium chloride equivalent is the weight of sodium chloride that will produce the same osmotic effect as 1 g of the specified chemical. For example, morphine hydrochloride has an E value of 0.15. This indicates that 1 g of morphine hydrochloride produces the same osmotic pressure (and depression of freezing point) in solutions, as 0.15 g of sodium chloride. *(1; 12)*

154. **(C)** *The Remington: The Science and Practice of Pharmacy* presents extensive tables of sodium chloride equivalents (E) and freezing point depression (D) values. *(1)*

155. **(C)** Any two solutions that have the same freezing points will have the same osmotic pressure and should be isotonic. Because blood freezes at −0.52°C, any aqueous solution that freezes at this temperature will be iso-osmotic. The use of freezing-point data for isotonicity adjustment for both ophthalmic and parenteral solutions is common in the pharmaceutical industry because freezing points can be measured easily. *(1; 12)*

156. **(D)** Aqueous solutions that freeze at the same temperature as blood have the same osmotic pressure as blood (ie, are iso-osmotic with blood and each other). However, to be isotonic a solution must maintain a certain pressure, or tone, with the RBCs. If the chemical in a solution passes freely through the RBC membrane, equalized pressure on both sides of the membrane is not possible without changes in the cell volume. Tone will not be maintained, and the solution will not be isotonic, though it might be iso-osmotic with blood. *(1; 12)*

157. **(A)** The capacity of the cul-de-sac is estimated to be not more than 0.03 mL, with a normal tear volume of approximately 0.007 mL. Probably less than 0.02 mL of an ophthalmic solution can be placed successfully in an eye at one time. This volume is less than the nominal 0.05 mL (1 drop) usually requested in

prescription directions. This implies that a portion of the dose is lost through drainage or overflow onto the cheek. *(1)*

158. **(E)** In spite of its name, Veegum is not an organic gum but is an inorganic clay. It is water insoluble and would probably be unsuitable for ophthalmic administration since insoluble particles could be deposited in the ocular areas. *(1)*

159. **(B)** Increasing the contact time between a drug and the cornea will often increase the amount of drug absorption that will occur. *(1; 4)*

160. **(B)** Fluorescein sodium is an ophthalmic diagnostic agent. It is instilled into the eye to delineate scratches and corneal lesions. It would be very dangerous to place a contaminated solution on a damaged cornea through which microorganisms may easily pass. If *P. aeruginosa* enters the interior of the eyeball, blindness may occur quickly. Pharmacists should not prepare fluorescein sodium solutions extemporaneously unless sterility can be guaranteed. Pharmaceutical manufacturers supply fluorescein as unit-dose solutions or individual paper strips. *(1)*

161. **(A)** *Acanthamoeba* keratitis has been identified in solutions used by contact lens wearers. These solutions were either home-made or commercial solutions that were recycled. Thermal disinfection is effective in eliminating microbial contamination including *Acanthamoeba*. *(2)*

162. **(A)** The combination of benzalkonium chloride and edetate (0.01% of each) is effective against those microorganisms likely to contaminate ophthalmic solutions. These include some strains of *P. aeruginosa* that are resistant to benzalkonium chloride alone. *(4; 24)*

163. **(D)** Papain and subtilisin are proteolytic enzymes that aid in the removal of proteinaceous residues that slowly build up on soft lenses during wear. Allergan markets Enzymatic Contact Lens Cleaner as tablets containing papain. Subtilisin is present in Bausch &

Lomb's ReNu series of products. A third enzyme that has been used is pancreatin. Once weekly, the soft lenses are soaked overnight in solutions prepared from the previously mentioned products. Hydrogen peroxide is the active ingredient in a number of soft lens disinfecting products. *(2)*

164. **(C)** Sodium bisulfite and sodium metabisulfite are included in pharmaceutical solutions as antioxidants. For example, the oxidation of epinephrine may be retarded by the presence of sodium bisulfite, which is preferentially oxidized. Unfortunately, some individuals are sensitive to the bisulfites and must avoid products containing them. The labels of many wines caution about the presence of bisulfites. *(1; 4)*

165. **(A)** One of the first signs of sensitivity to bisulfites is difficulty in breathing. Also, the patient may experience hives, abdominal pain, and wheezing. Bisulfites are one of the few ingredients that must be included on the labels of wines. *(24)*

166. **(C)** Because membrane filtration does not involve heat, it is suitable for drug solutions that either are sensitive to heat or have not been studied sufficiently concerning their heat stability. The pharmacist may purchase presterilized filter units such as Millipore's Millex through which 15 to 100 mL of solution can be filtered. However, autoclaving is still considered the most reliable sterilization procedure. *(13)*

167. **(D)** Since the ophthalmic solution is heat stable, steam autoclaving (121°C/15 lb of pressure per 15–30 minutes) is suitable. Depending upon the total volume of solution, membrane filtration into sterile bottles is feasible. Ethylene oxide gas is not practical since the gas must be in direct contact with the microbes. The gas could not penetrate the glass walls of the bottles and, if it did, it would contaminate the solution. *(1; 24)*

168. **(C)** Lyophilization or freeze-drying is a procedure by which water is sublimed from a frozen product. The remaining drug powder (cake) is more stable than the original solution. Although a second advantage is that the powder will dissolve quickly when diluent is added for reconstitution, which is not the main purpose for the procedure. The process of freeze-drying is relatively expensive and is usually reserved for drugs that have limited stability in aqueous solutions. *(1)*

169. **(B)** Often the weight of active drug in a lyophilized powder is very low and difficult to observe by the pharmacist attempting to reconstitute the dry powder. To obtain a larger, more visible cake, a bulking agent such as mannitol may be included in the formula so that the pharmacist may more readily ascertain when dissolution is completed. *(1)*

170. **(A)** Benzyl alcohol is used in many parenterals, especially in bacteriostatic sterile water for injection as an antimicrobial agent. Although its relative toxicity is low, there are a few reports of hypersensitivity. Also, it is contraindicated for use in premature infants because of reports of fetal toxic syndrome. *(13)*

171. **(D)** By definition. *(1; 12)*

172. **(C)** The Henderson–Hasselbalch equation, or buffer equation for a weak acid and its corresponding salt, is represented by

$$pH = pK_a + \log\left(\frac{[salt]}{[acid]}\right),$$

where pK_a is the negative log of the dissociation constant of the weak acid and salt/acid is the ratio of the molar concentrations of salt and acid in the system. The volume of the solution is not critical because the chemical concentrations are already expressed in terms of molar concentration. *(12)*

173. **(E)** According to the Henderson–Hasselbalch equation, pH will equal pK_a when the expression log([salt]/[acid]) is equal to zero. This can occur only when the salt/acid ratio equals 1, because the log of 1 is 0. The point at which the salt concentration equals the acid

concentration is the half-neutralization point. It is also the pH at which a buffer system, based on the weak acid's pK_a, has the best buffering capacity. *(12)*

174. **(C)** Hydrochloric acid is classified as a strong acid. Strong acids ionize almost completely into hydronium ions and the corresponding anions. Other strong acids are sulfuric and nitric. These acids do not have pK_a values listed because the values would be close to 0. The fact that all of the other acids listed in the question have pK_as indicates that they are weaker acids (with less ionization) than hydrochloric acid. *(12)*

175. **(C)** Strong acids have larger ionization constants than weak acids. Because the pK_a is the reciprocal of the log of the ionization constant, stronger acids have lower pK_as than weaker acids. Of the acids listed, boric acid has the highest pK_a; thus, it is the weakest of these acids. Salicylic acid, which has the lowest pK_a on the list, is the strongest. *(12)*

176. **(D)** A buffer system consists of a weak acid or base and its corresponding strong salt. In preparing a buffer system, one should choose an acid or a base with a pK_a close to the desired pH. For example, lactic acid and sodium lactate can be combined to obtain a pH of exactly 4.0. The needed molar concentration of each may be calculated by using the Henderson–Hasselbalch equation. *(1; 12)*

177. **(C)** This problem may be solved using the Henderson–Hasselbalch equation knowing that the pK_a of boric acid is 9.24.

$$pH = pK_a + \log\left(\frac{salt}{acid}\right)$$

$$pH = 9.24 + \log\left(\frac{0.05 \text{ mol/dL}}{0.005 \text{ mol/dL}}\right). \quad (23)$$

$$pH = 9.24 + \log 10$$

$$pH = 9.24 + 1 = 10.24$$

178. **(B)** For determining the ratio of a weak acid to its salt present at a given pH, the Henderson–Hasselbalch equation is used.

$$pH = pK_a + \log\left(\frac{dissociated}{undissociated}\right),$$

or

$$pH = pK_a + \log (B/A)$$

(B = ibuprofen salt; A = ibuprofen).

Substituting the pK_a of ibuprofen (5.5) and the pH of the urine of 7.5

$$7.5 = 5.5 + \log (B/A) \qquad \log (B/A) = 2.0.$$

Thus, the ratio of the dissociated form of the drug (B) to the undissociated form (A) will be the antilog of 2, a numeric value of 100. *(24)*

179. **(A)** This problem is solved using the same thought process as for question 178.

$$pH = pK_a + \log\left(\frac{dissociated}{undissociated}\right)$$

or

$$pH = pK_a + \log (B/A)$$

(B = salt of aspirin; A = aspirin)

Substituting the pK_a of aspirin (3.5) and the pH of the urine of 4.5

$$4.5 = 3.5 + \log (B/A) \qquad \log (B/A) = 1.0.$$

Thus, the ratio of the dissociated form of the drug (B) to the undissociated form (A) will be the antilog of 1, a numeric value of 10 or 10/1. Since (A) represents the aspirin, only 1 of every 11 molecules will be aspirin (a percentage of 9%) and 10 molecules will be the salt of aspirin (a percentage of 91%). *(24)*

180. **(D)** Because of individual patient biological variation and the technologic limitations of the precise control of drug release, drugs with either short half-lives, or low therapeutic indexes are not suited for sustained-release products. A drug which requires a dosage of 500 mg t.i.d is usually not suitable since 1,500 mg would be needed in the sustained-release dosage form. Almost all sustained-release products are designed for the treatment of chronic conditions in which acute dosing adjustments are not necessary. Hopefully, sustained-release products will improve patient compliance by requiring less frequent dosing. *(24)*

181. **(C)** Sustained-release dosage forms are intended to reduce dosing frequency while maintaining relatively consistent blood levels of the drug. The duration of activity of drugs with half-lives between 2 and 8 hours can be extended to obtain convenient once- or twice-daily dosing. Although it would be desirable to increase the therapeutic duration of those drugs with half-lives of less than 2 hours, the required high drug-release rates and high drug concentration in the dosage form reservoir usually preclude sustained-release dosage formulation. Also, individual biological variation could result in either sub- or hypertherapeutic blood levels. Drugs with half-lives greater than 8 hours usually have long intervals between doses, making sustained-release formulations unnecessary. *(1; 24)*

182. **(C)** GlaxoSmithKline's Spansule formulation consists of medicated pellets in a capsule dosage form. Some pellets are uncoated to give almost immediate drug release, whereas other pellets have lipid coatings of various thicknesses. Thus, the initial dose is reinforced with additional drug release over a period of time. Examples of Spansule products include Compazine and Thorazine. Another group of products based on the same principle are Lederle's Sequels including Diamox and Ferro-sequels. *(1; 24)*

183. **(E)** To meet USP specifications, not more than one capsule in a batch of 100 may assay as low as 30% below the labeled claim. Also, one capsule may exceed the labeled claim by as much as 25%. Also, not more than 10 of 100 capsules may be outside the 85% to 115% limit of the labeled claim. These surprising liberal limits are necessary because of manufacturing difficulties. *(24)*

184. **(C)** The original oral osmotic pump drug delivery system was Alza's Oros system. A semipermeable membrane allowed water to enter the tablet without causing tablet disintegration. Instead, small amounts of dissolved drug would leave the tablet for activity in the body. Both Glucotrol XL and Procardia XL are examples of Pfizer's osmotic gastrointestinal therapeutic system. Ferro-sequels are examples of encapsulated active drug in a capsule dosage form. *(1; 24)*

185. **(C)** Effexor XR (venlafaxine) is an extended release product for treatment of depression. It is available in a capsule dosage form suitable to be either swallowed or sprinkled onto food. Depakote (divalproex sodium) is also available as sprinkle capsules and used in epilepsy therapy. Ditropan XL (oxybutynin chloride) is an extended release tablet formula which must be swallowed whole. Its mechanism is the osmotic pressure-controlled delivery. *(3; 10)*

186. **(C)** A container that reduces light transmission in the range of 290 to 450 nm to the level specified in the USP may be considered light resistant and affords suitable protection from light. The container may be constructed of glass or plastic. Although amber units are most common, other colored or opaque containers may meet the official requirements. *(4; 18c; 24)*

187. **(D)** Yellow ferric oxide is included in some tablet formulas as a coloring agent. The amount of iron present is a subtherapeutic dose. Red ferric oxide is mixed with white zinc oxide to prepare calamine, which has a pink color. *(1; 4)*

188. **(E)** The expiration date for a pharmaceutical is based on the length of time during which the product continues to meet the specified monograph requirements. Requirements are stated in terms of amount of active ingredient that is present as determined by suitable assay. Most drug products are considered usable until approximately 10% of the drug or drug activity has been lost. However, some monographs specify other ranges. For example, digoxin tablets must assay between 92% and 108% of label claim. *(1)*

189. **(B)** Pharmacists are using beyond-use dating quite often as guidelines when dispensing prescriptions to limit prolonged use of the drug by the patient. This date is usually a shorter time span than the manufacturer's expiration date found on the original package. The beyond-use date shall not be later than either the expiration date on the manufacturer's container or 1 year from the date of dispensing, whichever is earlier. For reconstituted products, the beyond-use date will be of a significantly shorter duration and is based on the manufacturer's recommendation in the package insert or on the package. *(4)*

190. **(B)** The drug solution lost 0.5 mg of its 2.0 mg/mL concentration in 24 hours. This represents a loss of

$$\frac{0.5}{2.0} = 0.25 \text{ or } 25\%.$$

Since first-order reaction rates are expressed as fraction per unit of time, the value will be 0.25/d. *(24)*

191. **(A)** This problem may be solved either by using an equation or by the simple relationship of

Original concentration = 2.0 mg/mL
After one half-life (4 days) = 1.0 mg/mL
After two half-lives (8 days) = 0.5 mg/mL
After three half-lives (12 days) = 0.25 mg/mL.
(24)

192. **(B)** First, determine the concentration after 3 days.

Original concentration = 10,000 units/mL
After one half-life (1 day) = 5,000 units
After two half-lives (2 days) = 2,500 units
After three half-lives (3 days) = 1,250 units

Next, determine the milliliters of the final solution that contains the required dose of 2,000 units.

$$\frac{1,250 \text{ units}}{1 \text{ mL}} = \frac{2,000 \text{ units}}{x \text{ mL}}.$$

$$x = 1.6 \text{ mL} \qquad (24)$$

193. **(E)** Not only do drugs that consist proteins undergo the normally expected decomposition due to heat, they also are susceptible to denaturation. This process may occur during excessive or vigorous shaking of the protein solutions. *(1; 10)*

194. **(D)** Chlorobutanol is included in some ophthalmic and parenteral solutions as an antimicrobial preservative. All of the other chemicals listed may serve as antioxidants. Ascorbyl palmitate, butylated hydroxytoluene, and vitamin E are oil soluble, thus limiting their use to lipophilic systems. Ascorbic acid is a water-soluble antioxidant. *(4)*

195. **(D)** For many years, the Curie (Ci) has been the basic unit for expressing radioisotope decay. Now the Becquerel is recognized as the official unit. One Becquerel equals one decay per second (dps).

$$1 \text{ curie} = 3.7 \times 10^{10} \text{ Bq (dps).}$$

The rad is a quantitative measure of radioactivity. *(24)*

196. **(B)** Decay rate is the rate at which atoms undergo radioactive disintegration. The rate of decay ($\sim dn/dt$) is proportional to the number of atoms (n) present at any time (t); thus, radioactive decay is a first-order process. *(1)*

197. **(C)** Gamma radiation, x-rays, and ultraviolet radiation are forms of electromagnetic radiation and are radiated as photons or quanta of energy. These forms of radiation differ only in wavelength and are the most penetrating types of radiation. Gamma rays are the most penetrating of all and can easily penetrate more than a foot of tissue and several inches of lead. *(1; 13)*

(A—incorrect) Alpha radiation is particulate radiation consisting of two protons and two neutrons. The range of alpha particles is about 5 cm in the air and less than 100 μm in tissue.

(B—incorrect) Beta radiation is also particulate radiation, but exists as two types, the negative electron (negatron) and the positive electron (positron). Both may have a range of over 10 feet in the air and up to about 1 mm in the tissue.

198. (B) ^{90m}Tc is available commercially as a technetium generator from various manufacturers in which molybdenum ^{99}Mo is the parent nuclide. The half-life of technetium (6 hours) is long enough to allow completion of usual diagnostic procedures for which it is used, yet short enough to minimize the radiation dose to the patient. Lack of a beta component in its radiation further decreases the dose delivered to the patient. The gamma energy is weak enough to achieve good collimation, yet strong enough to penetrate tissue sufficiently to permit deep-organ scanning. *(1; 13)*

199. (B) Although it is desirable to use isotopes with short half-lives to minimize the radiation dose received by the patient, it is evident that the shorter the half-life, the greater the problem of supply. Radioisotope generators, or cows, have been developed to deal with this problem. A radioisotope generator is an ion-exchange column containing a resin of alumina on which a long-lived parent nuclide is absorbed. Radioactive decay of the long-lived parent results in the production of a short-lived daughter nuclide that is eluted or milked from the column by means of an appropriate solvent such as sterile, pyrogen-free saline. *(1)*

200. (D) Although Alcohol USP (95% v/v ethanol) is usually used in the production of pharmaceuticals, labels stating alcohol concentration are based on 100% v/v ethanol (absolute alcohol). Proof strengths of products are easily calculated by simply doubling the % v/v ethanol concentration. *(1; 23)*

201. (C) The benzophenones are effective in screening out the harmful (skin burning) UVB wavelengths as well as some of the UVA spectra. The cinnamates will screen the UVB wavelengths, and a combination of the two categories of sunscreens are often incorporated into commercial formulas. Methyl salicylate (oil of wintergreen) is included in topical products mainly for its pleasant odor. It does not possess sunscreening properties. However, homomenthyl salicylate (homosalicylate) possesses sunscreen properties. *(2; 11)*

202. (C) The SPF is a numeric value that indicates the multiple length of time an individual may be exposed to the sun with minimal erythema as compared to the exposure time without any protection. In this example, 30 minutes × 12 = 6 hours is the maximum protection that may be expected. Obviously, there are many variables that affect the quantity of radiation received on any day. *(2; 11)*

203. (C) Both ophthalmic and nasal preparations should have only a mild buffer capacity so that the organ's natural buffer system can overcome any pH differences. Otherwise, irritation might result. *(1)*

(A—incorrect) Nasal preparations usually have a pH in the range of 5.5 to 6.5. Often, phosphate buffers are used.

(B—incorrect) Rendering the nasal solution isotonic will decrease potential for damage to the local tissue.

(D—incorrect) The presence of an antimicrobial preservative is important because there may be accidental contamination of the dropper or nasal spray tip.

204. (A) Singulair (montelukast) is available as 10 mg tablets, 4 and 5 mg chewable tablets, and 4 mg oral granules. *(25)*

205. (C) Coumadin is DuPont's brand of warfarin sodium and is available in several strengths for convenient dosage adjustments. Tablets containing 2, 2.5, 5, 7.5, and 10 mg are marketed. *(25)*

206. (D) The antidepressant, Prozac (fluoxetine) is available in several strengths and dosage forms including Pulvules (10, 20, and 40 mg), a 10 mg tablet, a liquid (20 mg/5 mL), and a 90 mg tablet intended for once a week dosing. *(3)*

207. (C) Januvia (sitagliptin) is intended for control of type 2 diabetes. Available strengths include 25, 50, and 100 mg. *(3; 25)*

208. (A) Tricor (fenofibrate) is used to reduce body cholesterol. It is available in strengths of 48 and 145 mg. *(3)*

209. **(C)** Augmentin consists of amoxicillin and clavulanate potassium. Ziac contains bisoprolol plus hydrochlorothiazide. Zithromax has only azithromycin as an active ingredient. *(3; 25)*

210. **(A)** Percodan contains aspirin plus oxycodone. *(3; 10)*

211. **(D)** Lidocaine (Xylocaine) is a (local) anesthetic available as a cream, an ointment, and an oral spray. Lidocaine HCl is administered by injection as well as topically. *(3; 25)*

212. **(C)** Procaine (Novocain) is available only for parenteral use. *(1; 6)*

213. **(B)** Both Avinza and Kadian are long release forms of morphine sulfate.

214. **(E)** All of the products contain levothyroxine. *(10)*

215. **(C)** Dilacor XR and Tiazac are available as extended-release forms of diltiazem. Verelan contains verapamil. *(10)*

216. **(D)** Sofarin and Panwarfin are brands of warfarin. Hytrin is an antihypertensive agent, terazosin. *(10)*

217. **(B)** Zydone contains hydrocodone plus acetaminophen. Oxycontin contains only oxycodone while Tylox contains a mixture of oxycodone and acetaminophen. *(10)*

218. **(A)** *(25)*

219. **(C)** *(25)*

220. **(B)** *(25)*

221. **(A)** *(25)*

222. **(G)** *(25)*

223. **(G)** *(25)*

224. **(E)** *(25)*

225. **(E)** MAbs are large protein molecules produced by WBCs. The MAbs are purified antibodies produced by a single source or clone of cells. Since these drugs will bind to a single specific antigen, they will target a particular protein or cell. Besides being used for laboratory tests such as pregnancy, injectable drugs have been marketed. Adalimumab (Humira) is used for rheumatoid arthritis, infliximab (Remicade) for Crohn's disease, trastuzumab (Herceptin) for cancer, and omalizumab (Xolair) for asthma. *(1; 24)*

226. **(A)** Efavirenz is a nonnucleoside reverse transcriptase inhibitor used for the treatment of HIV. *(1; 24)*

227. **(B)** CSFs are glycoprotein regulators that bind to specific surface receptors to control the proliferation and differentiation of marrow cells into macrophages, neutrophils, platelets, or erythrocytes. Hopefully the CSFs can stimulate the body to produce additional bone marrow and also slow the subdivision of cancer cells. Filgrastim (Neupogen) stimulates the production of neutrophils to treat chemotherapy-related neutropenia. A related product is pegfilgrastim (Neulasta) which will decrease infections and neutropenic fever during cancer therapy. The pegylation of filgrastim increases the drug's half-life by altering its clearance. *(1; 24)*

228. **(E)** Remicade is used for rheumatoid arthritis and Crohn's Disease in patients not responding to standard treatments. It is also approved for treatment of ulcerative colitis in patients not responding to first-line drugs such as aminosalicylates (Asacol) for inflammation or second choices such as the corticosteroids. *(10; 24)*

229. **(D)** The ILs are key immune system regulators that cause chain reactions that intensify the body's immune responses. Excessive amounts of IL-1 may cause inflammatory disorders; for example rheumatoid arthritis. However, several ILs have been engineered with beneficial effects. Opelvekin (Neumega) is used for treating neutropenia and thrombocytopenia associated with chemotherapy. The orphan drug, aldesleukin (Proleukin), is used in patients with metastatic renal carcinoma. *(24)*

230. **(C)** EPO is a glycoprotein that enhances erythropoiesis by stimulating formation of proerythroblasts and releasing reticulocytes from bone marrow. Lack of EPO is a leading cause of anemia. Products such as epoetin alfa (Epogen and Procrit) are used in anemic patients. *(1; 24)*

231. **(E)** Tissue plasminogen activators are substances produced by the inner lining of blood vessels and muscular wall of the uterus. Recombinant alteplase (Activase) is used in the management of acute myocardial infarction, acute ischemic stroke, and pulmonary embolism. A major use is the treatment of massive pulmonary embolisms. The lyophilized powder is reconstituted with sterile water for injection; the resulting foam is allowed to dissipate then the solution is administered intravenously. The reconstituted solution is stable for only 8 hours at room temperature. *(24)*

232. **(A)** The antihyperlipidemic drug, Zetia (Ezetimibe) is marketed as a 10-mg tablet. *(10)*

233. **(C)** Ultram (tramadol) is classified as a central analgesic. *(10)*

234. **(A)** Strattera (atomoxetine) is a psychotherapeutic agent available as 10, 18, 25, 40, and 60 mg capsules. *(10)*

235. **(A)** The nonbenzodiazepine, zolpidem (Ambien), may be classified as a hypnotic, sedative, or tranquilizer. *(10)*

236. **(B)** The antidepressant Paxil (paroxetine) is available as 10-, 20-, 30-, and 40-mg tablets. *(10)*

237. **(B)** Prilosec (omeprazole) is available as both a 10- and 20-mg delayed-release capsule. It is intended for the short-term treatment of active duodenal ulcers. *(10)*

238. **(D)** The antihistamine, Allegra (fexofenadine) is marketed as 60-mg tablets. *(10)*

239. **(B)** Claritin (loratadine) is available as a non-prescription drug antihistamine. There are several dosage forms including a regular 10-mg tablet and as Claritin Reditabs that contain 10 mg of micronized drug for faster dissolution by placement on the tongue. Claritin-D contains 5 mg loratadine and 120 mg of pseudoephedrine. *(10)*

240. **(B)** Zyrtec (cetirizine HCl) is available as both 5 and 10 mg tablets and a syrup (5 mg/5 mL). It is an antihistamine. *(10)*

241. **(A)** *(10)*

242. **(B)** *(10)*

243. **(E)** *(10)*

244. **(C)** *(10)*

245. **(G)** *(10)*

246. **(F)** *(10)*

247. **(I)** *(10)*

248. **(H)** *(10)*

249. **(J)** *(10)*

250. **(E)** *(10)*

251. **(C)** *(10)*

252. **(A)** *(10)*

253. **(D)** *(10)*

254. **(A)** Aluminum hydroxide is a commonly used antacid because of its nonabsorbability, demulcent activity, and ability to adsorb pepsin. It is somewhat slow in respect to the onset of action. A second antacid product with just aluminum hydroxide is Basaljel. *(2; 11)*

255. **(E)** Sodium bicarbonate is an effective antacid in its capacity to neutralize hydrochloric acid in the stomach. Unfortunately it tends to raise

the pH of stomach contents too high, thus resulting in acid rebound. Long-term use in patients with hypertension should be discouraged because of the sodium ion. Other products containing sodium bicarbonate are Brioschi, BiSoDol, and Soda Mint. *(1; 2; 11)*

256. **(D)** Calcium carbonate is often considered the antacid of choice because of the rapid onset of action, high neutralizing capacity, and relatively prolonged action. Side effects include constipation, which may be prevented by combining calcium carbonate with either magnesium carbonate or magnesium oxide. Prolonged use of calcium carbonate may result in the formation of urinary calculi. Also, increased blood levels of calcium have been reported. *(2; 11)*

257. **(B)** Magnesium hydroxide is mixed with aluminum hydroxide in order to reduce the incidence of constipation attributed to the aluminum ion, and to reduce the incidence of diarrhea due to the magnesium ion. Most antacid products on the market consist of this combination. *(2; 11)*

258. **(A)** *(2; 11)*

259. **(A)** Although both products contain mesalamine (5-aminosalicylic acid) as the active ingredient, they are available in different dosage forms. *(10)*

260. **(D)** Active ingredient is levothyroxin. *(10)*

261. **(C)** Active ingredient is fluticasone. *(10)*

262. **(B)** Active ingredient is verapamil. *(10)*

263. **(A)** Celebrex is available as 100 and 200 mg capsules for either once daily or twice a day dosing. It is intended for treatment of rheumatoid arthritis and osteoarthritis. *(10)*

264. **(E)** Cerebyx injection is intended as a replacement for parenteral Dilantin for both the prevention and treatment of seizures. *(10)*

265. **(B)** Celexa is available as 20- and 40-mg tablets for depression and is given once a day. *(10)*

266. **(D)** *(2; 11)*

267. **(E)** *(2; 11)*

268. **(B)** Besides Afrin, both Dristan 12-hour and Neosynephrine 12-hour sprays contain 0.05% oxymetazoline. *(2; 11)*

269. **(E)** *(1, 2)*

270. **(C)** *(1, 2)*

271. **(B)** *(1, 2)*

272. **(A)** *(1, 2)*

273. **(B)** The injectable form of Vitamin B_{12} is a slightly pink to light red color, which does not indicate decomposition. The solution is stable at room temperature. While injected either subcutaneously or intramuscularly, the dosing intervals should be clarified since the injections may be given daily, every other day, or weekly depending on the severity of the disease. *(2; 10)*

274. **(C)** Mineral oil consists of low-molecular-weight, short-chained hydrocarbons which would not be assimilated by body tissue. All of the other choices are vegetable oils, which would break down in the body. *(2)*

275. **(A)** An example is NovoLog Mix 70/30. *(25)*

276. **(B)** An example is Permapen containing Penicillin G Benzethine Suspension. *(13)*

277. **(E)** An example is Heparin Lock Flush System. *(13)*

278. **(D)** An example is Imitrex. *(25)*

279. **(D)** Stevia is available as Truvia, PureVia, and Sun Crystals as a sweetener.

Its intensity of sweetness is approximately 250 to 300 times that of sugar. Some customers claim a slight aftertaste of licorice. Other agents include saccharin (Sweet'N Low) that is 200 to 700 sweeter than sugar. Some customers complain of a bitter aftertaste. The warning that saccharin is associated with bladder tumor growth was revoked in 1970. Aspartame (Equal, Nutrasweet, Nata Taste) has an intensity of 180 to 200× and no after-taste. However, it contains phenylalanine, to which some patients are sensitive and is also sensitive to heat. Another choice is sucralose (Splenda) which is 600× sweeter than sugar but may cause a lingering aftertaste. *(1; 10)*

280. **(A)** Abbott Labs has a number of products under the Lifecare name including IV pumps. *(1)*

281. **(B)** *(1)*

282. **(C)** The needle hub can be made of plastic or metal. It is fitted onto the syringe body either by a locking system such as the Luer-Lok or by a simple friction fit. *(13)*

283. **(A)** The bevel is ground to sharpness, but the back portion (heel) of the bevel is left dull. A dull heel has been shown to decrease the incidence of coring of the rubber closure and the skin. *(13)*

284. **(B)** Needle cannulas are made of various grades of steel. Both shaft strength and flexibility are needed. *(13)*

285. **(E)** The hole in the shaft is also called the bore. *(13)*

286. **(D)** *(1)*

287. **(A)** *(1)*

288. **(E)** Many OTC products intended for assisting in the removal of warts contain the keratolytic agent, 17% salicylic acid, in a collodion vehicle. Examples of products include Compound W, Duofilm, and Clear-Away. *(11)*

289. **(C)** Coal tar, at levels of 0.5% to 5%, may help relieve mild attacks of psoriasis. *(11)*

290. **(E)** The normal pH range for the blood is 7.36 to 7.40 for venous samples and 7.38 to 7.42 for arterial samples. It is essential that the blood

pH remains within the range of 7.35 to 7.45. Normal acid–base balance is generally maintained by three homeostatic mechanisms using endogenous chemical buffers (eg, bicarbonate and carbonic acid), respiratory control, and renal function. An impairment in any of these mechanisms can result in either acidosis or alkalosis. *(1; 24)*

291. **(E)** The pH of the lacrimal fluid is approximately 7.4 but varies with certain ailments. The eye can tolerate a pH of 6 to 8 with a minimum of discomfort. The buffering system of the lacrimal fluid is efficient enough to adjust the pH of most ophthalmic solutions. However, some solutions, particularly those containing strongly acidic drugs, will cause discomfort. *(24)*

292. **(B)** The pH of the skin is usually based on measurements of the lipid film that covers the epidermis. Although the value varies greatly between individuals and in various areas of the body, the average value is reported to be 5.5, with a range of 4.0 to 6.5. *(1)*

293. **(A)** The acidic pH (3.5–4.2) of the vagina discourages the growth of pathogenic microorganisms while providing a suitable environment for the growth of acid-producing bacilli. *(24)*

294. **(C)**

295. **(D)**

296. **(E)** Allegra-D 24-hour tablets are a combination of fexofenadine HCl 180 mg and pseudoephedrine HCl 240 mg. The tablet's unique Osmodex delivery system regulates 24-hour release. Take once a day swallowing tab whole either on empty stomach or with full glass of water

297. **(B)**

298. **(A)**

299. **(C)** Echinacea, is believed to stimulate the immune system thus reducing the severity of

cold and flu symptoms especially if consumed during the early stages of the exposure. *(1; 2; 11)*

300. **(B)** Some studies have indicated that gingko extracts improve blood perfusion. There is hope that the herb will improve memory. A problem may occur if gingko is taken by individuals being treated with the anticoagulants. *(2; 11)*

301. **(A)** St. John's wort may help cases of mild depression. Its active ingredient, hypericin, is believed to cause photodermatitis if light-skinned clients are exposed to direct sunlight. *(2; 11)*

302. **(D)** Saw palmetto may be useful in treating symptoms of benign prostatic hyperplasia (BPH). It appears to improve urinary flow in men with enlarged prostates. *(2; 11)*

303. **(A)** Health authorities have accepted valerian as an effective treatment for restlessness and sleep disturbances. Some classify the herb as a mild tranquilizer. *(1)*

304. **(E)** Transdermal drug delivery systems deliver drugs at an optimal rate through the skin and avoid the hepatic first-pass effect. Since the patch needs replacement only once daily or up to once a week depending upon the drug involved, patient compliance improves. Since most of the drug is in the patch reservoir, relatively large amounts of drugs with short half-lives can be formulated into transdermal patches. One criteria is the ability of the drug to diffuse through the skin. *(24)*

305. **(C)** Bupropion (Zyban) is used to aid in smoking cessation. It is available as 100 and 150 mg sustained-release tablets but not as a dermal patch. However, there are a number of nicotine patches on the market for smoking cessation. Scopolamine (Transderm Scop) is used to prevent motion sickness. Estradiol (Estraderm, Vivelle, and Climara) patches reduce postmenopausal symptoms. Also, there is an estrogen progestin combination (Evra) for use as a contraceptive patch. Fentanyl

(Duragesic) reduces chronic pain. Testosterone patches (Testoderm and Androderm) are used when there is a deficiency of testosterone. *(24)*

306. **(C)** Most nasal solutions are mildly buffered at pHs between 5.5 and 7.5 to prevent interference with normal cilia motion. The solutions should also be isotonic if possible. *(19)*

307. **(B)** Coenzyme Q10 is an endogenous substance in the body. Abnormal low levels in the myocardium have been associated with cardiac heart failure. It has good antioxidant properties and is a cofactor for ATP in oxidative respiration. It is available in OTC products in doses of 50, 75, 100, and 200 mg. The usual dose is one 100 mg tablet daily with a meal or may be given in divided doses. *(2)*

308. **(B)** Cranberry juice appears to prevent UTIs perhaps by preventing the causative agent, *Escherichia coli*, from adhering to the bladder and urinary tract walls. Unfortunately, large amounts are needed: 5 to 10 ounces of cranberry juice or three times as much of cranberry juice cocktail. Although TMZ (trimethoprim/sulfamethoxazole) is standard treatment for UTIs, it is inadvisable to use it every day as a preventative measure. Antibiotics such as penicillin should be reserved for specific microbial cultures not with shotgun therapy. *(1; 2)*

309. **(C)** Garlic in the dosing ranges of 600 to 900 mg may be beneficial in counteracting hyperlipidemia and hypertension. The herb does not appear to have significant antioxidant properties. The strong odor of garlic may be reduced by using "odorless" garlic products, but some of these have reduced levels of the active ingredient, alliin. Use of enteric-coated tablets or capsules may be advantageous since the alliin will be protected from decomposition by gastric acid. *(2)*

310. **(E)** Finasteride (Proscar or Propecia) is a prescription drug used for treating BPH. The herb, Saw palmetto, has had some success in relieving this condition. *(2)*

311. **(B)** Long-term use of laxatives should be discouraged since a chronic "laxative habit" develops. The pharmacist may advise the affected individual to increase his/her water intake and switch to bulk-forming laxatives. These exert a milder laxative effect in the body usually in 12 to 24 hours and are less habit forming. Examples include Metamucil, Fiber-Con, and Fiberall. *(2)*

312. **(B)** Regular Zyrtec tablets have the word, Zyrtec, and the strength, 5 or 10, impressed on them. The chewable form of Zyrtec also has a C5 or C10. *(10; 25)*

313. **(A)** Valerian has been suggested as a mild tranquilizer and/or sedative for insomnia. One advantage is the absence of a residual effect the following morning. Safe use during pregnancy has not been confirmed. If used with other sedatives or alcohol, one would expect an additive effect. One or two 400 mg capsules is the usual dose. *(1; 2)*

314. **(A)** Controlled studies of ginger root in the form of capsules indicate its ability to counteract mild cases of nausea and vomiting and also to prevent motion sickness. *(2; 11)*

315. **(B)** The USP/NF recognizes Eleuthero root or Siberian ginseng as a distinct entity different from Asian or American ginseng. Commission E has approved its use as a tonic for fatigue and debility, declining capacity for work, or poor concentration. The term ADAPTOGEN is used to describe a product's ability to increase "nonspecific" resistance to stress. This may result in better selective memory and feelings of well-being. (18)

316. **(C)** Milk thistle contains a group of compounds known as the silymarins. The herb appears to provide protection to the liver that has been exposed to chemicals such as carbon tetrachloride, and drugs such as acetaminophen. *(1)*

317. **(A)** Echinacea has not been reported as having significant effects on blood coagulation times, perhaps because it is not intended for long-term use. Its main use is to prevent or reduce the severity of the common cold and other upper respiratory infections. Its efficacy depends upon consumption when the symptoms of the cold first appear. All of the other herbs in the question may affect blood coagulation and the patient taking warfarin should be informed of potential problems. *(2)*

318. **(C)** There are numerous chemical types of ingredients in crude drugs, which make extraction of the actives an exacting science. The use of alcohol as a solvent (menstruum) is common since many actives such as alkaloids are readily soluble and evaporation of some of the alcohol allows a standardization of the product. Extraction may be accomplished by soaking (macerating) the crude plant in the menstruum or by slowly passing the menstruum through the crude plant; a process known as percolation. Historically, pharmacists prepared extracts and fluid extracts as final dosage forms. Today, pharmaceutical companies perform extractions with more accurate assays and standardization. Reverse osmosis is not used for crude drug extraction. Instead the process is used for purification of liquids such as water. *(1; 24)*

319. **(A)** The dietary supplement glucosamine is a natural building block of cartilage. Pure glucosamine is available in products such as Aflexa tablets. However, the most popular type of product is combinations with chondroitin which have been found effective in providing symptomatic relief from osteoarthritis. *(1; 2)*

320. **(E)** St. John's wort contains several active ingredients and is usually labeled based on its concentration of hypericin or hyperforin. The herb is used for the treatment of mild depression. However, patients consuming oral contraceptive tablets should be informed of a potential reduction in the effectiveness of the birth control tablets. The herb also tends to cause a photosensitivity in fair-skinned people. *(1; 2)*

321. **(A)** Black cohosh has been shown to be successful for reducing the severity of PMS symptoms in some women. However, its

greatest use today is to replace hormone replacement therapy in the postmenopausal female. One product is Remifemin, which contains 20 mg of black cohosh and is dosed twice a day. *(2; 24)*

322. **(D)** There is a multitude of active constituents in feverfew. Probably the major therapeutic use is in the prevention of migraines. Usually 50 to 100 mg of feverfew extract is needed. It is not effective for acute attacks. *(2)*

323. **(E)** The maximum strength of hydrocortisone available OTC in the United States is 1%. All of the products listed in this question contain 1%. *(2; 11)*

324. **(A)** SAMe, S-Adenosylmethionine is a naturally occurring substance in the human body. It appears to possess antidepressant activity with only minor side effects such as heartburn. *(2)*

325. **(C)** Aloe vera gel from the leaf of *Aloe vera* appears to possess both antibacterial and antifungal properties. Many households use the fresh mucilaginous gel for minor burns and soft-tissue injuries. Several companies have marketed commercial products with aloe vera as the featured ingredient. One caution is the avoidance of concomitant use of topical steroids and aloe vera because of potential increase in systemic absorption of the steroid. Tea tree oil has similar properties but its main use has been for athlete's foot at a 5% concentration. It is also used at a 100% concentration for toenail fungal infections. *(2)*

326. **(A)** The prescription-only drug, orlistat (Xenical), is now available OTC as 60 mg capsules under the brand name of Alli. Being a lipase inhibitor, it is classified as an antiobesity agent. *(10)*

327. **(B)** Indications for Children's Pepto are stomach problems such as heartburn, acid indigestion, sour stomach, and upset stomach. The chewable tablets contain 400 mg calcium carbonate (161 mg calcium) and are intended for children between 2 and 12 years of age. *(2)*

328. **(D)** Both products contain natural vegetable senna ingredients, the sennosides. However, Senokot-S also contains 50 mg docusate sodium. *(2)332. (D)*

329. **(A)** Both 10 units and 100 units/mL strengths of heparin are used as flush solutions.

330. **(E)** Levothyroxine products are best taken first thing in the morning on an empty stomach.

331. **(B)** For some individuals, the facial flushing that may occur with niacin may be limited by administering a 325 mg aspirin tablet approximately 30 minutes before the niacin. Usually niacin is best taken near bedtime.

332. **(D)** Although Ambien is very useful in some patients who have difficulty falling asleep, many patients will benefit with Tylenol PM which contains APAP 500 mg and the sleep aid diphenhydramine 25 mg. The pharmacist should caution the patient that these products are intended for occasional use only. Other patients may benefit from the use of herbal products such as St. John's Wort as a sleep sedative. *(2; 9; 11)*

333. **(B)** Lovaza contains omega-3 fatty acids which lower high triglyceride levels. It is available as a 1-g capsule. Omega-3 fish oil is available from several reputable suppliers as a dietary supplement. Fish oil supplements are effective in reducing several cardiovascular disease risks factors and may help with some aspects of rheumatoid arthritis. Active ingredients are eicosapentaenoic acid (EPA) and docosahexaenoic (DHA) which while very safe, may cause GI complaints in some patients. Such patients may better tolerance Lovaza. *(2; 9; 11)*

334. **(C)** The prescription only Nexium (esomeprazole) is very popular for controlling peptic acid production as a proton pump inhibitor. OTC products such as Pepcid AC have similar activity at a lower cost. *(2; 9; 11)*

335. **(D)** Vitamin B_3 (niacin) may be effective in controlling elevated lipid levels in patients who cannot tolerate statins. *(2; 9; 11)*

336. **(C)** Cutting most transdermal patches before application to the skin will result in abnormal high release of active drug. Most patches are constructed with a reservoir membrane-modulated systems and drug release controlled by the membrane. The reservoir system will be disrupted when cut. Probably the most dangerous drug release upon cutting will occur with the Duragesic transdermal system which would likely result in an overdose of the potent opioid, fentanyl.

There are a few exceptions to the "no cutting" rule, namely, Lidoderm, Flector, and oxybutynin which will still have normal release of the impregnated drug. These patches have a micro-reservoir system with the drug in multiple, smaller drug reservoirs. *(3; 10)*

337. **(A)** The letters "HFA" represent hydrofluoroalkane propellants which have replaced the chlorofluorocarbon (CFC) propellants in order to further protect the ozone layer. HFA products taste different, are less forceful, and are warmer and mistier than the CFC sprays. Some consumers may notice the difference compared to the older products. Examples include Albuterol HFA, Nasacort HFA, and Proventil HFA. *(3; 10)*

338. **(B)** Ginseng (Panax ginseng) is subclassified into two major types—Asian and North American. Both are considered to be "adaptogens," which implies that consumption will make the client feel better or improve his/her "QOL" (quality of life). Eleutherococcus is sometimes called Siberian ginseng, an entirely different species (*Eleutherococcus senticosus*). It also is considered to be an adaptogen with some use as a tonic for invigoration due to fatigue or debility or for convalescence. It should not be used for more than 3-month duration and is contraindicated in hypertensive patients. *(2)*

CHAPTER 4

Pharmaceutical Compounding

Compounding is considered an intrinsic skill of the pharmacist. Although the number of extemporaneously compounded prescriptions is steadily declining, some pharmacists have experienced professional satisfaction in their ability to prepare products that would otherwise not be available to the patient. Pharmacists in institutional settings are expected to prepare parenteral admixtures, reconstitute parenteral powders, and advise other health professionals in the handling, storage, administration, and potential incompatibilities of sterile products. The emerging field of home health care has called on both community and institutional pharmacists to prepare sterile chemotherapeutic, analgesic, and nutritional formulations.

This chapter reviews some of the compounding techniques, ingredients, and calculations that the practicing pharmacist may need to use.

Questions

1. The prescription balance needed for weighing chemicals is currently designated as a Class _____ balance by the National Bureau of Standards (NBS).

   (A) I
   (B) II
   (C) III
   (D) P
   (E) Q

2. Which one of the following statements concerning single-pan electronic balances as replacements for the Class III balance is true?

   (A) They cannot be used since they are too accurate for routine weighing.
   (B) They are not suitable since the official shift and rider balance tests cannot be performed.
   (C) They may be used if they have a sensitivity requirement (SR) of 6 mg or better.
   (D) They are not recommended since their total weight capacity is often less than 120 g.
   (E) They may be used if their total weight capacity is not greater than 120 g.

3. A technician weighs 140 mg of a potent drug on an electronic balance, which is claimed suitable for weighing up to 100 g with an error of only ± 10 mg. What is the error in the above weighing?

   (A) 0.01%
   (B) 0.5%
   (C) 5%
   (D) 7%
   (E) 10%

4. Pharmacists performing extemporaneous compounding should select chemical grades that meet specifications found in which of the following references?

   I. *Remington Science and Practice of Pharmacy*
   II. *USP/DI*
   III. *USP/NF*

   (A) I only
   (B) III only
   (C) I and II only
   (D) II and III only
   (E) I, II, and III

5. A topical formula for compounding includes Carbomer 934. What is the purpose of this ingredient?

   (A) antimicrobial preservative
   (B) antioxidant
   (C) sunscreening agent
   (D) surfactant
   (E) thickening agent

Questions 6 through 9 relate to the following prescription:

For: James Latimer	Age: 3
Rx	
Sodium fluoride	500 µg
M & Ft cap DTD # LX	
Sig: one cap QD	

6. How many milligrams of sodium fluoride are required to prepare this prescription?

   (A) 0.5
   (B) 30
   (C) 50
   (D) 300
   (E) 500

7. Problem(s) that the pharmacist should anticipate in preparing this prescription include which of the following?

   I. caustic nature of sodium fluoride
   II. poor water solubility of sodium fluoride
   III. difficulty in weighing a small quantity of powder

   (A) I only
   (B) III only
   (C) I and II only
   (D) II and III only
   (E) I, II, and III

8. What is the best choice of a diluent for stock powders, especially when preparing capsules?

   (A) ascorbic acid
   (B) lactose
   (C) sodium chloride
   (D) starch
   (E) talc

9. The pharmacist fills a #2 capsule and finds that the net weight of the powder is 40 mg less than needed. What may she elect to do?

   I. use a #1 capsule
   II. place additional powder into the head of the capsule
   III. use a #3 capsule

   (A) I only
   (B) III only
   (C) I and II only
   (D) II and III only
   (E) I, II, and III

Questions 10 through 12 refer to the following prescription:

For: Daniel Cummins	Age: 16
Rx	
Codeine sulfate	210 mg
Dimenhydrinate	1,000 mg
ASA	3,000 mg
M & Ft cap #20	
Sig: one cap q.i.d. prn for pain	

NOTE: The pharmacist has 50-mg dimenhydrinate tablets, each weighing 200 mg, and 30-mg codeine sulfate tablets, each weighing 100 mg. Aspirin is available as a powder.

10. Which of the following statements concerning the prescription is (are) true?

   I. The amount of codeine being consumed per day is an overdose.
   II. There is a chemical incompatibility between dimenhydrinate and codeine.
   III. The patient should be cautioned about the possibility of drowsiness from the capsules.

   (A) I only
   (B) III only
   (C) I and II only
   (D) II and III only
   (E) I, II, and III

11. When compounding this prescription, what must the pharmacist do?

   I. use a rubber spatula rather than a stainless steel spatula
   II. add lactose to the formula
   III. take into consideration the weight of the excipients in the codeine and dimenhydrinate tablets

   (A) I only
   (B) III only
   (C) I and II only
   (D) II and III only
   (E) I, II, and III

12. What is the approximate final weight of each capsule?

   (A) 150 mg
   (B) 210 mg
   (C) 235 mg
   (D) 360 mg
   (E) 385 mg

Answer questions 13 through 15 based on the following prescription:

```
Name: James McMaster          Age: 4
                              Wt.: 44 lb
Rx
   Ondansetron HCl        0.15 mg/kg/tsp
   Cherry syrup                  qs 60 mL

Sig: one tsp before therapy
```

13. How many 4-mg commercial tablets are needed to prepare this order?

   (A) 3
   (B) 6
   (C) 9
   (D) 12
   (E) 15

14. Which of the following statements concerning compounding this prescription is (are) true?

   I. It is necessary to dissolve the crushed tablets in alcohol before adding it to the syrup.

   II. The pH of the final product should be adjusted to a neutral pH.
   III. It is possible to use ondansetron injectable solution in place of the tablets.

   (A) I only
   (B) III only
   (C) I and II only
   (D) II and III only
   (E) I, II, and III

15.

```
Rx Resorcinol                    1.2 g
   Pur. water                    15 mL
   Aquaphor                      15 g
   White pet.                 qs 100 g
```

The technician prepares this topical product by dissolving 1.2 g of resorcinol in 15 mL of purified water and then incorporating this solution into 15 g of Aquaphor. However, he then uses 20 g of white petrolatum. What is the percent concentration of resorcinol in the final product?

   (A) 0.8
   (B) 1.0
   (C) 1.2
   (D) 1.5
   (E) 1.7

16. The following formula has been used as an oral solution for prevention of motion sickness:

```
Dimenhydrinate                 250 mg
Glycerin                          qs
Ora-Plus                       50 mL
Ora-Sweet SF               qs 100 mL
```

Which of the following is (are) accurate?

   I. The inclusion of glycerin is as a solvent for dimenhydrinate.

   II. Ora-Plus has properties as a suspending agent.

   III. The formula is intended for diabetics.

(A) I only

(B) III only

(C) I and II only

(D) II and III only

(E) I, II, and III

Questions 17 through 21 relate to the following parenteral admixture order as received in a hospital pharmacy:

Patient: Ronald Hazelton	Room no. 614
	DOB: 4/28/44
Aminophylline	400 mg
KCl	20 mEq
Thiamine HCl	100 mg
Heparin	2,000 units
D₅W	500 mL

Infuse over 4 h at 1,000, 1,400, and 1,800

17. Which ingredient in the above parenteral admixture may present a compatibility problem?

    (A) aminophylline

    (B) potassium chloride

    (C) thiamine HCl

    (D) heparin

    (E) dextrose

18. Aminophylline is available in 20-mL ampules (25 mg/mL). How many ampules are needed daily for this order?

    (A) 1

    (B) 2

    (C) 3

    (D) 4

    (E) 5

19. What does the correct method(s) for preparing the previously shown admixture include?

    I. adding the potassium chloride solution to the D₅W, followed by the aminophylline solution

    II. adding the aminophylline solution to the D₅W first, then add the potassium chloride solution

III. mixing the aminophylline solution and the potassium chloride solution, then add this mixture to the D₅W

(A) I only

(B) III only

(C) I and II only

(D) II and III only

(E) I, II, and III

20. What is the total amount (mg) of potassium administered in each admixture bottle? (K = 39.1, Cl = 35.5)

    (A) 780 mg

    (B) 1,180 mg

    (C) 2,340 mg

    (D) 4,480 mg

    (E) 2,240 mg

21. After removing the aminophylline solution from the ampule, the pharmacist should pass the solution through a device such as a filter needle. What is the filter needle intended to remove?

    I. particulate matter

    II. microorganisms

    III. pyrogens

    (A) I only

    (B) III only

    (C) I and II only

    (D) II and III only

    (E) I, II, and III

22. When instructing a technician concerning aseptic techniques, she should stress that certain portions of a syringe are "critical." These areas include which of the following?

    I. collar

    II. ribs

    III. tip

    (A) I only

    (B) III only

    (C) I and II only

    (D) II and III only

    (E) I, II, and III

23. Which of the following techniques is (are) appropriate when using a filter needle for removing glass from an opened 10-mL glass ampule?

  I. Place filter needle on 10-mL syringe, draw up the solution, and add to LVP bag.

  II. Place filter needle on 10-mL syringe, draw up the solution, replace the needle with a regular needle, and add the solution to LVP bag.

  III. Draw up the solution using a regular needle, replace with a filter needle, and add the solution to LVP bag.

  (A) I only
  (B) III only
  (C) I and II only
  (D) II and III only
  (E) I, II, and III

24. Which of the following laminar flow hoods is (are) considered a suitable working area for preparing the previously mentioned admixture order?

  I. convergent
  II. horizontal
  III. vertical

  (A) I only
  (B) III only
  (C) I and II only
  (D) II and III only
  (E) I, II, and III

25. Which of the following is (are) appropriate techniques when preparing most parenteral admixtures?

  I. Work within 6 in of the high-efficiency particulate air (HEPA) filter.

  II. Use a vertical laminar flow hood.

  III. Work in an area at least 6 in from the edge of the benchtop.

  (A) I only
  (B) III only
  (C) I and II only

  (D) II and III only
  (E) I, II, and III

26. Which of the following would the pharmacist consider as suitable agents for disinfecting a laminar flow hood?

  I. alcohol 70%
  II. acetone
  III. betadine

  (A) I only
  (B) III only
  (C) I and II only
  (D) II and III only
  (E) I, II, and III

27. The American Society of Health-System Pharmacists (ASHP) has developed a risk level classification with the strictest controls. What is the designation?

  (A) risk level 1
  (B) risk level 3
  (C) risk level X
  (D) risk level A
  (E) risk level F

Questions 28 through 30 relate to the following medication order:

Patient: Constance Morehead

Age: 57

Room: CCU

Morphine sulfate 15 mg + hydroxyzine HCl 25 mg STAT

28. Which of the following consultations between the pharmacist and the nurse is (are) appropriate?

  I. The two solutions may be mixed together in a syringe in order to administer a single injection.

  II. The morphine injection may be administered by either the IM or the SC route.

III. A precipitate may occur if either drug solution is injected into a heparinized scalp vein infusion set.

(A) I only
(B) III only
(C) I and II only
(D) II and III only
(E) I, II, and III

29. Which of the following steps is INCORRECT when the pharmacist removes 1.5 mL of solution from a 30-mL multidose vial of morphine sulfate injection (10 mg/mL)?

(A) Draw up 1.5 mL of air into the syringe.
(B) Place point of syringe needle onto the vial's rubber closure at a 45° angle.
(C) Rotate needle so that the bevel opening is facing upward.
(D) Raise the needle angle to 90° and insert needle through the rubber closure.
(E) After injecting the air, remove 2 mL of solution and aspirate excess solution into an alcohol swab.

30. When obtaining a 3-mL dose from a 5-mL ampule, which one of the following steps is incorrect?

(A) Draw up 3 mL of air into the syringe.
(B) Disinfect the neck of the ampule using an alcohol swab.
(C) Break ampule neck by snapping neck toward the side of the laminar flow hood.
(D) Place needle tip into solution while holding the ampule almost horizontally.
(E) After drawing up approximately 4 mL of solution, aspirate excess solution into the alcohol swab.

Answer questions 31 through 33 in reference to the following medication order:

Medication Order—Carefree Hospital

Patient: James Gardner   Room 314

Potassium Pen G 2 megaunits in 100-mL minibottles q6h ATC for 4 days

---

NOTE: The pharmacy has vials containing 5 million units of potassium penicillin G that, when reconstituted with diluent, will contain 750,000 units/mL. The label on the vial states that the powder contains a citrate buffer to maintain a pH of 6 to 6.5.

31. What is the total number of minibottles needed for Mr. Gardner's therapy?

(A) 3
(B) 4
(C) 10
(D) 12
(E) 16

32. Which of the following parenteral vehicles is (are) suitable for the above order?

I. D_5W (pH 4.5)
II. Normal saline (pH 6.0)
III. $D_{2.5}W$/0.45 normal saline (pH 5.0)

(A) I only
(B) III only
(C) I and II only
(D) II and III only
(E) I, II, and III

33. Which of the following procedures should the pharmacist use in preparing the minibottles?

(A) Remove 2.7 mL of vehicle from the minibottle, then inject 2.7 mL of penicillin solution.
(B) Inject 2.7 mL of penicillin solution directly into the minibottle.
(C) Remove 6.7 mL of vehicle from the minibottle, then inject 6.7 mL of penicillin solution.
(D) Inject 6.7 mL of penicillin solution directly into the minibottle.
(E) Inject 4 mL of penicillin solution directly into the minibottle.

34. An admixture calls for 5 mL of a chemotherapeutic agent in 100 mL NS. Which of the following techniques is (are) appropriate?

   I. Prepare the admixture in a vertical laminar flow hood.

   II. Aseptically remove the 5 mL of drug solution from a 30-mL vial using a positive pressure technique.

   III. Remove 5 mL of normal saline from the bag before adding the additive solution.

(A) I only
(B) III only
(C) I and II only
(D) II and III only
(E) I, II, and III

Questions 35 through 37 refer to the following prescription:

> **Rx**
> Calamine
> Zinc oxide   aa qs 15 g
> Resorcinol   2 g
> Glycerin   15 mL
> Alcohol 70%   30 mL
> Purified water ad   120 mL
>
> Sig: Use as directed t.i.d.

35. How is the final dosage form of this prescription best described?

(A) colloidal solution
(B) elixir
(C) O/W emulsion
(D) W/O emulsion
(E) suspension

36. When preparing the prescription, what will the pharmacist do?

   I. use 15 g of calamine

   II. dissolve the resorcinol in the alcohol

   III. triturate calamine and zinc oxide together and wet with glycerin

(A) I only
(B) III only

(C) I and II only
(D) II and III only
(E) I, II, and III

37. Which of the following auxiliary labels should the pharmacist attach to the container when dispensing the previously mentioned product?

   I. for external use only

   II. shake well

   III. keep in a cool place

(A) I only
(B) III only
(C) I and II only
(D) II and III only
(E) I, II, and III

38. The following prescription is received:

> **Rx**
> Itraconazole   1%
> Propylene glycol   10 mL
> MC 1500   1.5%
> Purified water   qs 60 mL
>
> Sig: Apply to nail bed b.i.d. ut dict

When preparing this prescription, what should the pharmacist do?

   I. disperse 0.9 g of methylcellulose 1500 in hot water

   II. use the contents from six 100-mg Sporanox capsules

   III. wet the capsule powder with the propylene glycol

(A) I only
(B) III only
(C) I and II only
(D) II and III only
(E) I, II, and III

DIRECTIONS (Questions 39 through 44): Each group of items in this section consists of lettered headings followed by a set of numbered words or

phrases. For each numbered word or phrase, select the ONE lettered heading that is most closely associated with it. Each lettered heading may be selected once, more than once, or not at all.

Questions 39 through 45

    (A) hydrocarbon (oleaginous)
    (B) absorption (anhydrous)
    (C) emulsion (W/O type)
    (D) emulsion (O/W type)
    (E) water soluble

39. Cold cream

40. Hydrophilic petrolatum

41. Aquaphor

42. Petrolatum

43. Polyethylene glycol ointment

44. Hydrophilic ointment

45. An experimental drug appears to be sensitive to hydrolysis. Which of the following ointment bases may be suitable vehicles to make a topical dosage form of this drug?

    I. Hydrophilic petrolatum
    II. Nivea
    III. Hydrophilic ointment

    (A) I only
    (B) III only
    (C) I and II only
    (D) II and III only
    (E) I, II, and III

Questions 46 through 48 relate to the following prescription:

```
Rx
  Burow's solution
  Propylene glycol            aa 15 mL
  White petrolatum                 60 g
```

46. What is the active ingredient in Burow's solution?

    (A) acetic acid
    (B) aluminum acetate
    (C) aluminum chloride
    (D) alcohol
    (E) hydrogen peroxide

47. Assuming that the pharmacist does not use an excess of each ingredient and there is no loss during compounding, what will be the weight of the final preparation?

    (A) less than 60 g
    (B) 60 g
    (C) 75 g
    (D) 90 g
    (E) greater than 90 g

48. When preparing this prescription, what may the pharmacist wish to include?

    I. Aquaphor
    II. Alcohol USP
    III. Tween 80

    (A) I only
    (B) III only
    (C) I and II only
    (D) II and III only
    (E) I, II, and III

49. A prescription calls for 10% urea in Aquaphor base. Which of the following is the best technique to make a pharmaceutically elegant product?

    (A) Dissolve urea in water then incorporate into the Aquaphor.
    (B) Dissolve urea in alcohol then incorporate into the Aquaphor.
    (C) Finely powder the urea and incorporate directly into the Aquaphor.
    (D) Dissolve urea in small amount of mineral oil and incorporate into the Aquaphor.
    (E) Melt the Aquaphor and dissolve the urea in the hot liquid.

50. When being incorporated into ointment bases, fine powders such as calamine and zinc oxide are often wetted and smoothed with mineral oil. What name is given to this process?

(A) attrition
(B) levigation
(C) milling
(D) pulverization by intervention
(E) trituration

Questions 51 through 53 refer to the following prescription:

Rx	
Retinoic acid	0.02%
Ac. Sal.	2%
Emulsion base	qs 60 g
Sig: Apply small amount onto spots hs	

51. Which of the following statements concerning this prescription is (are) true?

    I. Another name for retinoic acid is tretinoin.
    II. The amount of aspirin needed is 1.2 g.
    III. The term "emulsion base" refers to a brand of ointment base.

(A) I only
(B) III only
(C) I and II only
(D) II and III only
(E) I, II, and III

52. How many grams of 0.05% Retin-A cream may be used to supply the retinoic acid?

(A) 0.012
(B) 1.2
(C) 2.4
(D) 15
(E) 24

53. Which of the following should the pharmacist use when compounding this prescription?

    I. pill tile for mixing
    II. rubber spatulas for weighing and incorporating the ingredients
    III. alcohol to dissolve the salicylic acid

(A) I only
(B) III only
(C) I and II only
(D) II and III only
(E) I, II, and III

54. A prescription reads "Dilute a 0.25% steroidal cream to 0.1% strength using a vanishing cream base." How many grams of diluent should the pharmacist add to 30 g of the 0.25% cream?

(A) 6.5
(B) 12
(C) 30
(D) 45
(E) 75

55. The request for a "vanishing cream" base is best fulfilled using which of the following bases?

(A) cold cream
(B) hydrophilic ointment
(C) lanolin
(D) Vaseline
(E) polyethylene glycol (PEG) ointment

Questions 56 through 60: From the lettered list, select the most appropriate official topical base that the pharmacist should select for the desired characteristic in the numbered list. Each letter heading may be selected once, more than once, or not at all.

(A) cold cream
(B) hydrophilic ointment
(C) hydrophilic petrolatum
(D) PEG ointment
(E) white petrolatum

56. For an ophthalmic drug

57. For an antibiotic with limited stability

58. For absorbing a large quantity of water

59. To aid in hydrating the skin

60. Water washable base that will absorb serous discharge

61. Which of the following types of topical bases require the inclusion of an antimicrobial preservative?

    I.   aqueous gels
    II. water in oil (W/O) emulsions
    III. oil in water (O/W) emulsion

    (A) I only
    (B) III only
    (C) I and II only
    (D) II and III only
    (E) I, II, and III

62. Which of the following commercial ointment bases is (are) considered to be water washable?

    I.   Eucerin
    II. Nivea
    III. Cetaphil

    (A) I only
    (B) III only
    (C) I and II only
    (D) II and III only
    (E) I, II, and III

63. Alcohol is suitable as a solvent for menthol or salicylic acid when preparing which of the following dosage forms?

    I.   lotions
    II. ointments
    III. suppositories

    (A) I only
    (B) III only
    (C) I and II only
    (D) II and III only
    (E) I, II, and III

Answer questions 64 through 67 based on the following prescription:

Rx	
Ephedrine sulfate	2%
Menthol	0.5%
Camphor	
Methyl salicylate	aa 0.2%
Mineral oil	qs 30 mL

Sig: gtt ii both sides t.i.d.

64. Where may this prescription be administered?

    I.   nose
    II. eyes
    III. ears

    (A) I only
    (B) III only
    (C) I and II only
    (D) II and III only
    (E) I, II, and III

65. Which of the following ingredients will NOT dissolve in the prescribed solvent?

    I.   ephedrine sulfate
    II. menthol
    III. methyl salicylate

    (A) I only
    (B) III only
    (C) I and II only
    (D) II and III only
    (E) I, II, and III

66. Which of the following statements is (are) NOT true for camphor?

    I.   It forms a eutectic mixture with menthol.
    II. It can be powdered by rubbing with a small amount of alcohol or ether.
    III. It dissolves readily in water.

    (A) I only
    (B) III only
    (C) I and II only
    (D) II and III only
    (E) I, II, and III

67. What is methyl salicylate also known as?

    (A) camphorated oil
    (B) peppermint oil
    (C) salicylamide
    (D) oil of wintergreen
    (E) sweet oil

Questions 68 through 71 are based on the following order received from a hospital outpatient EENT clinic:

Tetracaine	1.0%
Boric acid	0.5%
Purified water	qs 100%
Dispense	60 mL
Make sterile and label as "Ophthalmic Solution TET 1%"	

68. Which of the following characteristics concerning tetracaine in the previously mentioned formula is (are) true?

    I.   poor water solubility
    II. chemically incompatible with boric acid
    III. not effective as a local anesthetic

    (A) I only
    (B) III only
    (C) I and II only
    (D) II and III only
    (E) I, II, and III

69. Boric acid is present in the formula as which of the following?

    I.   antioxidant
    II. antimicrobial preservative
    III. buffering agent

    (A) I only
    (B) III only
    (C) I and II only
    (D) II and III only
    (E) I, II, and III

70. How many milligrams of sodium chloride are needed to adjust the tonicity of the formula?

The following "E" values are available: tetracaine HCl = 0.18; boric acid = 0.50; sodium borate = 0.42.

    (A) 260
    (B) 280
    (C) 440
    (D) 540
    (E) 640

71. What is the most practical method for sterilizing the previous ophthalmic solution?

    (A) autoclaving for 15 minutes
    (B) autoclaving for 30 minutes
    (C) membrane filtration through 0.2-μm filter
    (D) membrane filtration through 5-μm filter
    (E) the use of ethylene oxide gas

Questions 72 through 74 refer to the following formula:

Progesterone	20 mg
PEG 400	60%
PEG 6000	40%
To make one vaginal suppository	

72. Which of the following statements is (are) true with respect to this formula?

    I.   The weight of the individual suppository must be determined experimentally.
    II. A mold must be used to prepare this formula.
    III. The bulk density of the progesterone must be calculated.

    (A) I only
    (B) III only
    (C) I and II only
    (D) II and III only
    (E) I, II, and III

73. What is the approximate ideal weight for a vaginal suppository?

    (A) 1 g
    (B) 2 g

(C) 5 g

(D) 10 g

(E) 15 g

74. Which of the following suppository bases melt rather than dissolve when inserted into the rectum?

   I. Cocoa butter

   II. Fattibase

   III. PEGs

(A) I only

(B) III only

(C) I and II only

(D) II and III only

(E) I, II, and III only

75. An order in a nursing home calls for 30 g of ointment to contain 15,000 units of polymyxin B sulfate per gram. The pharmacist has 10 mL parenteral vials labeled as containing 500,000 units of polymyxin B sulfate. Which of the following statements is (are) accurate?

   I. The pharmacist will use 9 mL of the polymyxin B sulfate solution.

   II. It will be best to incorporate the solution into an absorption type base.

   III. The solution should be incorporated into 30 g of ointment base.

(A) I only

(B) III only

(C) I and II only

(D) II and III only

(E) I, II, and III

76. Which one of the following diluents is LEAST suitable for reconstituting a sterile powder packaged in single-dose vials?

(A) bacteriostatic sterile water for injection (BSWFI)

(B) D_5W injection

(C) normal saline injection

(D) 1/2 normal saline injection

(E) sterile water for injection (SWFI)

77. Which of the following authors is (are) associated with reference sources that contain compilations of data describing compatibilities between various parenteral drug products?

   I. Trissel

   II. King

   III. Remington

(A) I only

(B) III only

(C) I and II only

(D) II and III only

(E) I, II, and III

78. When dispensing amphotericin, which one of the following statements is NOT true?

(A) The original product was a powder that was reconstituted with SWFI.

(B) The resulting liquid is a colloidal solution.

(C) The solution is incompatible with most acidic drug solutions.

(D) The solution is intended to be infused into a patient within 60 minutes.

(E) There is a liposomal dosage form available.

79. Which one of the following injectable solutions may result in a precipitate if added to 50 mL of D_5W or normal saline?

(A) diazepam (Valium) 20 mg

(B) folic acid (Folvite) 1 mg

(C) furosemide (Lasix) 40 mg

(D) gentamicin sulfate (Garamycin) 20 mg

(E) succinylcholine chloride (Anectine) 100 mg

80. Which of the following drug solutions is (are) compatible when added to 500 mL of D_5W?

   I. Thiamine HCl 200 mg

   II. Potassium chloride injection 20 mEq

   III. Chlorothiazide sodium 250 mg

(A) I only

(B) III only

(C) I and II only

(D) II and III only

(E) I, II, and III

81. Which of the following solutions would be incompatible in an order for Dobutamine HCl 250 mg in 250 mL normal saline?

I. Ranitidine HCl 125 mg
II. Diltiazem HCl 50 mg
III. Furosemide 40 mg

(A) I only
(B) III only
(C) I and II only
(D) II and III only
(E) I, II, and III

82. Which of the following cautions must be considered when dispensing most parenteral liposomal products?

I. Do not reconstitute with sodium chloride injection.
II. Dosing may differ from that of the conventional drug solutions.
III. Infuse only through administration sets that have an in-line filter.

(A) I only
(B) III only
(C) I and II only
(D) II and III only
(E) I, II, and III

83. A physician is seeking a commercial parenteral amino acids solution that contains a specific amount of two amino acids. Which one of the following books presents direct comparisons of such products from different companies?

(A) *Drug Facts and Comparisons*
(B) *Merck Index*
(C) *Physicians' Drug Reference*
(D) *Remington: The Science and Practice of Pharmacy*
(E) *USP/NF*

84. When reviewing the amino acids present in various amino acids injection formulas, the pharmacist will note which of the following?

I. Some of the formulas do not contain the nonessential amino acids.

II. Formulas with the same overall concentrations of amino acids may vary in the relative amounts of a specific amino acid present.
III. Some of the formulas contain higher amounts of the branched chain amino acids.

(A) I only
(B) III only
(C) I and II only
(D) II and III only
(E) I, II, and III

85. Which of the following statements concerning the development of total parenteral nutrition (TPN) solutions is (are) true?

I. The total daily caloric density of the solution should not exceed the basal energy expenditure (BEE) of the patient.
II. It is desirable to avoid EFAD in the patient.
III. The final solutions may have osmolarities greater than 300 mOsm/L.

(A) I only
(B) III only
(C) I and II only
(D) II and III only
(E) I, II, and III

86. Other names given to TPN solutions that contain the intravenous fat emulsions include which of the following?

I. MCTs
II. total nutrition admixture (TNA)
III. 3 in 1s

(A) I only
(B) III only
(C) I and II only
(D) II and III only
(E) I, II, and III

87. What caloric density value (kcal/g) should be used when calculating the contribution of dextrose in infusion solutions?

(A) 3.4
(B) 4.0

(C) 5.5

(D) 6.0

(E) 10

88. What is the average weight in grams of nitrogen present in every 100 mL of a 10% amino acids injection?

(A) 1.0

(B) 1.6

(C) 10

(D) 16

(E) 50

Questions 89 through 104: Answer the following series of questions based on the availability of the following parenteral solutions and hospital medication order:

Patient: Danielle Howell	Room: Main 218
Aminosyn II 8.5%	
$D_{50}W$	aa 500 mL
Potassium chloride	40 mEq
Sodium chloride	20 mEq
Potassium phosphate	40 mEq
MVI-12	1 vial
Zinc chloride	2 mg
Insulin	40 units
Calcium gluconate	10 mL
Infuse above t.i.d. for 6 days Add 500 mL Liposyn III 10% every Monday and Thursday	

Available to the pharmacist are the following parenteral solutions:

Aminosyn II 8.5%	500-mL full bts
Dextrose 50% injection	500-mL full bts
Calcium chloride 10%	10-mL vials
Calcium gluconate 10%	10-mL vials
Intralipid 10%	250-mL bottles
Magnesium sulfate	20-mL vials
Sodium chloride injection	30-mL vials
MTE-4	10-mL vials
Potassium chloride injection	20-mL vials
Potassium phosphate	10-mL vials

89. How is the TPN formula best prepared?

(A) adding the $D_{50}W$ to the Aminosyn bottle

(B) adding the Aminosyn to the $D_{50}W$ bottle

(C) transferring both the Aminosyn and the $D_{50}W$ to an empty, sterile infusion bag

(D) hanging the Aminosyn and the $D_{50}W$ solutions separately on the patient

(E) piggybacking the $D_{50}W$ into the Y-tubing of the Aminosyn administration set

90. How many nonprotein kilocalories are present in every liter of the TPN solution?

(A) 850

(B) 1,000

(C) 1,250

(D) 1,700

(E) 2,000

91. The pharmacist must be cognizant of potential incompatibilities between which of the following?

(A) potassium chloride and calcium gluconate

(B) potassium chloride and insulin

(C) potassium phosphate and calcium gluconate

(D) potassium phosphate and zinc chloride

(E) insulin and zinc chloride

92. Which of the following techniques may reduce the danger of the incompatibility mentioned in Question 91?

I. Limit the levels of potassium + sodium salts

II. Gently warm the mixture if a fine precipitate appears

III. Include sodium bicarbonate in the formula

(A) I only

(B) III only

(C) I and II only

(D) II and III only

(E) I, II, and III

93. To avoid the possibility of a precipitate, the pharmacist may choose to do which of the following?

    I. place the calcium gluconate and potassium phosphate into separate, alternate containers
    II. use sodium phosphate rather than potassium phosphate
    III. use calcium chloride rather than calcium gluconate

    (A) I only
    (B) III only
    (C) I and II only
    (D) II and III only
    (E) I, II, and III

94. What is the prime reason for including potassium phosphate in the formula?

    (A) source of phosphorus
    (B) source of potassium
    (C) buffer
    (D) antioxidant
    (E) stabilizer

95. The prescribing physician should be encouraged to order the potassium phosphate using which of the following concentration expressions?

    (A) milliequivalents
    (B) milligrams
    (C) milliliters
    (D) millimoles
    (E) milliosmoles

96. It is convenient and accurate for the pharmacist to measure the insulin required for this order by using which of the following?

    I. tuberculin syringe
    II. low-dose insulin syringe
    III. a 10-mL regular syringe

    (A) I only
    (B) III only
    (C) I and II only
    (D) II and III only
    (E) I, II, and III.

97. The pharmacist may consider contacting the physician to inform him that

    I. approximately half of the insulin will be adsorbed onto the walls of the glass container
    II. a strength of insulin is needed
    III. insulin is available as both a solution and a suspension

    (A) I only
    (B) III only
    (C) I and II only
    (D) II and III only
    (E) I, II, and III

98. The addition of Liposyn to the TPN

    I. causes the final solution to be cloudy
    II. is intended to prevent EFAD
    III. will adversely affect the osmolarity of the already hypertonic solution

    (A) I only
    (B) III only
    (C) I and II only
    (D) II and III only
    (E) I, II, and III

99. Before placing a patient onto IV fat emulsions, the pharmacist should confirm that the patient does not have

    (A) egg allergies
    (B) sensitivities to bisulfate
    (C) milk intolerance
    (D) lactose intolerance
    (E) sensitivities to tartrazine

100. Approximately how many additional kilocalories is the patient receiving when a 500-mL bottle of Liposyn 10% is included in the TPN?

    (A) 500
    (B) 1,000
    (C) 1,500
    (D) 1,700
    (E) 2,000

101. What is Ms. Howell's daily intake of nitrogen from the amino acids solution?

    (A) 7 g
    (B) 20 g
    (C) 42 g
    (D) 60 g
    (E) 130 g

102. What is a trace metal that the physician is likely to include in the TPN formula?

    (A) lithium
    (B) sodium
    (C) selenium
    (D) silicon
    (E) fluoride

103. Which of the following metals is (are) NOT present in the MTE-4 or in other multiple trace element solutions?

    I. aluminum
    II. manganese
    III. zinc

    (A) I only
    (B) III only
    (C) I and II only
    (D) II and III only
    (E) I, II, and III

104. To reduce the amount of chloride ion being consumed, the physician requests that the acetate salts of potassium and sodium be used. What information must the pharmacist utilize when making these changes?

    I. the molecular weights of both acetate salts
    II. the valences of the ions
    III. the concentrations of the salt solutions in mEq/mL

    (A) I only
    (B) III only
    (C) I and II only
    (D) II and III only
    (E) I, II, and III

105. A nurse reports that a previously clear TPN solution now appears to be slightly cloudy. What should the pharmacist advise the nurse to do?

    (A) discontinue the infusion
    (B) gently warm the solution
    (C) slow the infusion rate
    (D) continue with the infusion
    (E) use an administration set that has an in-line filter

106. Estimate the total kilocalorie count in the following TPN formula.

$D_{50}W$	500 mL
Veinamine 7%	400 mL
Liposyn 10%	100 mL

    (A) 320
    (B) 850
    (C) 950
    (D) 1,100
    (E) 1,230

107. What is the calorie to nitrogen ratio in the above formula?

    (A) 34/1
    (B) 100/1
    (C) 190/1
    (D) 214/1
    (E) 240/1

108. A home infusion pharmacy receives an order for 5-fluorouracil 400 mg in a disposable infusion pump for 1-hour delivery. Which of the following equipments would the pharmacist use in compounding this order?

    I. primary administration set
    II. volumetric burette
    III. plastic syringe

    (A) I only
    (B) III only
    (C) I and II only
    (D) II and III only
    (E) I, II, and III

Questions 109 through 111: Answer the following series of questions based on receiving the following order in a home infusion pharmacy.

For Robert Graves	Diagnosis: term. CA bone
Hydromorphone HCl	300 mg
Rx	
Normal saline	qs 100 mL
Place in PCA device with flow rate of 0.5 mL/h	

109. Which of the following should be the pharmacist's assessment(s) of the above order?

    I. The solubility of the drug is too low for the requested concentration.

    II. The drug is available as Dilaudid in several dosage forms.

    III. The dosing is high; confirm with prescriber.

    (A) I only
    (B) III only
    (C) I and II only
    (D) II and III only
    (E) I, II, and III

110. Which of the following methods may be utilized in preparing the above order?

    I. Prepare a solution using Dilaudid nonsterile powder.

    II. Use Dilaudid-HP Injection (10 mg/mL).

    III. Use 20-mL vials containing 2 mg/mL of drug.

    (A) I only
    (B) III only
    (C) I and II only
    (D) II and III only
    (E) I, II, and III

111. Into which ASHP risk category would compounding the above solution belong?

    (A) 1
    (B) 2
    (C) 3
    (D) 4
    (E) X

112. Describe techniques by which a pharmacist would compound 1 L of the following order.

Betadine surgical scrub	20 mL
Alcohol, USP	
Purified water	aa 40 mL

    I. Place 400 mL alcohol in a graduate and add sufficient purified water to measure 800 mL then add 200 mL of betadine solution.

    II. Place 400 mL purified water in a graduate and add sufficient alcohol to measure 800 mL then add 200 mL of betadine solution.

    III. Add 200 mL of betadine solution to 400 mL purified water then add sufficient alcohol to measure 1,000 mL.

    (A) I only
    (B) III only
    (C) I and II only
    (D) II and III only
    (E) I, II, and III

113. Infusion of morphine sulfate solutions to an ambulatory hospice patient in a home setting is best accomplished by the use of which system?

    (A) PCA
    (B) PVP
    (C) Homepump
    (D) Implant
    (E) ADD-Vantage

114. Which of the following statements is (are) true concerning the elastomeric balloon pumps such as Intermate or Homepump?

    I. Unit may be used in the home for ambulatory patient.

    II. Unit is refillable.

    III. Bolus dosing is possible with the unit.

    (A) I only
    (B) III only
    (C) I and II only
    (D) II and III only
    (E) I, II, and III

115. Which of the following actions is likely to result in a parenteral incompatibility?

    I. Dilution of 2 mL of an injection with a pH of 8 into 100 mL D_5W (pH of 5.5)

    II. Dilution of an injection that has a non-aqueous solvent into 50 mL D_5W

    III. Dilution of 2 mL of an injection with a pH of 8 into 100 mL D_5W solution containing an acidic drug (pH 3.5)

(A) I only

(B) III only

(C) I and II only

(D) II and III only

(E) I, II, and III

116. A hospital pharmacist is responsible for preparing syringes containing two injection solutions for Y-Site administration. Which one of the following injection combinations is unsuitable for such mixing?

(A) Fentanyl citrate + diphenhydramine HCl

(B) Phenytoin + lidocaine

(C) Morphine sulfate + hydroxyzine HCl

(D) Lidocaine + meperidine HCl

(E) Vitamin B complex with C + hydroxyzine HCl

Answers and Explanations

Numbers within parentheses at the end of the answers refer to the numbered references that are listed in the front matter.

1. **(C)** The prescription torsion balance designated by NBS as Class III must have a SR of not greater than 6 mg. Most Class III balances have a maximum capacity of 60 g rather than the usual 120 g for the Class A. The pharmacist should check the serial plate on the back of the balance to ascertain the limits of the balance. Obviously, a balance with a SR of 6 mg is more accurate than one with a SR of 10 mg. The USP/NF specifies that more accurate balances, such as certain electronic balances, may be used. *(1; 4)*

2. **(C)** Although free-swinging pan balances based on the torsion principle are traditional in pharmacy, the more sophisticated electronic balances are suitable provided that they meet USP/NF standards of a SR of 6 mg or less (better). While the usual largest quantity to be weighed on the torsion balance without causing damage was 120 g, this is not an absolute quantity. The most important value for compounding is the allowable error, which should be not more than ±5%. *(19)*

3. **(D)** The imperceptible weighing error could be up to 10 mg, too high or too low. When 10 mg is divided by the desired weight of 140 mg = 7% error. While electronic balances are easy to use and are perceived as being accurate, the pharmacist must still recognize their limitations especially when weighing small amounts. Many of the newer electronic balances have a weighing error of only ±1 mg. *(1; 24)*

4. **(B)** The primary designation that the pharmacist seeks when selecting a chemical for compounding is USP/NF grade. This indicates that the chemical meets standards described in official monographs, which are recognized by the FDA. If there is no official monograph for a specific chemical, the pharmacist must carefully evaluate available grades and select one that is of high quality. For example, American Chemical Society (ACS) grade or analytical reagent (AR) grade may be suitable. It is important to consider the quantity of active moiety present since some official chemical designations do not indicate 100% pure chemical. For example, waters of hydration, a certain amount of moisture, or other impurities must be taken into consideration. *(4; 19)*

5. **(E)** The carbomers such as Carbopol 934 will increase the viscosity of topical products such as lotions. They will also form gels. One potential disadvantage is that their viscosity will decrease at low pHs especially below pH of 4. *(1; 4; 19)*

6. **(B)** Five hundred micrograms is equivalent to 0.5 mg, and 60 capsules were requested

   $$0.5 \text{ mg} \times 60 \text{ capsules} = 30 \text{ mg} \qquad (23)$$

7. **(B)** The minimum quantity that can be weighed accurately on the Class III (Class A) prescription balance with an error of not more than 5% is 120 mg (assuming a SR of 6 mg). In order to weigh the required 30 mg of sodium fluoride, a stock powder of NaF is needed. In this problem, mixing 120 mg of NaF with 360 mg of diluent and using 120 mg of this stock powder will deliver the required 30 mg of

sodium fluoride. Because of its strong ionic bonds, sodium fluoride is not caustic. A stainless steel spatula can be used for the weighing procedure. Sodium fluoride has good water solubility. *(1; 23)*

8. **(B)** Lactose is a relatively inert water-soluble substance that also packs well into capsules. An alternative would be the use of starch. For the sodium fluoride prescription, the pharmacist will have to include additional lactose to raise the content of the capsule to a quantity that is weighable and convenient to pack into capsules. For example, a net weight of 300 mg may be selected arbitrarily. *(24)*

9. **(A)** Empty capsules are sized by a numbering system, the largest being a #000 and the smallest a #5. If the #2 capsule is too small, the pharmacist should try the next largest, the #1. The correct capsule filling procedure is to place powder only into the body or base of the empty capsule. It is not good technique to place powder into the head of the cap because the fit of the head onto the body may not be tight. *(1; 24)*

10. **(B)** Both codeine and dimenhydrinate have a tendency to produce drowsiness as a side effect. Codeine is a weak organic base whereas dimenhydrinate is a combination of diphenhydramine and 8-chlorotheophylline. No chemical reaction between the two drugs would be expected. The amount of codeine consumed per dose is 10 or 40 mg daily. This is within the therapeutic dosage range for a 10-year-old child. *(1)*

11. **(B)** If only pure chemicals were available, the weight of powder in each capsule would be 210 mg (4,210 mg divided by 20 capsules). However, if the pharmacist has to use commercial tablets when preparing this prescription, the contributory weight of the additional ingredients (excipients) present in the tablets must be included in the calculations. Although lactose is a popular diluent when making capsules, the high weight of each capsule precludes its use. Weighing the aspirin with a rubber

spatula is not necessary because aspirin is not as reactive as salicylic acid. *(4)*

12. **(E)** The total amount of ingredients may be calculated as follows:

Drug	Total Weight of Powder
Codeine, seven tablets each weighing 100 mg	700 mg
Dimenhydrinate, 20 tablets each weighing 100 mg	4,000 mg
Aspirin powder	3,000 mg
Total weight	7,700 mg

7,770 mg divided into 20 capsules = 385 mg each. *(4)*

13. **(C)** The weight of the child in kg is

$$44 \text{ lb} \times \frac{1 \text{ kg}}{2.2 \text{ lb}} = 20 \text{ kg}$$

Each teaspoon dose will contain 0.15 mg × 20 kg = 3 mg; number of doses = 60 divided by 5 mL = 12 doses (12 doses = 3 mg/dose = 36 mg); therefore, nine tablets are needed. *(23)*

14. **(B)** Ondansetron HCl injection is available in vials containing 2 mg/mL. The solution contains both methyl and propyl paraben preservatives that will protect the prescription from microbial growth. Because ondansetron HCl has good water solubility, it is inadvisable to include alcohol in the prescription. As the pH of solutions of the drug is increased, a precipitate may occur. It is best to use acidic vehicles such as orange juice, Coca-Cola, or cherry syrup. *(3; 20)*

15. **(B)** Resorcinol 1.2 g + water 15 g + Aquaphor 15 g + 85 g white petrolatum = total weight of 116.2 g. 1.2 g ÷ 116.2 = 1% W/W (rather than the requested strength of 1.2% W/W) *(4; 23)*

16. **(C)** Dimenhydrinate is only slightly soluble in water but soluble in alcohol, glycerin, and propylene glycol. The drug should be added

to approximately 10 mL of glycerin, then further diluted with 50 mL of Ora-Plus and sufficient Ora-Sweet to make 100 mL. Ora-Plus is a mixture of celluloses with other gums and used as an oral suspending vehicle with thixotropic (sol–gel) properties. Ora-Sweet is a pleasantly flavored vehicle but contains sucrose, glycerin, and sorbitol. Since a sugar-free vehicle is needed, Ora-Sweet SF should be used since it is a sugar-free formula containing saccharin. *(1; 4)*

17. **(C)** Alkaline pHs may cause either a fine precipitation or decrease the vitamin activity of thiamine hydrochloride solutions, which have a pH of 2.5 to 4.5. Aminophylline injection has a very high pH of 8.5 to 9. Heparin sodium solutions have approximately a neutral pH (5–8) as does potassium chloride solutions. Although dextrose 5% injections have pH ranges of 4.0 to 5, they have virtually no buffering capacity. Thus, their pH values will quickly adjust to the pH of the aminophylline solution. *(21)*

18. **(C)** Each 20-mL ampule of aminophylline contains 500 mg of drug. Because the individual admixture order requires 400 mg, the pharmacist will have to open an ampule for each admixture and remove 16 mL of solution. Even if the pharmacist is preparing all three admixtures at one time, three ampules (48 mL total) will still be needed for the order. *(23)*

19. **(C)** Because no incompatibilities exist between the aminophylline and the potassium chloride, either could be added first to the D₅W container. It would be impractical and time consuming to mix the two solutions first in a syringe and then add them to the D₅W. Also, there would be an increased possibility of inaccurate measurements. For example, if only 9 mL of KCl solution was drawn up instead of the correct 10 mL, 17 mL rather than 16 mL of aminophylline solution may be drawn into a syringe to make the desired volume of 26 mL. *(21)*

20. **(A)** Each admixture container will contain 20 mEq of KCl or 20 mEq each of potassium and chloride ion. To determine the milligram of potassium present, use the following relationship:

$$mg\ (potassium) = \frac{(20\ mEq)\ (39.1)}{1}$$

$$x = 780\ mg$$

The above calculation is based on the atomic weight of potassium being 39.1 with a valence of +1. *(23)*

21. **(A)** The pore size of filter needles is approximately 5 μm, which is too coarse for removing either pyrogens or bacteria. Instead, the filter needle is intended to remove larger particulate matter such as glass fragments that may have fallen into the ampule during the breaking of the ampule's neck. *(13)*

22. **(D)** Both the syringe tip and ribs may be in contact with the parenteral solution, thus must not be touched by the operator. *(1: 13)*

23. **(D)** The filter needle contains a 5-μm filter and is intended to remove particulate matter; in this case, a small piece of glass that may have entered the solution when the ampule top was broken. Answer I is NOT correct since one may visualize that the glass particles would be drawn up onto the filter, then washed into the final solution. *(1; 13; 24)*

24. **(C)** Air in the horizontal laminar flow hood flows directly toward the operator, thereby preventing contaminants from entering the admixtures being prepared. This hood provides maximum protection for the parenteral admixture. Vertical hoods have downward air flow, which increases the risk of product contamination but protects the operator from droplets of product solution. These hoods should be used only for the preparation of products that pose a significant risk to the operator; for example, carcinogenic or mutagenic chemotherapeutic drugs. The newest concept for hood design is the convergent flow, which combines both vertical and horizontal flow. *(13)*

25. **(B)** As the air passing through the HEPA filter nears the edge of the benchtop, it becomes more turbulent, thus defeating the purpose of

the horizontal or convergent laminar flow hood. For this reason, many horizontal laminar flow hoods have a line drawn 6 in from the edge as a reminder to work further inside the hood. Usually hoods are left running 24 hours a day or are turned on and left running throughout the workday. Work should not commence until the hood has been running for at least 15 to 30 minutes. It is inadvisable to work within 6 in of the HEPA filter because airflow may be partially blocked. *(13)*

26. **(A)** Alcohol (70%) or isopropyl alcohol (70%) are the two disinfectant solutions usually used to disinfect laminar flow hoods before compounding admixtures. Both are effective antimicrobial agents and will evaporate within a few minutes. Acetone is never used because it is flammable and dangerous if inhaled. Betadine is an effective antimicrobial agent as a skin antiseptic or hand wash but would leave a residual buildup if used in hoods. It also is not very volatile. *(1)*

27. **(B)** Improvements in quality control for the preparation of sterile products by pharmacies have been advocated by several health groups including the ASHP and FDA. The ASHP "risk level classification" describes compounding, storage, and stability standards that should be followed. Of the three risk levels, level 3 is the strictest. Clean room standards have also been proposed to ensure tight standards, especially when manipulating unsterile ingredients. *(24)*

28. **(E)** Both morphine sulfate and hydroxyzine HCl solutions will have acidic pHs and are therefore expected to be compatible when mixed together in a syringe. However, if either solution is placed directly into a heparinized lock or infusion set, there may be a precipitate because heparin sodium has a higher pH. *(21)*

29. **(E)** It is preferable to aspirate excessive solution and air bubbles while the needle is still in the vial. This prevents accidental contamination of the hood and personnel. Also, it is inadvisable to waste 0.5 mL of drug solution, especially a controlled substance. It is neces-

sary to inject a volume of air equal to the volume of solution to be withdrawn. Otherwise, a vacuum would occur in the vial, making it difficult to remove liquid. *(13)*

30. **(A)** There is no reason to inject air into the opened ampule because no vacuum will form when an ampule is opened and solution is removed. All ampules are intended as single-dose units and should be discarded after opening. *(13)*

31. **(E)** The direction of "q6h ATC" indicates that a minibottle will be hung every 6 hours around the clock. Therefore, 4 bottles daily × 4 days = 16 bottles. *(23)*

32. **(E)** The citrate buffer system is intended to readily adjust the pH of each listed vehicle to a pH range in which the penicillin is stable. Although the dextrose 5% injection has a pH of 4.5, it has virtually no buffering capacity and does not influence the pH of admixtures. Some hospitals prefer to use dextrose solutions as the vehicle for most admixtures to limit the sodium intake by patients. Other hospitals use normal saline injection to avoid supplying the calories present in dextrose solutions. *(13; 21)*

33. **(B)** There is no need to remove vehicle solution when adding small volumes of drug additives. The final volume will always vary because the manufacturer places some excess of solution into each unit. To calculate the milliliter of penicillin, solution required

$$\frac{750{,}000 \text{ units}}{1 \text{ mL}} = \frac{2{,}000{,}000 \text{ units}}{x \text{ mL}}$$
$$x \text{ mL} = 2.7 \text{ mL} \qquad (23)$$

34. **(A)** Since many of the chemotherapeutic drugs are carcinogenic and possibly mutagenic, health professionals should work in the confines of vertical laminar flow hoods. These hoods direct air directly downward, thus protecting the operator from solution droplets.

Answer II is incorrect. When removing 5 mL of a drug solution from a vial, the negative pressure technique is appropriate especially when several doses of drug are being removed from a multidose vial. The pharmacist will introduce only 2 or 3 mL of the air into the vial, fill the syringe with 5 mL of drug solution, and remove the solution. Thus, a small vacuum is left in the vial, which will prevent droplet spray leaving the vial when the needle is withdrawn.

Answer III is incorrect. Since the volume of drug solution being added to the 100 mL of NS is low, the general policy is not to remove 5 mL of normal saline to compensate for the increased volume in the final dilution. *(1; 24)*

35. **(E)** A suspension must be prepared because there are water-insoluble powders present in the prescription. An emulsion is not possible because there is no oil indicated in the formula. *(1)*

36. **(D)** The designation "aa qs 15 g" translates as "of each enough to make 15 g." Therefore, 7.5 g of calamine and 7.5 g of zinc oxide are needed. The water-insoluble powders, calamine and zinc oxide, should be triturated together using a mortar and pestle, then wetted with the glycerin. Resorcinol is soluble in both water and alcohol, but it is more convenient to dissolve it in the alcohol and dilute the powder paste with the liquid. Finally, add portions of purified water to rinse out the mortar while placing the suspension into a precalibrated wide-mouth bottle. *(1)*

37. **(C)** Most of the ingredients in this preparation are intended for topical use only. Although the suspension may not separate or settle immediately, it may do so after a few days. It is standard procedure to place "shake well" labels on all suspension formulas. None of the ingredients decompose in the presence of moderate heat; therefore, a "store in a cool place" label is not required. *(24)*

38. **(E)** The easiest way to hydrate methylcellulose is to add the powder to hot water and allow the powder to hydrate for 10 to 15 minutes before adding cold water. Six itraconazole (Sporanox) capsules may be opened and the powder wetted by the propylene glycol.

The thickened methylcellulose solution can then be added to the powder followed by sufficient purified water to make 60 mL. *(1; 19)*

39. **(C)** Cold cream is a W/O emulsion base with good emollient properties. *(4)*

40. **(B)** Hydrophilic petrolatum is an anhydrous preparation that will absorb significant amounts of water forming a W/O emulsion. It contains cholesterol as the emulsifying agent. *(1; 24)*

41. **(B)** Large quantities of liquids may be incorporated into Aquaphor. The characteristics of this ointment base are similar to hydrophilic petrolatum. *(1; 4; 19)*

42. **(A)** *(1; 24)*

43. **(E)** *(1; 24)*

44. **(D)** *(1; 24)*

45. **(A)** Hydrophilic petrolatum is anhydrous, thus unlikely to support hydrolysis of the drug. Nivea is a water-in-oil ointment base. Hydrophilic ointment also has water in its formula. *(1; 4)*

46. **(B)** Burow's solution is officially known as aluminum acetate topical solution. It is classified as a topical astringent dressing. *(1; 24)*

47. **(E)** The prescription calls for 15 mL each of Burow's solution and propylene glycol. Burow's solution consists mainly of water; therefore 15 mL equals 15 g. However, propylene glycol has a specific gravity of 1.25 and 15 mL will weigh approximately 18.75 g. The total weight of the ointment will be 15 g + 18.75 g + 60 g = 93.75 g. *(1; 23)*

48. **(A)** Aqueous solutions such as Burow's solution cannot be incorporated directly into oleaginous bases such as petrolatum or white petrolatum. Aquaphor is an adjuvant that will absorb aqueous solutions and is miscible with petrolatum. Although smaller amounts could be used, 15 g of Aquaphor will readily pick

up the required amount of Burow's solution. The amount of white petrolatum must be decreased by 15 g to ensure the correct concentration of Burow's solution in the final preparation. Alcohol is seldom included in semisolid ointments or creams because it is likely to evaporate slowly. It is more likely to be included in lotion formulas. *(20)*

49. **(A)** Urea has good solubility in water. The resulting solution can readily be incorporated into the Aquaphor. *(4; 24)*

50. **(B)** Incorporating powders into ointment bases may be eased by first wetting the powders with a small amount of liquid that is miscible with the main vehicle. The wetted powder is rubbed with a spatula on an ointment tile to form a paste. Usually, mineral oil is employed when the vehicle is oleaginous. Glycerin or propylene glycol may be used for more hydrophilic bases. *(1; 4; 24)*

51. **(A)** Tretinoin is the official name for retinoic acid. The drug is commercially available under the trade name of Retin-A. The designation of Ac. Sal. refers to salicylic acid, not aspirin (acetylsalicylic acid). The term emulsion base is nondescript. It could refer to a number of ointment bases, including those with either W/O or O/W characteristics. Clarification of the type of ointment base desired should be made. Before compounding this prescription, the pharmacist should contact the prescriber concerning the inclusion of a keratolytic agent such as salicylic acid in a topical preparation containing tretinoin, a compound that exhibits keratolytic activity as a side effect. *(1; 19; 20)*

52. **(E)** An easy method for determining the amount of 0.05% cream is

$$60 \text{ g} \times 0.02\% = 0.012 \text{ g of pure retinoic acid}$$
$$\frac{0.012 \text{ g}}{x \text{ g}} = \frac{0.05 \text{ g}}{100 \text{ g}}$$
$$0.05x = 1.2$$
$$x = 24 \text{ g of } 0.05\% \qquad (23)$$

53. **(C)** Incorporating powders or liquids into relatively small amounts of ointment base is best accomplished on a pill tile (also known as an ointment tile). Because of the caustic nature of salicylic acid, rubber spatulas should be used rather than stainless steel, which would be discolored by the acid. While salicylic acid is soluble in alcohol, the use of alcohol as a levigating agent is discouraged since crystals of salicylic acid may form on the surface of the product when the alcohol evaporates. *(1; 4)*

54. **(D)** Let Q_1 and C_1 represent the quantity and concentration of new product desired and Q_2 and C_2 represent the original quantity and strength:

$$Q_1 \times C_1 = Q_2 \times C_2$$
$$[x \text{ g}] [0.1\%] = [30 \text{ g}] [0.25\%]$$
$$x = 75 \text{ g (total amount of ointment that can be prepared)}$$

Therefore, 75 g − the original 30 g = 45 g of diluent needed. *(1)*

55. **(B)** Hydrophilic ointment is an O/W emulsion base containing sodium lauryl sulfate, petrolatum, and stearyl alcohol. Of the listed bases, it is closest to a vanishing cream base because such a system is characterized by the presence of an O/W stearate emulsion. When placed on the skin, the ointment appears to "disappear" but a very thin layer of stearate remains. *(24)*

56. **(E)** White petrolatum is a bland base with a very low incidence of irritation to the eye. Also, because of the absence of water, it has low susceptibility to microbial growth. *(24)*

57. **(E)** Many antibiotics undergo decomposition by hydrolysis in the presence of water. White petrolatum is anhydrous and is very inert. *(1; 4)*

58. **(C)** Of all the bases listed, hydrophilic petrolatum will absorb the greatest quantity of water. *(1)*

59. **(E)** The occlusive characteristics of petrolatum will prevent further water loss through the stratum corneum. Thus, the skin will remain more hydrated and pliable. *(1)*

60. **(B)** Hydrophilic ointment is an oil-in-water emulsion base that is easy to apply onto the skin and will wash off the skin readily. It will absorb aqueous discharges yet retain its normal consistency. *(1; 24)*

61. **(E)** Any product containing water will be susceptible to the growth of microorganisms and should include an antimicrobial agent. *(4; 24)*

62. **(B)** Cetaphil is classified as an O/W base that is water washable. The other two choices are W/O emulsion bases, thus are not easily washed off the skin. *(1: 4)*

63. **(A)** Because of the volatility of alcohol, it is not suitable in dosage forms from which it may slowly evaporate. If ingredients were dissolved in alcohol and incorporated into either ointments or suppositories, crystals of the ingredients would slowly appear on the surface of the dosage unit. However, one would expect alcohol to remain within the lotion formula until placed on the skin. *(1)*

64. **(A)** This prescription uses mineral oil as the solvent. It is not suited for administration into the eye. Ephedrine is used as a topical decongestant when administered by the intranasal route. The product would be ineffective if placed in the ear. *(1; 24)*

65. **(A)** Ephedrine sulfate is water soluble. It is best to request the prescriber's permission to use ephedrine base, which is soluble in nonpolar solvents such as mineral oil. Solid chemicals such as phenol, camphor, and menthol will liquefy when mixed together even at room temperature without heating. This phenomenon is known as forming a eutectic mixture. *(1)*

66. **(B)** Camphor is soluble in alcohol or organic solvents but is only slightly soluble in water (1 g in 800 mL). *(1)*

67. **(D)** Methyl salicylate can be used in small quantities as a flavoring or perfuming agent. It is also included in many topical products such as rubbing alcohol, gels, and liniments as a counterirritant. *(1; 2)*

68. **(A)** Tetracaine is a weak organic base with poor water solubility (1 g in 1 L of water). The hydrochloride salt, which is very soluble (1 g needs less than 1 mL of water), should be used. Boric acid, which is a very weak acid, is chemically compatible with both tetracaine-free base and the HCl salt. Tetracaine, epinephrine (Adrenalin), and cocaine combinations are used as local anesthetics and are known as "TAC topical solutions." *(1; 20)*

69. **(D)** Boric acid is an effective buffer in ophthalmic solutions because it will maintain a slightly acidic pH, but when placed in the eye, it is quickly neutralized by the buffers in the lacrimal fluid. Boric acid has weak antimicrobial activity. *(1; 4)*

70. **(B)** This problem may be solved using the "*E*" values for the chemicals.

Drug	Wt. of Drug	×	"E" Values	Equiv. Amount of NaCl
Tetracaine	600 mg	×	0.18	= 108 mg
Boric acid	300 mg	×	0.50	= 150 mg
Total				= 258 mg

60 mL of solution × 0.9% NaCl = 540 mg of NaCl 540 − 258 mg = 282 mg of NaCl to adjust for tonicity. *(1; 23)*

71. **(C)** Membrane filtration represents one of the most convenient sterilization methods available to the pharmacist performing extemporaneous compounding. It involves the passing of solutions through a 0.2-μm filter using one of the commercially available sterile filter units such as Millipore's Millex or Swinnex units. The method does not involve heat, therefore, there is no decomposition of heat labile drugs as might occur with autoclaving. Ethylene oxide gas is not practical for solutions because it

would have to penetrate the solution and residues may be left behind. *(1; 13)*

72. **(C)** Because the exact density of the PEG 400/6,000 mixture is not known, the pharmacist must prepare a trial batch in a mold to determine the weight of an individual suppository. In this prescription, the volume occupied by 20 mg of progesterone is insignificant, and it is not necessary to determine its bulk density. However, when a drug represents a large proportion of the total suppository weight, one must prepare a trial suppository that includes the active drug to calculate its bulk density. For example, boric acid has been prescribed at a dose of 600 mg per suppository. Progesterone has been extemporaneously incorporated into vaginal suppositories for the maintenance of pregnancy in luteal phase dysfunction. The usual dose has been 25 mg. *(1; 4; 24)*

73. **(C)** Vaginal suppositories or pessaries are traditionally larger in size and weight (5 g) than rectal suppositories (2 g). However, a regular rectal suppository mold could be used if the larger vaginal mold is not available. For many suppository formulas, a water-soluble base, such as the PEGs or glycerinated gelatin, is preferred over oil bases such as cocoa butter. *(1; 24)*

74. **(C)** Cocoa butter, a mixture of triglycerides, has been used for more than 100 years as a suppository base. A disadvantage of cocoa butter is its inability to absorb aqueous solutions. It melts at slightly below body temperature, and its melting point might be affected by drugs. Fattibase is a mixture of triglycerides from palm, palm kernel, and coconut oils + glyceryl monostearate SE and polyoxylstearate emulsifiers. Other suppository bases that melt include the Witepsols and the Wecobees. Although cocoa butter suppositories can be hand rolled or prepared by fusion in molds, the other bases are intended for mold use. Different molecular weight PEGs can be blended and formed into suppositories by fusion using molds. However, the PEG suppositories do not melt in the body; instead, they slowly dissolve in the limited amount of water in the rectum. *(1; 4; 19)*

75. **(C)**

$$\frac{15{,}000 \text{ units}}{\text{g}} \times 30 \text{ g} = 450{,}000 \text{ units}$$

$$\frac{500{,}000 \text{ units}}{10 \text{ mL}} = \frac{450{,}000 \text{ units}}{x \text{ mL}}$$

$$x = 9 \text{ mL of solution}$$

The 9 mL of solution should be incorporated into 21 g of an absorption base such as hydrophilic petrolatum or Aquaphor. Hydrophilic ointment is probably a poor choice since the 9 mL of liquid will thin the base too much. The pharmacist would not incorporate 9 mL of antibiotic solution directly into 30 g of ointment base because the final concentration of drug would be incorrect. *(4; 23)*

76. **(A)** Product inserts are the best sources of information concerning appropriate diluents for a given drug powder. However, BSWFI should not be used for reconstituting single-dose units because the preservative present would serve no useful purpose, and large amounts of the preservative could increase the incidence or severity of toxicity. The use of BSWFI may be appropriate if a powder in a multidose vial is being reconstituted. *(13; 24)*

77. **(C)** Currently, there are two major reference sources in the United States that present detailed information concerning the compatibilities and incompatibilities of parenteral products. Trissel is the author of the *Handbook on Injectable Drugs*. The second book, King's *Guide to Parenteral Admixtures* presents similar material and is available in both print and on a regularly updated CD-ROM. Not only do the references describe mixing of drug solutions, but also compatibilities when mixing solutions in syringes and adding solutions into the Y-tubes on administration sets. *(1; 13; 21)*

78. **(D)** Amphotericin B is administered by slow intravenous infusion over a 2- to 4-hour period. The original product was available in vials containing 50 mg of drug as a powder with SWFI specified as the diluent. Other ve-

hicles such as NS may cause a precipitate. Because of the colloidal nature of the product, administration sets with in-line filters may not be used. Amphotericin is incompatible with most solutions having acidic pHs. The pharmacist must be cognizant that there is a liposomal dosage form of Amphotericin that has a different dosage regimen. *(21)*

79. **(A)** The pH of diazepam solution is slightly acidic (pH of 6.2–6.9). To solubilize diazepam, a mixed solvent system of 40% propylene glycol, 10% alcohol, and water is necessary. When diazepam solution is added to an aqueous solution, a portion of the diazepam may precipitate. *(21:333)*

80. **(E)** Thiamine HCl has a pH in the range of 2.5 to 4.5. Potassium chloride injection has a pH of 4 to 6 while chlorothiazide in solution has a high pH—approximately 9.5. Dextrose 5% Injection usually exhibits an acidic pH range between 4.3 and 6.

However, one must remember that these solutions have no buffering capacity. Even when very alkaline solutions such as chlorothiazide are added, the pH quickly adjusts to the alkaline range with no precipitation. Another example is an admixture of aminophylline 500 mg solution (pH of 8.6–9) and D_5W. The acid/base incompatibility is just theoretical. Naturally, D_5W and the acidic thiamine HCl solution are compatible. *(1; 21)*

81. **(B)** Furosemide injection has an alkaline pH of 8 to 9 and would form a precipitate if mixed with the acidic Dobutamine HCl. The other two solutions are hydrochloride salts and will be expected to have acidic pHs. Actually, Ranitidine HCl has a neutral pH of 6.7 to 7.3 but would be compatible with the acidic Dobutamine HCl. *(1; 21)*

82. **(C)** Liposomal powders are usually reconstituted using SWFI. Other diluents such as sodium chloride injection may cause breakage of the liposomal system. Since many of the liposomal products are formulated as "targeted drug delivery systems," the drug present will concentrate in areas of the body in which they are most active. Thus, the drug dose required is often less. Consequently, if the larger conventional dose is given, toxic levels of the drug may occur. Conversely, if the conventional drug is required and the liposomal drug dose is given, the dose may be subtherapeutic. *(24)*

83. **(A)** *Drug Facts and Comparisons* has a section that lists all commercial amino acid solutions by total concentration, individual amino acids present in each formula, and other pertinent information such as grams of nitrogen present, and other miscellaneous ingredients. *(3)*

84. **(E)** There is a large variety of parenteral amino acids formulas on the market. Some contain a mixture of both the essential and the nonessential amino acids while others contain almost exclusively the essential amino acids. Some formulas contain significantly higher levels of branched chained amino acids, which are believed to be more readily assimilated in the body. When comparing similar formulas containing the same total amino acids concentration, the relative amounts of the individual amino acids present may vary slightly. These minor differences may be ignored when selecting one company's product versus another. *(4; 10)*

85. **(D)** Most TPN solutions are hypertonic because of the high concentrations of dextrose present. This is not a problem if they are slowly infused through major blood vessels. Essential fatty acid deficiencies are avoided by including certain vegetable oils in the formulas. BEE is the calculated minimum calories that must be provided to a patient for his or her daily needs. However, in a malnourished patient, larger amounts of calories should be provided. *(4; 14)*

86. **(D)** Multicomponent admixtures that contain dextrose, amino acids, and fat oil emulsions are referred to as TNAs, or 3 in 1s. Although these combinations simplify administration of calories and protein, the cloudy nature of the product precludes examination of the product for fine precipitants. The designation MCT has been used to represent medium chain triglycerides, which may be

used in patients suffering from malabsorption. *(21; 24)*

87. **(A)** The concentration of dextrose in parenteral infusion solutions is based on the official form of hydrous dextrose. Its caloric density (or count) is 3.4 kcal/g. *(4)*

88. **(B)** Although the exact amount of nitrogen in an amino acid structure varies with the molecular weight of the amino acid, approximately 16% of any mixture of common amino acids will consist of nitrogen. Therefore,

100 mL of 10% amino acids injection

= 10 g amino acids

10 g amino acids × 16% = 1.6 g of nitrogen *(4)*

89. **(C)** Because the pharmacist has only $D_{50}W$ and Aminosyn II packaged in 500-mL bottles, it is most convenient to transfer each solution aseptically to an evacuated sterile glass bottle or plastic bag. *(3)*

90. **(A)** Each 1 L of the TPN solution contains 500 mL each of the Aminosyn II solution and 50% dextrose injection.

500 mL × 50% = 250 g of dextrose

Since the caloric density of hydrated dextrose = 3.4 kcal/g, 250 g × 3.4 kcal/g = 850 kcal. *(4)*

91. **(C)** Many calcium salts, such as the phosphate and carbonate, have limited water solubility. When calcium salts and phosphate salts are included in the same admixture, it is possible that the very insoluble calcium phosphates may form. The pharmacist must recognize the potential danger of infusing such solutions into patients. Several reference sources list the limits of each salt that is compatible with the other. However, the precipitate may form slowly and would be invisible if a fat emulsion is included in the TPN. *(4; 21)*

92. **(A)** Graphs in both Trissel's and King's books indicate the upper levels of sodium and potassium salts that may be mixed in the same TPN bottle with varying amounts of the phosphate salts. *(1; 4)*

93. **(A)** It is often possible to reduce the likelihood of a precipitation if the potassium phosphate is dissolved or mixed with the vehicle first followed by the calcium solution, which is added slowly while stirring. The pharmacist could also alternate the calcium and the phosphate solutions in the series of TPN containers. However, he or she should inform the prescriber, and double the amount of ion added each time. *(4)*

94. **(A)** Phosphorus is an essential mineral for the body and is readily available in the phosphate ion. When the potassium ion is required, the chloride or acetate salts are used. *(13)*

95. **(D)** Most electrolytes are ordered in terms of milliequivalents. The exceptions are the phosphates. Commercially available potassium phosphate injections consist of a mixture of monobasic (potassium) and dibasic (dipotassium) phosphates. Because body phosphate requirements are usually expressed in terms of millimoles (mM) per kilogram per day and the available solutions are mixtures of the two salts, it is more convenient to express the phosphate additive in terms of mM/L rather than mEq/L. The average adult needs 10 to 15 mmol of phosphorus per day. *(4; 13)*

96. **(C)** Low-dose insulin syringes are calibrated to contain 0.5 mL (50 units) of insulin. The 40 units of insulin (0.4 mL) could also be measured accurately using the tuberculin syringe, which has the capacity of 1 mL. The smallest calibrations on 10-mL syringes will not allow accurate enough measurements of 0.4 mL. *(13; 24)*

97. **(A)** When low concentrations of insulin are included in LVPs, the percentage of insulin adsorbed onto the walls of the containers and also onto the administration sets is significant. One can expect at least 50% insulin loss when only 40 units are added to the container. *(13; 24)* The other answers are incorrect. Because the insulin dosage is expressed in units, the strength of the insulin is not

needed. Most likely, the U-100 solution will be used. Only insulin solution is given intravenously; the suspension forms are intended for subcutaneous administration.

98. **(C)** Liposyn is a fatty acid emulsion with a physical appearance similar to that of milk. When included in TPN solutions, the resulting product will be somewhat cloudy. The intent of the Liposyn is to correct or prevent fatty acid deficiencies by providing linoleic and linolenic acids, which are present in either soybean or safflower oil. The fat emulsions also provide calories. For example, every milliliter of the 10% strength contributes 1.1 kcal, and a milliliter of the 20% provides 2.0 kcal. Because the fat emulsions have been adjusted for tonicity, they do not adversely affect the osmolarity of TPN solutions. *(4; 21)*

99. **(A)** Fatty oil emulsions are stabilized by the presence of egg phospholipids. As such they are usually contraindicated in those patients with serious allergies to eggs. *(4; 5)*

100. **(A)** Depending upon the reference source, the caloric density of the 10% fatty oil emulsions is reported as either 1 kcal/mL or probably the more accurate 1.1 kcal/mL. The 20% fatty oil emulsions use a value of 2 kcal/mL.

$$\text{Using 1 kcal/mL, 500 mL} \times 1 = 500 \text{ kcal}$$
$$\text{Using 1.1 kcal/mL 500 mL} \times 1.1 = 550 \text{ kcal}$$

101. **(B)** The TPN formula calls for 500 mL of 8.5% amino acids solution per bottle. Since three bottles are administered per day, the total amount of amino acids is 500 mL $\times$ 3 bts $\times$ 8.5% = 127.5 g. The average amount of nitrogen in amino acids is 16%, therefore,

$$127.5 \text{ g} \times 16\% = 20.4 \text{ g} \qquad (4)$$

102. **(C)** Selenium deficiencies may cause muscle pain, tenderness, and cardiomyopathy. *(3)*

103. **(A)** There are several sterile solutions that contain the most popular trace metals likely to be requested for TPNs. Aluminum is deliberately avoided since there is no bodily requirement for it. In fact, the USP has established

impurity limits for aluminum in large volume parenterals containers. Both manganese and zinc are essential trace metals. While iron is necessary for the body it is seldom included in TPN solutions because of compatibility problems. *(3)*

104. **(B)** Milliequivalent expressions allow direct comparisons of ions when different salt forms are being used. In other words, 40 mEq of sodium acetate will contain the same weight of sodium as will 40 mEq of sodium chloride. *(23)*

105. **(A)** Although the exact cause of the cloudy solution is unknown, it is likely due to a calcium/phosphate interaction. Under certain conditions, such as concentrations, calcium salts such as the chloride or the gluconate will react with phosphates forming the very water insoluble calcium phosphate. The precipitate may worsen as time elapses, especially if infused into the patient since calcium phosphate's solubility decreases with higher temperatures. Use of an in-line filter is not feasible since it will slow down the infusion with eventual clogging of the line. (4)

106. **(D)** $D_{50}W$ – 500 mL $\times$ 50% = 250 g $\times$ 3.4 kcal/g = 850 kcal

Veinamine – 400 mL $\times$ 7% = 28 g $\times$ 4 kcal/g = 112 kcal

Liposyn 10% 100 mL $\times$ 1.1 kcal/mL = 110 kcal

Total kcalories = 1,072 kcal *(1: 23)*

107. **(D)** The ratio of calories to grams of nitrogen in any TPN formula is important to ensure that sufficient energy is being provided to (1) provide energy to the body and (2) to allow conversion of the nitrogen to lean body mass (protein synthesis). Usually ratios of at least 125:1 up to 175:1 are desired. Calories provided by the amino acids are NOT included in the calculations.

Lower ratios indicate that not enough calories are being provided, and some of the amino acids will not be converted into lean body mass (anabolism). Very high ratios indicate that the excessive energy may be wasted.

In this question, 1. Determine the grams of nitrogen present in the Veinamine.

28 g × 16% (average percentage of N in mixture of amino acids) = 4.48 g

2. Divide total of nonprotein calories by gram of nitrogen

960 kcal to 4.48 g nitrogen = 214 to 1
Answer E is incorrect. This ratio is obtained if the calories of the Veinamine are included in the calculations. Answers A or B are incorrect. These answers may occur if one fails to convert total weight of amino acids present to gram of nitrogen. *(1; 23)*

108. **(B)** Disposable infusion pumps such as the Block Medical's Homepumps and Baxter's Intermates are ideal for home infusion of parenterals at intermittent intervals. The elastomeric balloon present gives constant flow of solution without the need of pump device or gravity flow. The usual volume capacity of the units varies from 50 to 250 mL. Pharmacists fill the units by drawing up active drug solution plus diluent into plastic syringes then injecting through a filling port on the unit. The units have small diameter tubing already attached, which allows the patient to attach the unit to a previously inserted infusion catheter. *(22)*

109. **(B)** Hydromorphone HCL is approximately eight times stronger than morphine with usual parenteral doses of 1 to 5 mg every 4 to 6 hours. Epidural administration results in longer durations of analgesia: 10 to 12 hours. It appears that the drug is being prescribed for a patient suffering from severe pain of terminal cancer. The dosing regimen is probably not unrealistic but should be confirmed with the prescriber. The chemical's water solubility is high, 1 g in 3 mL. There are several dosage forms of hydromorphone including multidose vials (2 mg/mL), high dose vials (10 mg/mL), and vials of nonsterile powder. After parenteral administration, the drug's analgesic effect occurs in 10 to 15 minutes and lasts 4 to 5 hours. Advantages over morphine are that it has less tendency to cause sleep, vomiting, and constipation. *(1; 21; 24)*

110. **(C)** Since hydromorphone has good water solubility (1 g in 3 mL), 300 mg of the Dilaudid powder may be dissolved in approximately 10 to 20 mL of NS. This solution should be filtered through a 0.22-μm filter into the PCA cassette and sufficient sterile normal saline added to make 100 mL.

A second alternative is to use 30 mL of Dilaudid-HP Injection and qs to 100 mL with sterile normal saline.

Answer III is incorrect since the volume of drug solution needed is too high.

$$\frac{2 \text{ mg}}{1 \text{ mL}} = \frac{300 \text{ mL}}{x \text{ mL}}$$

$x = 150$ mL, which is greater than the total volume requested in the order. *(1; 24)*

111. **(C)** The preparation of parenteral admixtures and compounding of other sterile products in pharmacies must be done under stringent conditions to ensure sterility of the final product. The ASHP has established guidelines consisting of three risk levels. Risk level 1 is most lenient while risk level 3 has the tightest controls. For example, compounding sterile products using nonsterile powders requires a terminal sterilization procedure. *(24)*

112. **(A)** The pharmacist recognizes that mixing equal volumes of alcohol and purified water will result in some shrinkage in final volume. The alcohol quantity is the controlling factor to obtain a certain percentage of ethanol in the final dilution. *(1)*

113. **(A)** PCA is the acronym for "patient-controlled analgesia," the name related to small devices worn outside the body, which can provide constant, slow infusion of analgesics into patients. Pharmacists compound these units by aseptically placing the analgesic solution plus diluent into the flexible plastic cartridge, which is then placed in an outer unit, which controls the flow rate and pumping mechanism. The solution is slowly infused into the patient at a constant preset rate. The drug reservoir provides several days of therapy. Many of the units have a mechanism for bolus dosing if the patient is experiencing

breakthrough pain. While the original units were used for strong analgesics such as morphine and Dilaudid, other drug solutions, such as 5-fluorouracil, may be infused through the PCA. Several companies manufacture these ambulatory infusion devices including Pharmacia's CADD. *(22)*

114. **(A)** The elastomeric balloon pumps flow by pressure not gravity. Thus, the patient may store the unit in his pocket or backpack even while infusing the solution. The individual units are not intended to be refilled, that is, they are considered disposable. Because the infusion is at a constant rate, there is no mechanism for obtaining a bolus dose. This curtails the use of these units for pain management. Instead the units are used for such purposes as home infusion of antibiotics. *(22)*

115. **(D)** Although the USP/NF monograph for D_5W specifies that the pH may be as low as 5.5, the solution has no buffering capacity.

Thus, either acidic or basic (alkaline) solutions may be added. On the other hand, answer III is incorrect since there will likely be an acid/base reaction with the formation of a precipitate. Answer II is also incorrect. Nonaqueous solvents such as propylene glycol and alcohol are employed when the active drug has limited water solubility. *(1; 4)*

116. **(B)** If uncertain of possible incompatibilities, the pharmacist should check both reference sources and product inserts. Mixing of two solutions in a syringe may present a serious situation since a concentrated mixture is formed. A general guideline is to determine the pHs of the two solutions involved cognizant that most reactions will involve acid–base interactions. In this problem, the pharmacist should recognize that Phenytoin injection has a high pH (≥ 10). Thus, it is incompatible with an acidic solution such as Lidocaine HCl. All of the other solutions in the choices have acidic pHs. *(21)*

CHAPTER 5

Biopharmaceutics and Pharmacokinetics

Biopharmaceutics is a scientific discipline concerned with the relationship between the physicochemical properties of a drug in a dosage form and the biological response observed after its administration. It includes the study of the release of the drug from its dosage form. Pharmacokinetics is the study of the absorption, distribution, metabolism, and elimination (ADME) of drugs. As more quantitative and sophisticated assay techniques have been developed, a better understanding of the therapeutic pathways for drugs has emerged. This chapter tests the reader's knowledge of the principles of biopharmaceutics and pharmacokinetics, which is fundamental to the rational selection of quality drug products, the determination of appropriate dose and dosing schedules, and the monitoring of therapy.

Questions

DIRECTIONS (Questions 1 through 110): Each of the numbered items or incomplete statements in this section is followed by answers or completions of the statement. Select the one lettered answer or completion that is most correct in each case.

1. A prime consideration in biopharmaceutics is a drug's "bioavailability" which refers to the relative amount of drug that reaches which area?

    (A) small intestine
    (B) stomach
    (C) systemic circulation
    (D) liver
    (E) kidneys

2. The areas under the curve (AUC) can be described as which of the following?

    I. a theoretic value
    II. a measure of drug concentration–time curve
    III. having units of weight and time/volume

    (A) I only
    (B) III only
    (C) I and II only
    (D) II and III only
    (E) I, II, and III

3. The AUC of a drug can be determined from a graph by using which of the following methods?

    I. law of diminishing returns
    II. rule of nines
    III. trapezoidal rule

    (A) I only
    (B) III only
    (C) I and II only
    (D) II and III only
    (E) I, II, and III

4. Based on graphic comparisons of AUCs, under which of the following criteria may a generic drug product be considered by the FDA to be bioequivalent with a trade name product?

    I. The generic's AUC may be superimposed on that of the brand name product.
    II. The generic's overall AUC is 15% lower than the brand name product.
    III. The generic's overall AUC is 18% higher than the brand name product.

    (A) I only
    (B) III only
    (C) I and II only
    (D) II and III only
    (E) I, II, and III

5. The relative bioavailability of a drug product can be determined by comparing which of the following values to similar control drug values?

    I. AUC
    II. total drug urinary excretion
    III. peak blood drug concentrations

    (A) I only
    (B) III only
    (C) I and II only
    (D) II and III only
    (E) I, II, and III

6. What is potentially the first rate-limiting process when a tablet dosage form is administered?

   (A) ionization of the drug
   (B) diffusion of the drug through the GI epithelium
   (C) dissolution of the drug in the GI fluids
   (D) dissolution of the drug in the blood
   (E) disintegration of the tablet

7. Which of the following could be the rate-limiting steps for drug absorption from an orally administered drug product?

   I. disintegration of the unit
   II. dissolution of the active drug
   III. diffusion of active drug through the intestinal wall

   (A) I only
   (B) III only
   (C) I and II only
   (D) II and III only
   (E) I, II, and III

8. Dissolution may be described by using which one of the following equations or laws?

   (A) Fick's second law
   (B) Fick's first law
   (C) Noyes–Whitney equation
   (D) Poiseuille's law
   (E) Stoke's law

9. The peak of the serum concentration versus time graph approximates the

   (A) point in time when the maximum pharmacological effect occurs
   (B) point in time when absorption and elimination of the drug have equalized
   (C) maximum concentration of free drug in the urine
   (D) time required for essentially all of the drug to be absorbed from the GI tract
   (E) point in time when the drug begins to be metabolized

10. In which of the following sites may drugs be metabolized?

    I. skin
    II. lungs
    III. liver

    (A) I only
    (B) III only
    (C) I and II only
    (D) II and III only
    (E) I, II, and III

11. When compared to their parent compound, metabolites usually have which of the following?

    (A) greater water solubility
    (B) lower water solubility
    (C) greater therapeutic activity
    (D) no therapeutic activity
    (E) greater diffusion through the blood–brain barrier

12. When graphed, nonlinear pharmacokinetics is characterized by data that can be described as which of the following?

    (A) does not yield a straight line at any time
    (B) exhibits a straight line only when plotted as log–log functions
    (C) is dose dependent
    (D) follows first-order kinetics
    (E) will have a negative slope

13. To what is the "F" value for a drug product ideally compared?

    (A) absolute bioavailability
    (B) dosing rate
    (C) clearance rate
    (D) relative bioavailability
    (E) route of administration

14. Determine the F value for a drug available as a 100-mg capsule with a calculated AUC of 20 mg/dL/h when a 100-mg IV bolus of the same drug exhibits an AUC of 25 mg/dL/h.

(A) 0.2
(B) 0.4
(C) 0.8
(D) 1.25
(E) 20

15. What is the F value for an experimental drug tablet based on the following data?

Drug Dosage Form	Dose	AUC (μg/mL/h)
Tablet	100 mg po	20
Solution (control)	100 mg po	30
Injection (control)	50 mg IV push	40

(A) 0.25
(B) 0.38
(C) 0.50
(D) 0.66
(E) 0.90

16. Assuming 100% ionization, what F value should be assigned to the salt form of a drug (mol. wt. = 240) when comparing it to the base form of the drug (mol. wt. = 180)? The valence of the molecule is 2.

(A) 0.375
(B) 0.667
(C) 0.75
(D) 1
(E) 1.33

17. To what does the term "therapeutic window" refer?

(A) time interval between administration and the beginning of activity
(B) concentration differential between drug's MTC and MEC
(C) concentration, which must be reached before activity begins
(D) concentration versus time curve

(E) time period before administration of the next dose

18. For two drug products to be considered "pharmaceutical equivalents," the products must have which of the following?

I. have the same active drug (therapeutic moiety)
II. consist of the same salt
III. contain the same excipients

(A) I only
(B) III only
(C) I and II only
(D) II and III only
(E) I, II, and III

19. Requirements for drug products to be considered "pharmaceutical alternatives" necessitate having which of the following characteristics be the same?

I. active drug or precursor
II. dosage form
III. salt or ester

(A) I only
(B) III only
(C) I and II only
(D) II and III only
(E) I, II, and III

20. Which one of the following is a guideline used by the FDA to evaluate bioequivalence for multisource drug products?

(A) dimensional analysis
(B) 80/20 rule
(C) first in/first out principle
(D) law of diminishing returns
(E) rule of the thumb

21. Based on the pH partition theory, why are weakly acidic drugs more likely to be absorbed from the stomach?

(A) the drugs will exist primarily in the unionized, more lipid-soluble form

(B) the drugs will exist primarily in the ionized, more water-soluble form

(C) weak acids are more soluble in acid media

(D) the ionic form of the drug facilitates dissolution

(E) weak acids will further depress pH

22. Gastric emptying is slowed by all of the following EXCEPT which of the following?

(A) vigorous exercise

(B) fatty foods

(C) hot meals

(D) hunger

(E) emotional stress

23. Protein binding in the blood is most significant with drugs that possess which of the following characteristics?

   I. easily displaced from protein-binding sites

  II. therapeutic action occurs within cells

 III. high therapeutic indexes

(A) I only

(B) III only

(C) I and II only

(D) II and III only

(E) I, II, and III

24. When comparing three structurally related antihypertensive agents, which of the following activities would be predicted for the drug that is most highly protein-bound?

   I. faster and more complete urinary excretion

  II. faster metabolism in the liver

 III. a longer half-life

(A) I only

(B) III only

(C) I and II only

(D) II and III only

(E) I, II, and III

25. Which of the following statements concerning the blood protein albumin is (are) true?

   I. It is a very site-specific binding agent.

  II. It will generally bind acidic drugs.

 III. Blood levels are approximately 3.5–5.0 g/dL.

(A) I only

(B) III only

(C) I and II only

(D) II and III only

(E) I, II, and III

26. Which one of the following drugs is unlikely to bind to blood albumin?

(A) lidocaine

(B) naproxen

(C) penicillin

(D) phenytoin

(E) warfarin

27. Which of the following conditions may significantly reduce blood albumin levels?

   I. extensive body burns

  II. cystic fibrosis

 III. chronic renal failure

(A) I only

(B) III only

(C) I and II only

(D) II and III only

(E) I, II, and III

28. Drugs that are absorbed from the GI tract are generally

(A) absorbed into the portal circulation and pass through the liver before entering the general circulation

(B) filtered from the blood by the kidney, then reabsorbed into the general circulation

(C) absorbed into the portal circulation and are distributed by an enterohepatic cycle

(D) not affected by liver enzymes

(E) stored in the liver

29. What is true about the biological half-life of a drug?

    (A) It is a constant physical property of the drug.
    (B) It is a constant chemical property of the drug.
    (C) It is the time for one-half of the therapeutic activity to be lost.
    (D) It may be decreased by giving the drug by rapid IV injection.
    (E) It depends entirely on the route of administration.

30. The biological half-life of a drug that is eliminated by first-order kinetics is represented mathematically by _____, where k is the first-order rate constant for elimination.

    (A) $1/k$
    (B) $\log k$
    (C) $0.693/k$
    (D) $2.303/k$
    (E) peak serum concentration/$2k$

31. A specific drug has a first-order biological half-life of 4 hours. What is true about the half-life value of this drug?

    (A) It will be independent of the initial drug concentration.
    (B) It will increase when the concentration of the drug increases.
    (C) It will decrease when the concentration of the drug increases.
    (D) It will decrease if the patient has renal impairment.
    (E) It will be the same whether the drug level is determined in the blood or by observing the pharmacological action.

32. A drug that follows linear pharmacokinetics has a half-life of 4 hours. How many milligrams of the drug will remain in the body 12 hours after the administration of a 400-mg dose?

    (A) 10
    (B) 25
    (C) 50

    (D) 100
    (E) 200

33. Determine the half-life of furosemide if it appears to be eliminated from the body at a rate constant of 46% per hour. Assume that first-order kinetics occurs.

    (A) <1 hour
    (B) 1.5 hours
    (C) 3.0 hours
    (D) 4.0 hours
    (E) >5 hours

34. Which one of the following drugs has the longest elimination half-life?

    (A) acetaminophen
    (B) digoxin
    (C) ibuprofen
    (D) nitroglycerin
    (E) ranitidine

35. What is the volume of distribution of a drug?

    I. a mathematical relationship between the total amount of drug in the body and the concentration of drug in the blood
    II. a measure of an individual's blood volume
    III. a measure of an individual's total body volume

    (A) I only
    (B) III only
    (C) I and II only
    (D) II and III only
    (E) I, II, and III

36. The volume of distribution (V_d) of a particular drug will be which of the following?

    (A) greater for drugs that concentrate in tissues rather than in plasma
    (B) greater for drugs that concentrate in plasma rather than in tissues
    (C) independent of tissue concentration
    (D) independent of plasma concentration
    (E) approximately the same for all drugs in a given individual

37. What can you do with the knowledge of V_d for a given drug?

(A) estimate the elimination rate constant
(B) determine the biological half-life
(C) calculate a reasonable loading dose
(D) determine the best dosing interval
(E) determine the peak plasma concentration

38. Estimate the plasma concentration of a drug when 50 mg is given by IV bolus to a 140-lb patient if her volume of distribution is 1.6 L/kg.

(A) 0.1 mg/L
(B) 0.5 mg/L
(C) 1 mg/L
(D) 5 mg/L
(E) 31 mg/L

39. What does the time needed to achieve a steady-state plasma level for a drug administered by infusion depend upon?

I. amount of drug being infused
II. volume of distribution of the drug
III. half-life of the drug

(A) I only
(B) III only
(C) I and II only
(D) II and III only
(E) I, II, and III

Questions 40 through 44: The following graph represents drug blood level curves. Answer the next five questions based on this graph.

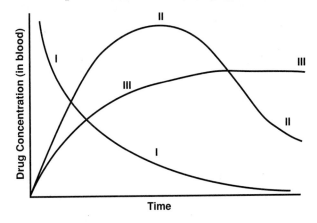

40. Curve I represents the blood level concentration of a drug administered by which method?

I. the oral route
II. intramuscular injection
III. intravenous injection

(A) I only
(B) III only
(C) I and II only
(D) II and III only
(E) I, II, and III

41. What could the upward slope of curve II represent?

I. increased absorption of drug from a capsule dosage form
II. absorption of drug from an intramuscular injection
III. absorption of drug from a sustained-release tablet

(A) I only
(B) III only
(C) I and II only
(D) II and III only
(E) I, II, and III

42. Which one of the following statements concerning the graph is completely true?

(A) Once the peak in curve II has been reached, no further drug absorption is likely to occur.
(B) Doubling the administered dose will double the height of curve II.
(C) The Y-axis (concentration of drug in the blood) is being expressed as a log function.
(D) The X-axis (time) is being expressed as a log function.
(E) The curves in lines II and III indicate that the absorption rate (k_a) is greater than the elimination rate (k_e).

43. Which method best illustrates drug administration in curve III?

    (A) intravenous push
    (B) intravenous infusion
    (C) intramuscular injection
    (D) intrathecal injection
    (E) either intravenous push or infusion

44. What is the time needed to reach optimum drug blood levels (the plateau portion of curve III) during constant-rate intravenous infusion?

    (A) directly proportional to the rate of infusion
    (B) inversely proportional to the rate of infusion
    (C) independent of the rate of infusion
    (D) independent of the biological half-life
    (E) not related to either the infusion rate or the biological half-life

45. What factor besides the desired steady-state concentration (C_{ss}) is most important for determining an infusion rate of a parenteral solution?

    (A) half-life of the drug
    (B) metabolism rate
    (C) renal elimination
    (D) total clearance
    (E) volume of distribution

46. Compartmental models are often used to illustrate the various principles of pharmacokinetics. How is "compartment" best defined?

    (A) any anatomic entity that is capable of absorbing drug
    (B) a kinetically distinguishable pool of drug
    (C) specific body organs or tissues that can be assayed for drug
    (D) any body fluid, such as blood or urine, that may contain drug
    (E) any component of the blood, including blood proteins that would have a tendency to absorb drug

47. When evaluating data concerning a drug exhibiting two-compartment modeling, which of the following will be reported with two values?

    I. clearance
    II. half-life
    III. volume of distribution

    (A) I only
    (B) III only
    (C) I and II only
    (D) II and III only
    (E) I, II, and III

48. When reviewing the literature, a pharmacist observes that a drug exhibiting two-compartment modeling has an initial volume of distribution of 0.3 L/kg and a final volume of distribution of 0.88 L/kg. If the clearance rate of this drug is 6 mL/min/kg, what loading dose should be injected? A steady-state concentration of 0.5 mg/L is desired. The 60-year-old patient weighs 60 kg.

    (A) 9 mg
    (B) 18 mg
    (C) 36 mg
    (D) 72 mg
    (E) 360 mg

49. Which of the following is (are) true of nonlinear pharmacokinetics?

    I. follows zero-order kinetics
    II. elimination half-life will change as the dose is increased
    III. half-life is expressed in terms of fraction per unit of time

    (A) I only
    (B) III only
    (C) I and II only
    (D) II and III only
    (E) I, II, and III

50. Which of the following dosage forms is (are) likely to follow zero-order kinetics?

    I. transdermal patches
    II. delayed release tablets
    III. suppositories

(A) I only

(B) III only

(C) I and II only

(D) II and III only

(E) I, II, and III

51. The difference between peak and trough concentrations is greatest when a drug is given at dosing intervals that are which one of the following?

(A) much longer than the half-life

(B) about equal to the half-life

(C) much shorter than the half-life

(D) equal to the half-life times serum creatinine

(E) equal to the time it takes to reach peak concentration following a single oral dose

52. When conducting clinical trials, low values for which of the following parameters is (are) desired?

  I. p or P value (probability)

  II. placebo effect

  III. standard deviation

(A) I only

(B) III only

(C) I and II only

(D) II and III only

(E) I, II, and III

53. What is the pharmacokinetic parameter known as "clearance" essentially?

(A) rate at which the plasma is cleared of all waste materials and foreign substances (eg, drugs)

(B) volume of blood that passes through the kidneys per unit of time

(C) volume of blood that passes through the liver per unit of time

(D) rate at which a drug is removed (cleared) from its site of absorption

(E) volume of blood that is completely cleared of drug per unit of time

54. Why is the knowledge of the clearance (CL) of a given drug useful?

(A) It allows the calculation of the maintenance dose required to sustain a desired average steady-state plasma concentration.

(B) It allows the determination of a loading dose but not the maintenance dose.

(C) It allows the determination of the ideal dosing interval.

(D) It allows the decision whether a loading dose is necessary.

(E) It allows the determination if the drug is metabolized or excreted unchanged.

55. In dosing drugs that are primarily excreted by the kidneys, one must have some idea of the patient's renal function. What is a calculated pharmacokinetic parameter that gives us a reasonable estimate of renal function?

(A) blood urea nitrogen (BUN)

(B) serum creatinine (Sr_{cr})

(C) creatinine clearance (CL_{cr})

(D) urine creatinine (U_{cr})

(E) free water clearance (CL_{fw})

56. If the rate of elimination of a drug is reduced because of impaired renal function, what is the effect on the drug half-life and the time required to reach steady-state plasma levels (steady-state concentrations, C_{ss})?

(A) They both increase

(B) They both decrease

(C) There will be an increase in half-life and a decrease in the time to reach C_{ss}

(D) There will be a decrease in half-life but an increase in the time to reach C_{ss}.

(E) It will be negligible

57. For many drugs, bioavailability can be evaluated using urinary excretion data. What assumption is this statement based on?

(A) Bioavailability studies can be done only on drugs that are completely excreted unchanged by the kidneys.

(B) Drug levels can be measured more accurately in urine than in blood.

(C) A drug must first be absorbed into the systemic circulation before it can appear in the urine.

(D) All of the administered dose can be recovered from the urine.

(E) Only drug metabolites are excreted in the urine.

58. Estimating bioavailability from urinary excretion data is less satisfactory than estimates based on blood level data because accurate urinary excretion studies require which of the following?

   I. complete urine collection
   II. normal or near-normal renal function
   III. that the drug be completely excreted unchanged by the kidney

(A) I only
(B) III only
(C) I and II only
(D) II and III only
(E) I, II, and III

Questions 59 through 61 are to be answered using the following data collected by testing various dosage forms of the same drug manufactured by two companies.

Product by Company	Dosage Form	Dose Administered	Cumulative Urinary Amount (mg)
A	Parenteral injection	10 mg IV	9.4
A	Tablet	20 mg po	12.0
B	Tablet	20 mg po	8.2
B	Capsule	15 mg po	6.8

59. What is the best estimate of absolute bioavailability of Company B tablets?

(A) 25%
(B) 40%
(C) 44%
(D) 68%
(E) 87%

60. What is the relative bioavailability of Company B tablets?

(A) 25%
(B) 40%
(C) 44%
(D) 68%
(E) 76%

61. What is the relative bioavailability of Company B tablets when compared to the capsule formula?

(A) 44%
(B) 68%
(C) 76%
(D) 90%
(E) 120%

62. Company A conducts a study comparing the AUCs for its generic version of a drug with Company B's tradename product. The respective AUCs for each company's 10-mg oral tablets were 80 and 76 μg h/mL. Which of the following statements is (are) true?

   I. The absolute bioavailability of Company A's product cannot be determined from this data.

   II. The relative bioavailability of Company A's product is 0.95.

   III. The study is flawed since Company A's drug has a higher AUC than Company B's.

(A) I only
(B) III only
(C) I and II only
(D) II and III only
(E) I, II, and III

63. The above drug follows linear pharmacokinetics and has a half-life of 8 hours with complete renal clearance. What is the elimination rate for this drug when a 10-mg dose is given?

    (A) 0.087/h
    (B) 0.33/h
    (C) 1.25 mg/h
    (D) 4 mg/h
    (E) 5.5 L/h

64. An antibiotic has clearance rates of renal 0.06/h and nonrenal 0.02/h. What is the approximate half-life of this drug if the patient's volume of distribution is estimated to be 28 L?

    (A) 8.7 hours
    (B) 11 hours
    (C) 35 hours
    (D) 245 hours
    (E) 580 hours

65. The latest lab report indicates that the above patient has 40% renal impairment. What is the estimate of the new half-life of the drug in this patient?

    (A) 9 hours
    (B) 12 hours
    (C) 16 hours
    (D) 19 hours
    (E) 32 hours

66. The half-life of an antibacterial drug has been reported as being approximately 4 hours. What is the estimated clearance of this drug in a patient.having received 50-mg bolus dose 10:00 if the blood sample drawn at 14:00 assays at 10 mg/L?

    (A) 0.8 L/h
    (B) 1.25 L/h
    (C) 1.6 L/h
    (D) 2.5 L/h
    (E) 5 L/h

67. Which of the following factors is (are) included in the Cockcroft and Gault equation for estimating creatinine clearance?

    I. patient's age
    II. patient's height and weight
    III. patient's calculated BEE

    (A) I only
    (B) III only
    (C) I and II only
    (D) II and III only
    (E) I, II, and III

68. What is the approximate creatinine clearance in a 140-lb, 50-year-old patient if the lab reports a serum creatinine value of 1.5 mg/dL?

    (A) 50–55 mL/min
    (B) 100–105 mL/min
    (C) 110–118 mL/min
    (D) 120–125 mL/min
    (E) 130–140 mL/min

69. The patient in the previous problem is a female. What correction, if any, should be made in calculating her creatinine clearance value?

    (A) The value will be 50% of the male value.
    (B) The value will be 75% of the male value.
    (C) The value will be 80% of the male value.
    (D) The value will be 85% of the male value.
    (E) No correction is needed.

70. When converting a patient from theophylline to aminophylline, which of the following is true about a dose adjustment?

    (A) it is not needed
    (B) an increase of 20% is suggested
    (C) an increase of 50% is suggested
    (D) a decrease of 20% is suggested
    (E) a decrease of 50% is suggested

71. Determine the loading dose of aminophylline needed in a 55-year-old male patient weighing 70 kg if the targeted theophylline plasma level is 10 mg/L. What is the patient's estimated volume of distribution in 0.5 L/kg?

    (A) 150 mg
    (B) 350 mg
    (C) 400 mg
    (D) 500 mg
    (E) 800 mg

72. What maintenance dose is appropriate in the above patient if the clearance is estimated to be 0.35 mL/min/kg?

    (A) 10 mg/h
    (B) 14 mg/h
    (C) 17 mg/h
    (D) 20 mg/h
    (E) 25 mg/h

73. A drug with a half-life of 6 hours has a targeted steady-state concentration of 1 mg/dL. What infusion rate (mg/min) should be established on a patient if the total clearance is approximately 0.04 L/h?

    (A) 0.007
    (B) 0.07
    (C) 0.04
    (D) 0.4
    (E) 4

Questions 74 and 75 are to be answered using the following data for an experimental antibiotic administered by injection: desired steady-state concentration = 40 mg/L, half-life of drug = 2 hours, Vd = 8 L, patient's weight and age = 55 kg and 44 years.

74. Assuming that the drug follows linear pharmacokinetics, what is the estimated clearance rate of this drug?

    (A) 0.35/h
    (B) 0.5/h
    (C) 0.7/h
    (D) 1.4 L/h
    (E) 2.8 L/h

75. What approximate infusion rate (mg/min) should a pharmacist suggest for this patient?

    (A) 2
    (B) 4
    (C) 10
    (D) 15
    (E) 110

76. Which of following statements is (are) accurate when pharmacokinetic data refers to the "extraction ratio"?

    I. The major organ involved is the liver.
    II. A high value indicates a large amount of drug being extracted.
    III. The values range from 0 to 1.

    (A) I only
    (B) III only
    (C) I and II only
    (D) II and III only
    (E) I, II, and III

77. What does the metabolism of drugs generally result in?

    (A) less acidic compounds
    (B) more acidic compounds
    (C) compounds having a higher oil/water partition coefficient
    (D) more polar compounds
    (E) compounds with lower aqueous solubility

78. The pharmacist may suspect that a drug undergoes a significant First-Pass effect when which of the following occurs?

    I. The average oral dose is significantly higher than the parenteral bolus dose.
    II. The drug is marketed in a sustained-release dosage form.
    III. The drug is contraindicated when renal impairment is present.

    (A) I only
    (B) III only
    (C) I and II only

(D) II and III only

(E) I, II, and III

79. All of the following drugs are believed to undergo significant First-Pass hepatic bio-transformation except which of the following?

(A) lidocaine

(B) morphine

(C) propranolol

(D) phenytoin

(E) verapamil

80. Dosage forms of nitroglycerin that are minimally affected by the First-Pass effect include which of the following?

I. intravenous

II. transdermal patches

III. sublingual tablets

(A) I only

(B) III only

(C) I and II only

(D) II and III only

(E) I, II, and III

81. The product literature states that a drug has a reported extraction ratio of 0.7. This value indicates which one of the following?

(A) 70% of the drug is being absorbed from the GI tract

(B) 30% of the drug is being absorbed from the GI tract

(C) 70% of the drug is removed by the liver

(D) 30% of the drug is removed by the liver

(E) The drug salt contains 70% active drug

82. All of the following drugs have shown an increase in their bioavailability with the coadministration of concentrated grapefruit juice EXCEPT?

(A) coumadin

(B) cyclosporine

(C) felodipine

(D) phenytoin

(E) saquinavir

83. Which of the following is (are) appropriate communications to present to a patient who insists on drinking her 8 oz of grapefruit juice while taking a drug known to be metabolized by the CYP3A group of enzymes?

I. To avoid enzyme interference, be sure to separate the two by at least 1 hour.

II. It is better to take the juice in the morning and the drug in the evening to avoid the interference.

III. Realize that the juice will slow the metabolism of the drug, so do not change your habits while consuming both.

(A) I only

(B) III only

(C) I and II only

(D) II and III only

(E) I, II, and III

84. Which one of the following drugs is most likely to be affected by pharmacogenetics?

(A) ampicillin

(B) ascorbic acid

(C) citalopram

(D) nitroglycerin

(E) warfarin

85. The rate of diffusion of drugs across biological membranes is most commonly which of the following?

(A) independent of the concentration gradient

(B) directly proportional to the concentration gradient

(C) dependent on the availability of carrier substrate

(D) dependent on the route of administration

(E) directly proportional to membrane thickness

86. Which one of the following statements concerning active transport systems is NOT correct?

    (A) They are also known as carrier-mediated transport.
    (B) They may be adversely affected by certain chemicals.
    (C) They are structure specific.
    (D) They reach equilibrium faster than passive transport systems.
    (E) They consume energy.

87. When the active transport system described in Question 86 becomes saturated, what will be the rate process?

    (A) zero order
    (B) pseudo-zero order
    (C) first order
    (D) pseudo-first order
    (E) second order

88. When comparing a highly protein-bound drug to its less- or nonprotein-bound analog, what will the highly bound drug probably have?

    I. faster metabolism rate
    II. a longer biological half-life
    III. slower diffusion into tissue

    (A) I only
    (B) III only
    (C) I and II only
    (D) II and III only
    (E) I, II, and III

89. Which one of the following drugs does NOT bind to plasma protein to any significant extent?

    (A) allopurinol (Zyloprim)
    (B) furosemide (Lasix)
    (C) phenytoin (Dilantin)
    (D) propranolol (Inderal)
    (E) warfarin (Coumadin)

90. Which of the following is (are) likely to occur with highly protein-bound cephalosporin drugs?

    I. The drug's half-life will be longer.
    II. The renal clearance value will be greater.
    III. Transfer into tissue will be easier.

    (A) I only
    (B) III only
    (C) I and II only
    (D) II and III only
    (E) I, II, and III

91. Dialysis is most successful with drugs that are characterized by which of the following?

    I. relatively low molecular weights
    II. protein bound
    III. high volumes of distribution

    (A) I only
    (B) III only
    (C) I and II only
    (D) II and III only
    (E) I, II, and III

92. Which of the following drugs is (are) poor candidates for removal from the body by hemodialysis?

    I. digoxin
    II. amphotericin B
    III. doxycycline

    (A) I only
    (B) III only
    (C) I and II only
    (D) II and III only
    (E) I, II, and III

93. Why will the excretion of a weakly acidic drug (eg, pK_a of 3.5) be more rapid in alkaline urine than in acidic urine?

    (A) All drugs are excreted more rapidly in alkaline urine.
    (B) The drug will exist primarily in the unionized form, which cannot be reabsorbed easily.
    (C) The drug will exist primarily in the ionized form, which cannot be reabsorbed easily.

(D) Weak acids cannot be reabsorbed from the kidney tubules.

(E) Active transport mechanisms function better in alkaline urine.

94. Lidocaine is commonly administered for patient exhibiting cardiac arrhythmias. Its pharmacokinetics include:

half-life = 2 hours; clearance = 9 mL/min/kg; and volume of distribution = 70 L.

How many hours will pass before a 70-kg patient will reach 87.5% of steady-state concentration?

(A) 2
(B) 4
(C) 6
(D) 8
(E) 10

95. Why may the rectal route of administration be preferred over the oral route for some systemic-acting drugs?

(A) The drug does not have to be absorbed.

(B) Absorption is predictable and complete.

(C) A portion of the absorbed drug does not pass through the liver before entering the systemic circulation.

(D) Inert binders, diluents, and excipients cannot interfere with absorption.

(E) The dissolution process is avoided.

96. Which statement is true pertaining to when a drug appears in the feces after oral adminis-tration?

(A) The drug cannot have been completely absorbed from the GI tract.

(B) The drug must not have completely dissolved in the GI fluids.

(C) The drug must have complexed with materials in the GI tract.

(D) Parenteral administration of the drug may determine the contribution of the biliary system to the amount of drug in the feces.

(E) Parenteral administration of the drug will be useful to determine the bioavail-ability of the oral formulation.

97. Drugs that are poorly lipid soluble, polar, or extensively ionized at the pH of blood generally do which of the following?

(A) penetrate the CNS very slowly and may be eliminated from the body before a significant concentration in the CNS is reached

(B) penetrate the CNS very slowly but are centrally active in much lower concentration

(C) achieve adequate CNS concentrations only if given IV

(D) must be metabolized to a more polar form before they can gain access to the CNS

(E) can gain access to the CNS if other drugs are used to modify blood pH

98. What does the term "prodrug" refers to?

(A) chemical substance that is part of the synthesis procedure in preparing a drug

(B) compound that liberates an active drug in the body

(C) compound that may be therapeutically active but is still under clinical trials

(D) drug that has only prophylactic activity in the body

(E) drug that is classified as being "probably effective"

99. Which of the following drugs is (are) classi-fied as prodrugs?

I. clorazepate (Tranxene)
II. enalapril (Vasotec)
III. lisinopril (Zestril)

(A) I only
(B) III only
(C) I and II only
(D) II and III only
(E) I, II, and III

100. For which one of the following purposes is haloperidol formulated as the decanoate?

(A) better water solubility
(B) longer duration of therapeutic activity
(C) greater stability
(D) immediate activity
(E) sustained release from a capsule

101. Which of the following agents may be utilized as targeted drug delivery systems?

I. lyophilized powders
II. liposomes
III. MABs

(A) I only
(B) III only
(C) I and II only
(D) II and III only
(E) I, II, and III

102. Which of the following properties of a drug may preclude its formulation into a sustained-release dosage form?

I. half-life less than 2 hours
II. erratic absorption from the GI tract
III. low therapeutic index

(A) I only
(B) III only
(C) I and II only
(D) II and III only
(E) I, II, and III

103. Which one of the following oral dosage forms is likely to exhibit the longest lag time?

(A) delayed-release tablet
(B) elixir (20% alcohol)
(C) enteric-coated tablet
(D) osmotic tablet
(E) sustained-release capsule

104. Why is the biological half-life of many drugs often prolonged in newborn infants?

(A) a higher degree of protein binding
(B) microsomal enzyme induction
(C) more complete absorption of drugs
(D) incompletely developed enzyme systems
(E) incompletely developed barriers to the distribution of drugs in the body

105. Which of the following pharmacokinetic parameters is (are) likely to decrease in the geriatric population when compared to the average population?

I. renal elimination
II. drug metabolism
III. volume of distribution

(A) I only
(B) III only
(C) I and II only
(D) II and III only
(E) I, II, and III

106. A drug has an elimination half-life of 3 hours and its apparent volume of distribution is 100 mL/kg. What is the total body renal clearance of this drug in a 70-kg male in terms of L/h?

(A) 0.5 L/h
(B) 1.6 L/h
(C) 8 L/h
(D) 14.6 L/h
(E) 16.3 L/h

107. For which one of the following situations will reducing drug particle size enhance drug absorption?

(A) Absorption process occurs by active transport.
(B) Absorption process is rate limited by the dissolution of drug in GI fluids.
(C) Drug is very water soluble.
(D) Drug is very potent.
(E) Drug is irritating to the GI tract.

108. An experimental drug is administered as a continuous IV infusion at a rate of 1 mg/min. The drug is known to have a half-life of 2 hours, and a clearance of 0.5 L/min. What will be the drug's steady-state concentration in terms of mg/L?

(A) 0.02

(B) 0.4

(C) 1

(D) 2

(E) 4

109. A research group determines that the volume of distribution of an experimental drug is 80 L and its clearance appears to be 4 L/h. What is the estimated half-life of this drug?

(A) <7 hours

(B) 7 hours

(C) 14 hours

(D) 21 hours

(E) >21 hours

110. An antibiotic with a molecular weight of 300 has an active moiety of 220. When a dose of 300 mg in 500 mL D_5W is infused over 6 hours, a steady-state concentration of 20 µg/mL is obtained. Determine the clearance rate of this drug if the patient's volume of distribution for the drug is 20 L.

(A) 0.09/h

(B) 0.125/h

(C) 0.18/h

(D) 0.54/h

(E) 0.9/h

Answers and Explanations

1. **(C)** For most drugs, a dose–response relationship can be correlated with the amount of drug that gains access to the general circulation. In many cases, the amount of drug that is present in the blood (blood level) directly relates to the intensity and duration of the pharmacological effect. The relative amount of drug that is biologically available compared to the total amount of drug in the dosage form administered is a measure of bioavailability. Usually, bioavailability is expressed as the fraction or percentage of the administered drug that is absorbed. The term "absolute bioavailability" compares the amount of drug absorbed with the "gold standard" of the amount present in the blood after administration by an IV bolus. *(15)*

2. **(D)** The AUC can be calculated mathematically by the use of equations or evaluation of a graph when concentration (drug wt./vol.) is plotted on the Y-axis and time is plotted on the X-axis. Units for AUC are weight and time/volume. *(17)*

3. **(B)** By employing the mathematical technique known as the trapezoidal rule, one may calculate an AUC. The AUC is subdivided into individual segments and the area of each is determined. By totaling these areas, an accurate estimate of the total AUC is obtained. *(17)*

4. **(E)** The area under the plasma level time curve (AUC) is a measurement that allows comparisons of similar drug products. For two products of the same drug to be considered bioequivalent, their AUCs must be similar in size and shape. However, the FDA does allow some leeway for overall AUCs. Differences of less than 20% in either the AUC or the maximum concentration (C_{max}) are unlikely to be clinically significant in patients. Thus, a generic house may present data illustrating that their product has an AUC of 1,800 µg h/mL while the trade named product has an AUC of only 1,600 µg h/mL. *(17; 29)*

5. **(C)** The availability of a drug from a specific formulation is compared to a reference standard administered at the same dose level. The standard for oral drugs is usually a solution of the pure drug. The relative bioavailability is then calculated by dividing either the AUC of the drug or the total amount of the drug excreted in the urine by respective values for the reference standard. The absolute bioavailability can be calculated by comparing similar data for the drug product to an IV bolus dose. *(17)*

6. **(E)** The surface area of a drug is so limited in the intact tablet that dissolution of drug from the intact tablet is negligible except for very water-soluble drugs. Therefore, although a drug must dissolve before it can be absorbed, a tablet must generally disintegrate before the drug can dissolve. *(17)*

7. **(E)** The rate-limiting step is considered the slowest step in the kinetics of drug absorption. For some drugs, especially tablet dosage forms, the slow release of the drug from the dosage form may be due to slow tablet

disintegration due to excessive tablet hardness or excessive amounts of water-insoluble lubricant. Once disintegration has occurred, a poorly water-soluble drug may only slowly dissolve, thus limiting absorption. If a drug has high water solubility and the tablet has disintegrated rapidly, the rate-limiting step may be the ability of the drug to diffuse through the GI tract wall. *(17)*

8. **(C)** Terms in the Noyes–Whitney equation reflect the rate at which a drug dissolves from the surface of a solid mass followed by diffusion through the stagnant layer that surrounds the solid particle. The Noyes–Whitney equation is a modified form of Fick's first law used to describe diffusion. *(17)*

9. **(B)** Prior to the peak time, the rate of absorption is greater than the rate of elimination, and the curve ascends. After the peak, the rate of elimination is greater than the rate of absorption, and the curve descends. If these rates are equal for some time interval, the curve will show a plateau rather than a distinct peak. *(1; 17)*

10. **(E)** Drug metabolism or biotransformation is usually associated with the liver and its numerous enzymes. However, enzymes present in other body organs and tissues may metabolize some drugs. These sites include the lungs, skin, kidney, and small intestine. *(7; 15)*

11. **(A)** Drug metabolites such as the glucuronides, sulfates, or glycine conjugates are more polar, that is, water soluble than their parent compound. There are exceptions such as the acetylated compounds, which are less polar. The greater water solubility results in more rapid excretion through the kidneys. Some metabolites are less therapeutic than the original compound but others are more active. In fact, some drugs must first metabolize in the body before biological activity occurs. These are known as prodrugs. *(17; 24)*

12. **(C)** Linear pharmacokinetics is characterized by straight-line (linear) relationships when plotted as a log function (Y-axis) versus time

(X-axis). Some drugs deviate from this straight line, especially when their doses are increased or multidoses are given. Such drugs are described as following dose-dependent or nonlinear pharmacokinetics. The classic example is a drug that demonstrates a saturable elimination process. *(17)*

13. **(A)** F values are calculated for drugs in their dosage forms by comparing AUCs, or total amount of drug excreted, to the control reference of an IV bolus dose, as outlined in Question 5. An ideal F value would be 1.0, which indicates complete absorption of the drug and no losses from other mechanisms such as hepatic First-Pass effect. The F value is also known as the bioavailability factor. *(17; 23)*

14. **(C)** As outlined in Question 13, the F value can be estimated by using the following equation:

$$F = \frac{AUC_{cap}}{AUC_{IV}} = \frac{20}{25} = 0.8$$

Because in this example the comparison of AUCs relates to the absolute standard of an IV bolus dose, the drug's absolute bioavailability was calculated. If the comparison had been to another standard, such as to an oral solution or another product of the same drug, the F value would be the relative bioavailability. *(17)*

15. **(A)** This problem is similar to Question 14, except that a correction factor is necessary since different amounts of drug were given by tablet versus IV. If 50 mg IV had an AUC of 40, 100 mg IV would theoretically have an AUC of 80. The F ratio would be

$$F = \frac{AUC_{tab}}{AUC_{IV}} \quad \frac{20}{80} = 0.25 \qquad (17)$$

16. **(C)** The salt portion of the drug molecule does not contribute to the therapeutic activity of the actual drug. Thus, the portion that is active will be 180 divided by 240 = 0.75. *(1; 17)*

17. **(B)** The therapeutic window is calculated by determining the minimum toxic concentration (MTC) and the minimum effective concentration (MEC). The difference between these

two concentrations is usually referred to as the "therapeutic window" of the drug. *(15; 17)*

18. **(C)** Pharmaceutical equivalents are considered to be drug products that are almost identical in all aspects and are expected to exhibit almost identical therapeutic activity. Bioavailablity data submitted to the FDA must show that similar values for onset of action, duration, peak concentrations, and time to peak concentration are obtained. One of the few variables allowed is the choice of excipients. These excipients, or "inactive ingredients," include binders, diluents, lubricants, and so on. Naturally, the manufacturers must include data proving that these excipients do not adversely affect the performance of their product. *(17; 24)*

19. **(A)** Drug products considered to be pharmaceutical alternatives are allowed greater variation from each other. Although they must contain the same active drug or its precursor, they may consist of different dosage forms, strengths, or contain a different salt of the drug. *(17; 24)*

20. **(B)** When comparing a generic product with the standard brand name product for bioequivalence, the FDA recognizes that it is unlikely that both products will exhibit identical pharmacokinetic data. A guideline referred to as the 80/20 rule is applied. If it can be shown that there will not be more than a 20% difference in the two products with a certainty of 80%, the two products will be considered bioequivalent. *(1; 24)*

21. **(A)** The ionic equilibrium that is established in the acid contents of the stomach will favor a relatively higher concentration of unionized drug in solution. The unionized molecule, because of the absence of a charge, is more lipid soluble than the ionic species and will be able to cross biological membranes more easily. If the drug reaches the more alkaline contents of the intestines before absorption is complete, the higher pH will then favor the ionic form of the drug, which has considerably less lipid solubility and is much less readily absorbed. It should be pointed out,

however, that because of the extremely large surface area of the intestine, weakly acidic drugs can be absorbed from the intestine in spite of the unfavorable ion/molecule ratio. *(15)*

22. **(D)** Gastric emptying appears to be a process with a normal half-life of between 20 and 60 minutes. However, many factors can influence the rate of this process. It is slowed by the A, B, C, and E choices and is speeded by hunger, mild exercise, cold meals, dilute solutions, and lying on the right side. Because some drugs and some dosage forms (eg, enteric-coated tablets) are absorbed at rather specific sites along the GI tract, alterations in the rate of gastric emptying may lead to erratic and unpredictable absorption. For example, if an acid-labile drug that is preferentially absorbed from a portion of the small intestine is consumed as an enteric-coated tablet, a greatly reduced gastric emptying rate may permit the tablet to dissolve in the stomach and be degraded by the acid fluids of the stomach. Similarly, if the gastric emptying rate is greatly increased, the tablet may not dissolve before it reaches its primary site of absorption. *(17)*

23. **(C)** Drugs that form relatively weak bonds with protein have a greater tendency to be displaced when a second drug bound to the same sites is introduced into the blood. Usually, the portion of a drug that is protein bound will not pass through cell membranes because of the large size of the macromolecules nor exhibit therapeutic action. For example, the fraction bound of warfarin is estimated to be about 97% with the remaining unbound 3% being active. Protein binding is most critical with a drug possessing a low therapeutic index since displacement of the drug from sites by another drug will greatly increase the therapeutic action. *(15; 17; 29)*

24. **(B)** The macromolecules consisting of the protein-bound fraction of the drug will probably be excreted and metabolized at a much slower rate than the unbound drug. Also, the protein-bound portion of the drug serves as a reservoir. Assuming that the equilibrium is reversible, portion of bound-drug will be

released to reestablish a balance as the unbound drug is utilized. Thus, the apparent half-life will be expected to be longer. *(15; 17; 29)*

25. **(D)** Albumin will bind numerous drugs that have an acid functional group. Because of its nonspecificity and high blood levels (3.5–5%), the loading doses of some drugs must be high to at least partially saturate the protein-binding sites. *(1; 15)*

26. **(A)** All five of the listed drugs are significantly bound to plasma proteins. Acidic drugs have the tendency to bind to albumin. Lidocaine is a basic drug and will bind to other proteins such as alpha 1-acid glycoprotein. *(1; 24)*

27. **(E)** All three situations may significantly reduce blood albumin levels. Adjustment of drug dosing may be necessary especially for drugs known to have a high degree of protein binding. *(1; 24)*

28. **(A)** Drugs are generally absorbed from the GI tract through capillaries that empty into the portal vein. This vessel carries the absorbed drugs to the liver, where they are subjected to varying degrees of metabolism before they are carried into the general circulation. This initial passage through the liver is therapeutically significant, primarily for drugs that are metabolized to a less active or inactive form by the liver. *(17)*

29. **(C)** Generally, when a particular drug has a half-life of 6 hours, there is reasonable certainty that in spite of as much as a one- to twofold intersubject variation, the mean biological half-life in any group of subjects will be approximately 6 hours. Alterations in biological half-life can be expected when a particular drug is primarily excreted unchanged by the kidneys. The presence of renal impairment slows the process of excretion and thereby increases the biological half-life of the drug in the blood. *(1; 24)*

30. **(C)** *(1; 24)*

31. **(A)** Most drugs have biological half-lives that follow first-order kinetics. A basic characteristic

of first-order kinetics is that the rate constants for metabolism or excretion are independent of the initial drug concentration. That is, a specific fraction of drug will be lost in a given time period. Doubling the drug concentration will not change the rate constant, even though the amount of drug lost in a given time period would increase.

(D, incorrect)—Renal impairment may affect the biological half-life of drugs eliminated by the kidneys. However, the half-life would be expected to increase (not decrease), because the drug remains in the circulation for longer periods of time.

(E, incorrect)—Two methods for determining half-life are (1) to determine drug blood levels with respect to time, and (2) to quantify with respect to time actual biological responses to the drug. Ideally, the half-life values determined by each method should be identical. However, they will be identical only when there is a direct and measurable relationship between drug blood concentrations and the biological response. *(17)*

32. **(C)** One-half (200 mg) of the administered dose will be eliminated in 4 hours. Of the remaining 200 mg, one-half (100 mg) will be eliminated in the second 4-hour period. In the next 4-hour span, an additional 50 mg of drug will be lost. Therefore, after 12 hours (or three half-lives), only 50 mg of drug remains. If graphed as log percent of drug remaining (*Y*-axis) versus time (*X*-axis), the data will appear as a straight line (first-order kinetics). *(1; 23)*

33. **(B)** A rate constant of 46% per hour refers to a fractional loss of 0.46 per hour. The equation for determining half-lives for first-order reactions is

$$t_{0.5} = \frac{0.693}{k} \text{ or } \frac{0.693}{0.46} = 1.5 \text{ h} \quad (23)$$

34. **(B)** Digoxin has an elimination half-life between 1.5 and 2 days. The values for the other choices are as follows: acetaminophen = 1–4 hours; ibuprofen = 2 hours; nitroglycerin = 3 minutes; ranitidine = 2.5–3 hours. A clue to the correct answer is realizing that digoxin is administered only once a day because of its

long half-life while the other drugs are given several times a day to obtain desired therapeutic action. Obviously, there are increased dangers of toxicity if digoxin accumulates in the body. *(1; 24)*

35. **(A)** Volume of distribution (V_d) is an "apparent volume" measured in terms of a reference compartment, usually the blood, because of the accessibility of this compartment to sampling. Because the drug dose is known and the blood concentration can be determined, the V_d may be calculated by

$$V_d = A_b/C_b$$

where A_b is the total amount of unchanged drug in the body and C_b is the concentration of drug in the blood. Knowledge of the V_d for a particular drug permits calculation of the total amount of drug in the body (A_b) at any time by measuring the drug concentration in the blood (because $A_b = V_d$) accumulation in specific body areas. Also, because only the unbound fraction of drug is available for biotransformation and excretion, protein-bound drugs have a tendency to remain in the body longer (ie, delayed elimination and longer half-lives). *(1; 17)*

36. **(A)** Following a given dose of a drug, the greater its concentration in various tissue compartments, the smaller its concentration in plasma. Therefore, according to the relationship Dose $= C_{ss} \times V_d$, the volume of distribution of a particular drug will be greater for those drugs that tend to concentrate in tissues than remain in the plasma. *(1; 15)*

37. **(C)** Because the V_d is a parameter that allows accountability for all of the drug in the body, it can be used to calculate the loading dose that would rapidly result in a desired plasma concentration (C_p).

$$\text{Loading dose} = \frac{V_d \times C_p}{S \times F}$$

where S is the portion of the salt form that is active drug and F is the fraction of dose absorbed. *(15; 17)*

38. **(B)** One can easily picture that the plasma concentration of the drug (C_p) will be equal to the amount of drug (D) administered or absorbed divided by the body volume (V_d) in which it is distributed.

$$\text{Dose} = C_p \times V_d$$

In this problem,

Step 1: 140 lb $\times$ 1 kg/2.2 lb = 64 kg (body weight)
Step 2: V_d = 64 kg $\times$ 1.6 L/kg = 102 L
Step 3: 50 mg = (C_p) (102 L)
Step 4: C_p = 0.5 mg/L   *(6; 23)*

39. **(B)** For any drug that is eliminated by first-order kinetics, the time required to achieve steady-state plasma levels is dependent only on the biological half-life of that drug in a given individual. As a drug is repeatedly administered in constant dosage and at constant time intervals (that are short enough to preclude complete elimination of the drug), the elimination rate of the drug increases as the concentration of drug in plasma increases. The tendency of a drug to accumulate on repeated dosing is, therefore, balanced by increased amounts of drug being eliminated. Eventually, a steady state will be reached in which the amount of drug absorbed will equal the amount of drug being eliminated. The time to reach steady state corresponds to about four to five half-lives and is more completely described in the following table:

Time Plasma (Half-Lives)	Concentration (% of Steady-State Level)
1	50
2	75
3	88
4	94
5	97
6	98
7	99

40. **(B)** Curve I shows an initial high concentration of drug in the blood with a steadily decreasing concentration. This curve is characteristic of drugs administered by rapid intravenous injection. *(17)*

41. **(E)** Any of the listed dosage forms could exhibit blood level curves similar to curve II. The first portion of the curve shows an increasing concentration of drug in the blood. This pattern would be expected whenever there is steady drug absorption (ie, when absorption is greater than elimination), either from the GI tract or from a tissue injection site. Curve III is also a good representation for a sustained-release product as it illustrates a plateau effect. *(17)*

42. **(E)** For any drug to exhibit high blood levels it must be absorbed at a rate significantly greater than the rate by which it is eliminated. That is, K_a must be greater than K_e, at least in the early period of its therapeutic curve. Obviously, the manufacturer bases dosing amounts on the relative speed and extent of absorption versus how quickly the drug is being eliminated. *(15)*

    (A, incorrect)—Blood levels of drug increase until a peak occurs where the rate of absorption equals the rate of elimination. Drug absorption will usually continue to occur even after the peak blood concentration has been reached. However, the blood level curve is then declining, because the rate of elimination is greater than the rate of absorption.

    (B, incorrect)—Because most of the factors affecting pharmacokinetics are first order, doubling a drug dose will seldom double the height of a blood level curve. However, the total area under the drug curve can be expected to double, because the AUC is directly proportional to the dose.

    (C, incorrect)—The pharmacokinetics of most drugs follow a first-order pattern. Therefore, if the concentration of drug in the blood is plotted as a log function on the Y-axis, a straight line will be obtained rather than a curve, as shown on the graph.

    (D, incorrect)—The time factor is a constant variable plotted at regular intervals (hours, days, etc). It is very seldom expressed as a log function.

43. **(B)** Administration of drugs by intravenous infusion, which implies slow flow into a vein, will result in a plateau effect in respect to drug blood levels. The resulting steady-state levels are directly proportional to the infusion rate.

    (A, incorrect)—An intravenous push (bolus dose) will give a curve similar to curve I on the graph.

    (D, incorrect)—The blood level curve for an intrathecal (spinal) injection will probably resemble curve II as the drug slowly diffuses into the blood. *(15)*

44. **(C)** The time in which the optimum drug blood level is obtained is independent of the infusion rate. It is dependent only on the biological half-life of the particular drug. The time required to reach the plateau (steady state) is approximately four to five half-lives. At the blood concentration plateau, the K_e equals the infusion rate. *(15)*

45. **(D)** Determination of the rate of infusion of a parenteral solution may be accomplished using the following equation:

$$R \text{ (infusion rate)} = C_{ss} \times CL$$

    It is obvious that the higher the total clearance rate, the faster the infusion rate to maintain a specific steady-state concentration. Although renal clearance predominates for many drugs, hepatic metabolism, or other elimination processes may be present. *(15; 17)*

46. **(B)** Although various organs, tissues, and fluids in the body can be considered to be compartments for a specific drug, a compartment does not necessarily have to be an anatomic entity. Any body site or fluid that appears to contain the drug may be described as a compartment or "pool" in the model. *(17; 24)*

47. **(D)** Drugs exhibiting two-compartment modeling will have two distinct, relatively straight lines when the drug's blood concentration is plotted against time. These two portions are often referred to as the alpha and beta phases. With intravenous bolus dosing, the alpha phase is the first portion of the graph and represents the initial half-life with fast distribution of the drug out of the blood into tissue. The second portion, the beta phase, represents the longer half-life or elimination of the drug

from the body. Thus, there are two half-lives and two volumes of distribution but only one clearance. *(1; 15; 17)*

48. **(A)** Loading dose = $[C_{ss}]\,[V_d]$

    Using the initial volume of distribution of $0.3 \text{ L/kg} \times 60 \text{ kg} = 18 \text{ L}$

    $$x = [0.5 \text{ mg/L}]\,[18 \text{ L}]$$
    $$x = 9 \text{ mg}$$

    If a maintenance dose or infusion was requested, the pharmacist would use the final volume of distribution. *(1; 15; 17)*

49. **(C)** Nonlinear pharmacokinetics follows zero-order kinetics in which the half-life changes as the drug dose is changed. It usually reflects the effect of enzymes or the presence of carrier-mediated systems. In these situations, the elimination half-life of the drug will increase when the dose is increased. *(15; 17)*

50. **(A)** Zero-order kinetics implies a steady, constant change in drug concentration per unit of time. For example, the constant loss of drug from a solution. Transdermal patches should be releasing a constant amount of drug over a period of time. Delayed release tablets usually release a set amount of drug at time zero followed by another bulk release at a later period of time. Suppositories will either melt or dissolve releasing the drug following first-order kinetics. *(1; 24)*

51. **(A)** Drugs (eg, aminoglycosides) given at intervals that are much longer than one half-life are almost completely eliminated from the body before the next dose is given. This results in a large difference between peak and trough drug concentrations, thus timing of blood sample(s) becomes crucial to interpretation of results. At the other extreme, drugs given at intervals that are much shorter than one half-life (eg, phenobarbital) are slowly cleared from the body; consequently, their peak-to-trough concentration differences are relatively small. *(17)*

52. **(E)** Probability (p) may be defined as the fraction of a population in which a given result would occur by random sampling or chance.

Thus, a high value indicates a high possibility of random results that is undesirable. For most medical experiments p values of 0.05 or lower are desired. The standard deviation ($\pm$) reflects the spread of individual values around the arithmetic mean of a bell-shaped curve. Low $\pm$ values indicate that most experimental values are close to the mean. Most clinical studies include a placebo usually a dosage unit without any drug or a procedure not expected to have a beneficial effect. A high placebo effect indicates that many patients are benefiting from the control. *(1; 15; 17)*

53. **(E)** This is the definition of total systemic (whole body) clearance, which is the sum of all the separate clearances (ie, renal and hepatic). *(17)*

54. **(A)** When the clearance (CL) of a drug is known, the maintenance dose required to sustain a desired average steady-state plasma concentration can be calculated by

    $$\text{Maintenance dose} = \frac{\text{CL} \times C_p \times \tau}{S \times F}$$

    where C_p = average steady-state plasma concentration
    τ = dosing interval (tau)
    S = portion of salt that is active drug
    F = fraction of dose absorbed *(17)*

55. **(C)** Drug elimination by the kidneys can often be correlated with BUN, serum creatinine (Sr_{cr}), and creatinine clearance (CL_{cr}). The BUN and Sr_{cr}, however, are less useful indices of renal function than the CL_{cr} because they are influenced by other factors (eg, state of hydration and age). For example, as patients age, both the production and the clearance of creatinine decrease. Therefore, an elderly patient with a normal serum creatinine of 1 mg/dL may have a CL_{cr} of much less than 100 mL/min (normal CL_{cr} is 100–120 mL/min for a 70-kg adult). There are a number of methods used to calculate CL_{cr}. One equation, the Cockcroft and Gault equation, reads

    $$CL_{cr} \text{ (for a male)} = \frac{(140 - \text{age})(\text{weight})}{72(Sr_{cr})}$$

Units include age in years, weight in kilograms, and serum creatinine measurements in mg/dL. For females, the calculated CL value is reduced by multiplying by 0.85. *(17; 23)*

56. **(A)** If the biological half-life of a drug increases in patients with impaired renal function, the time required to reach steady-state plasma levels will also be increased. This time factor is only dependent on the biological half-life of a given drug in a given individual. *(17)*

57. **(C)** Once a drug gains access to the systemic circulation, it may be metabolized to varying degrees and/or be excreted unchanged. For most drugs and their metabolites, the kidneys are the primary organ of excretion. The presence of a drug and/or its metabolites in the urine must be preceded by the presence of drug in the blood. When an appreciable amount of drug is excreted in the urine, it is often possible to use urinary excretion data—such as cumulative amount of drug in the urine and maximum urinary excretion rate—to evaluate the systemic availability of various drug formulations. *(17)*

58. **(C)** Urinary excretion studies require complete urine collection so that the total quantity of drug that is excreted in the urine can be determined. Normal or near-normal renal function is also a prerequisite for accurate urinary excretion studies because sufficiently impaired renal function can alter the composition of various body fluids that, in turn, can alter the pharmacokinetic properties of many drugs. Although urinary excretion studies are usually conducted on drugs that are primarily excreted unchanged by the kidney, it is not necessary that a drug be completely excreted unchanged by the kidney. *(17)*

59. **(C)** The best measure of absolute bioavailability is considered to be AUC data obtained after a bolus IV injection of a drug. Because AUC data are not available for these drug products, the next best comparison will be the use of cumulative drug amounts found in the urine. Because the IV injection dose was 10 mg

whereas the oral tablet dose was 20 mg, a correction factor of $2\times$ is needed. Cumulative amount if 20 mg had been injected will be $9.4 \times 2 = 18.8$. Dividing 8.2 mg by 18.8 mg = 0.44, or 44%. *(17)*

60. **(D)** Relative bioavailability of Company B's tablet when compared to Company A's tablet will be 8.2 mg divided by 12 mg = 0.68, or 68%. *(17)*

61. **(D)** To determine the relative bioavailability of Company B's tablet when compared to the capsule formula, one must correct for the fact that the capsule dose was 15 mg. That is, determine the milligram of drug that would accumulate in the urine if a 20-mg capsule dose had been administered.

$$\frac{15 \text{ mg cap}}{6.8 \text{ mg (in urine)}} = \frac{20 \text{ mg}}{x \text{ mg (in urine)}}$$

$$x = 9.1 \text{ mg}$$

Relative bioavailability of the tablet will equal 8.2 divided by 9.1 mg or 0.90 (90%). One may expect higher amounts of drug from a capsule to reach the urine since most capsules disintegrate in the GI tract faster. Neither of Company B's dosage forms, tablet, or capsule, can be considered bioequivalent to Company A's tablet because neither is within 80% of the cumulative amount of drug in the urine. This 80% guideline has been accepted by the FDA for determining bioequivalency of similar drug products. *(17)*

62. **(A)** Since there are no data based on calculated AUCs after intravenous bolus dosing the absolute bioavailability of Company A's drug cannot be determined. The relative bioavailability can be determined by

$$\text{Relative bioavailability} = \frac{\text{AUC (Company A)}}{\text{AUC (Company B)}}$$

$$= \frac{80 \text{ } \mu\text{g h/mL}}{76 \text{ } \mu\text{g h/mL}} = 1.05$$

As shown above, it is possible for the experimental drug to have greater bioavailability than the standard or control drug. *(17)*

63. (A) Linear pharmacokinetics indicate first-order rates, thus half-life $= 0.693/k$.

$$8\,\text{h} = \frac{0.693}{k} = 0.087/\text{h} \qquad (17)$$

64. (A)

$$\text{Half-life} = \frac{0.693}{[\text{Cl}_r + \text{CL}_{nr}]} = \frac{0.693}{[0.06 + 0.02]}$$

$$= \frac{0.693}{0.08} = 8.7\,\text{h}$$

65. (B) Obviously, only the renal clearance value will change and the total clearance will be $0.036 + 0.02/\text{h}$

$$\text{Half-life} = \frac{0.693}{[\text{Clr} + \text{Clnr}]} = \frac{0.693}{[0.036 + 0.02]}$$

$$= \frac{0.693}{0.056k} = 12.4\,\text{h}$$

66. (B) The fastest estimation of clearance may be obtained using the following equation:

$$\text{Dose} = C_{ss} \times \text{CL}$$

$$\frac{50\,\text{mg}}{4\,\text{h}} = \frac{10\,\text{mg}}{\text{L}} \times \text{CL} \qquad (17)$$

$$\text{CL} = 1.25\,\text{L/h}$$

67. (A) The Cockcroft and Gault equation allows estimations of a patient's creatinine clearance. It reads

$$\text{CL}_{cr} = \frac{[140 - \text{age}][\text{body wt.}]}{72[\text{serum creatinine conc.}]}$$

The age is expressed in years and the body weight in kilograms.

　　Although the patient's weight is needed, his or her height is not. A patient's BEE refers to basal energy expenditure, a useful measurement in determining caloric needs of a patient. *(17; 23)*

68. (A)

$$\text{CL}_{cr} = \frac{[140 - \text{age}][\text{body wt.}]}{72[\text{serum creatinine conc.}]}$$

Body weight of $140\,\text{lb} \times 1\,\text{kg}/2.2\,\text{lb} = 63.6\,\text{kg}$

$$\text{CL}_{cr} = \frac{[140 - 50][63.6\,\text{kg}]}{72\,[1.5\,\text{mg/dL}]}$$

$$\text{CL}_{cr} = 52.9\,\text{mL/min}$$

69. (D) Female creatinine clearance values are approximately 85% of the values calculated for a male. Other factors that affect creatinine clearance values include relative obesity. For these patients the lean body mass should be used in the equation rather than the total body weight. *(15; 17; 23)*

70. (B) The water solubility of theophylline is enhanced by combining it with ethylenediamine, forming the drug aminophylline. Because the active moiety, theophylline, contributes 80% of the molecular weight of aminophylline, a correction factor is needed to convert between the two drugs when predicting therapeutic activity. This conversion factor is often referred to as the "S" factor, and is expressed as a fraction. In some books, a correction of 85% is used instead of 80%. This minor discrepancy is based on whether the hydrous or anhydrous form of aminophylline is present. *(1; 5; 17)*

71. (C) *(F)* (Loading dose) = (plasma conc.) × (volume of distribution)

1. Patient's total V_d will be $0.5\,\text{L/kg} \times 70\,\text{kg} = 35\,\text{L}$
2. Since aminophylline consists of 85% theophylline, its F value will be 0.85.

$$(0.85)\,(\text{LD}) = (10\,\text{mg/L})\,(35\,\text{L})$$
$$\text{LD} = 412\,\text{mg} \qquad (5; 17)$$

72. (C) Convert the clearance to L/h and eliminate the kg weight,

$$0.35\,\text{mL/min/kg} \times 60\,\text{min/h} \times 70\,\text{kg}$$
$$= 1{,}470\,\text{mL/h or } 1.47\,\text{L/h}$$

(F) (maintenance dose)
$$= (\text{plasma conc.})(\text{clearance})$$

$$(0.85)\,x = (10\,\text{mg/L})\,(1.47\,\text{L/h}) \qquad (5)$$

$$x = 17.3\,\text{mg/h}$$

73. (A) Using the equation R (infusion rate) $= [C_{ss}][\text{CL}]$

Infusion rate $(R) = C_{ss} \times \text{CL}$

$$R = \frac{1\,\text{mg}}{\text{dL}} \times \frac{0.4\,\text{dL}}{\text{h}}$$

$$R = 0.4 \text{ mg/h} \quad \text{and} \quad \frac{0.4 \text{ mg}}{60 \text{ min}} = \frac{x \text{ mg}}{1 \text{ min}} \quad (15; 17)$$

$$x = 0.0067 \text{ mg/min}$$

74. **(A)**

$$\text{Half-life} = \frac{0.693}{\text{Cl}} \qquad 2h = \frac{0.693}{\text{Cl}}$$

$$\text{Cl} = 0.35/h \qquad\qquad (15; 17)$$

75. **(A)** $R = C_{ss} \times \text{Cl} \times V_d$

$$R = 40 \text{ mg/L} \times 0.35/h \times 8 \text{ L}$$

$$R = 112 \text{ mg/h} \text{ or } 1.87 \text{ mg/min} \quad (15; 17)$$

76. **(E)** The hepatic extraction ratio or fraction of drug metabolized is determined by measuring the C_a (arterial plasma drug concentration) and the C_v (venous plasma drug concentration), then using the following equation:

$$\text{Extraction ratio} = \frac{C_a - C_v}{C_a}$$

The resulting ratio may vary from 0 (no extraction) to 1 (100% extraction). Thus, high values indicate a large percentage of the drug is being metabolized. *(1; 24)*

77. **(D)** Drug metabolites are usually more polar and less lipid soluble than the parent compound. Because of these changes, metabolites are usually not as tightly nor as extensively protein bound. They are ionized to a greater degree and are less likely to cross biological membranes than the parent compound. Drug metabolism, therefore, is generally a process that inactivates a drug and changes it to a form that can be excreted more easily and rapidly. For some drugs, however, metabolism may result in activation of an inactive substance, or an active substance may be transformed into (an) active metabolite(s). In these cases, either further biotransformation takes place to inactivate the metabolite(s), or it (they) is (are) excreted unchanged. *(1)*

78. **(A)** The term "First-Pass" refers to the first passage of drug molecules through a designated organ such as the lungs or the liver. Biotransformation will often occur at this site, thereby altering the absolute bioavailability of a drug. Commercial preparations of such drugs are formulated to contain sufficient quantities of drug to compensate for loss due to First-Pass biotransformation. *(17)*

79. **(D)** Only 5% of phenytoin is metabolized in the liver; most of the drug is excreted unchanged. When significant amounts of a drug are metabolized by the liver immediately after absorption through the GI tract wall (First-Pass effect), manufacturers may compensate by increasing the dose present in oral dosage forms. For example, propranolol is available as 40- and 80-mg tablets, whereas the parenteral form is 2-mL ampules containing 2 mg/mL. *(17; 24)*

80. **(E)** All three routes of administration are used for delivering nitroglycerin. In each case, the drug enters systemic blood before significant loss occurs due to the First-Pass effect. *(17)*

81. **(C)** A drug's extraction ratio (ER) usually indicates the amount of drug being removed during its first pass through the liver

$$\text{ER} = \frac{C_a - C_v}{C_a}$$

where C_a = drug concentration in blood entering liver and C_v = drug concentration leaving liver.

If 100 mg of a drug enters the liver and only 30 mg is emitted, the

ER will be: $\dfrac{100 - 30}{100} = 0.7$ (or 70% removal)

One may assume that drugs with high ERs usually undergo high first-pass effects in the liver. *(12, 29)*

82. **(D)** The other listed drugs have shown improvement in their bioavailability when administered with grapefruit juice. Most notable is saquinavir, which normally has only a 4% bioavailability, but demonstrated a 150% to 220% increase with the juice. It is believed that the bioflavonoid naringin, found in grapefruit juice, inhibits the liver cytochrome P450 enzyme. *(17)*

83. **(B)** Liver enzymes such as the P450 and CYP3As will interfere with drug metabolism, thus increasing body levels of the drug. The activity of the grapefruit lasts for at least 24 hours; so the interaction cannot be avoided by separating the times between the drug and consumption of the grapefruit juice. However, with the permission of the prescriber, the patient may consistently take both and adjust to the increased drug activity. *(1; 24)*

84. **(E)** Pharmacogenetics studies how genetics variation may affect drug response. There have been many reports of wide variations in the anticoagulant properties of warfarin in individual patients. Another popular drug whose metabolism may be affected by genetic factors in some patients is clopidogrel (Plavix). *(12, 29)*

85. **(B)** The greater the difference between the drug concentrations on each side of a biological membrane, the greater the rate of transfer from the side having the higher concentration to the side having the lower concentration. *(24)*

86. **(D)** As the name implies, carrier-mediated or active transport involves active participation of a membrane in transferring molecules from one side to the other. The "carrier," such as an enzyme in the membrane, aids in transporting the molecules of drug across the membrane. Because this transfer process is continuous, it can work against a concentration gradient and continue until all of the drugs have been transported. Therefore, equilibrium does not occur.

   (E, incorrect)—Active transport requires energy. Facilitated diffusion is a carrier-mediated transport process that does not require energy.

   (B, incorrect)—Certain chemicals, known as poisons, can reduce active transport, probably by destroying, or inactivating the drug carriers.

   (C, incorrect)—Carriers are often very specific in respect to the drug they will transport. Only a certain chemical structure or similar chemical structures may be actively transported by a given carrier. Because of the chemical specificity and limited capacity of carriers, active transport systems may become saturated. When this occurs, the active transport rate becomes a constant value until the drug concentration is reduced. *(6; 23; 17)*

87. **(A)** A characteristic of a zero-order process or reaction is a constant rate of change. When the active transport system is saturated, there are not enough carriers to handle the large number of transferable molecules. Therefore, the carriers work at maximum capacity, transferring molecules at a constant rate until the drug concentration is reduced to less than the capacity of the carrier system. At this time, the number of molecules transferred will be a fraction of those present for transfer (ie, a first-order rate will exist). *(1)*

88. **(D)** Only the unbound fraction of a drug is available for biotransformation and excretion. Protein-bound drugs have a tendency to remain in the body longer because they do not readily enter hepatocytes for metabolism by the liver. Protein-bound drugs are larger molecules and cannot as readily diffuse through the renal glomeruli for eventual excretion, thus their half-lives will be longer. *(17; 24)*

89. **(A)** When administered in therapeutic doses, allopurinol does not appear to bind to plasma proteins. All of the other choices are drugs known to undergo significant protein binding. The pharmacist should carefully monitor drug therapy when two or more drugs that exhibit significant protein-binding properties are prescribed. Relatively small changes in the degree of protein binding caused by competition for binding sites can result in significant changes in plasma concentration of free drug and in the intensity of the clinical response. *(1; 17)*

90. **(A)** Cephalosporins are mainly eliminated from the body by renal excretion. The greater the degree of protein binding, the slower the excretion clearance, thus increasing both the body half-life and the elimination half-life. For example, ceftriaxone is 96% protein bound

with a half-life of 8 hours and a clearance of 10 mL/min/1.73 m². Cefazolin that is 70% protein bound has values of 2.7 hours half-life and 56 mL/min/1.73 m² clearance. Since a protein-bound drug is less able to diffuse through membranes, the elimination through the kidneys will be less resulting in a longer half-life. *(17)*

91. **(A)** Drugs that can be dialyzed include those that are water soluble and have relatively low molecular weights. Protein bound drugs do not readily diffuse through membranes. A high volume of distribution indicates that the drug is distributed throughout the body or concentrated in certain organs or tissue, therefore not readily available for fast dialysis. *(17)*

92. **(E)** It is unlikely if any of the drugs in this question will be removed by hemodialysis to any significant extent. Digoxin has a very high volume of distribution meaning that it is distributed throughout the body. Amphotericin B and doxycycline are large molecules and will not diffuse readily through membranes. *(1: 17)*

93. **(C)** Just as shifting the ionic equilibrium in favor of the ionic species reduces the probability that a weakly acidic drug will be absorbed from the alkaline fluids of the intestines, it also reduces the probability that the drug will be reabsorbed from the renal tubules into the blood. Consequently, a greater fraction of drug in the tubules cannot be reabsorbed and will be excreted in the urine. *(15; 17)*

94. **(C)** When the half-life of a drug is given, the easiest method for estimating times to reach steady state is:

    One half-life = 50% of steady state
    Two half-lives = 75%
    Three half-lives = 87.5%
    Four half-lives = 94%

Therefore, a drug with a half-life of 2 hours will take three half-lives to reach 87.5%. Thus, 2 × 3 hours = 6 hours. Based on half-lives, the therapeutic effects of drugs with very long values (4 days and more), will not occur for a long time.

A classic example is carbamazepine with a theoretical half-life of 20 to 28 days. During therapy, carbamazepine induces its own metabolism through hepatic enzymes. This lead to a reduction in half-life to about 15 hours. Thus, steady state may be expected after 3 to 4 days. However, if an intern requests a blood level after only two doses q8h, the blood levels will not be at steady state. *(15; 17; 29)*

95. **(C)** Although it is desirable for drugs that are rapidly metabolized by the liver to bypass absorption into the portal circulation, the value of using the rectal route for this purpose is limited. This is due to the fact that while three principal veins drain the blood supply to the rectum, only the middle and inferior hemorrhoidal veins actually bypass the liver. The superior hemorrhoidal vein enters the portal circulation via the inferior mesenteric vein. *(17; 24)*

96. **(D)** If an orally administered drug appears in the feces, it might be desirable to determine whether this is the result of incomplete absorption or secretion of the drug into the GI tract via biliary excretion. The clinical significance of biliary excretion or enterohepatic cycling of the drug depends on the fraction of the dose excreted in the bile. By administering the drug parenterally, this fraction can be determined. *(15; 17)*

97. **(A)** The "blood–brain barrier" appears to behave as a lipid membrane toward foreign compounds. This barrier may be due to a sheath of glial cells surrounding the capillaries of the brain. The rate of entry of a drug can often be correlated with its oil/water partition coefficient and degree of ionization at plasma pH. *(17)*

98. **(B)** In order to take advantage of certain desirable characteristics, some drugs are marketed as prodrugs. These are chemical modifications of biologically active drugs and are not active themselves. However, the active form of the drug, the metabolite, is liberated in the body by biotransformation. Prodrugs may be better absorbed, possess better water

solubility, be more stable, have a less objectionable taste, or give higher blood levels than the parent compound. *(17; 24)*

99. **(C)** Clorazepate (Tranxene) is rapidly decarboxylated in the acidic stomach to an active metabolite that possesses antiepileptic properties. Enalapril (Vasotec) is hydrolyzed to enalaprilat, which is the active angiotensin-converting enzyme (ACE) inhibitor for hypertension. However, lisinopril (Zestril) does not undergo metabolism, instead, is excreted unchanged in the urine. Other drugs, such as verapamil (Calan) form a large number of metabolites. *(10; 24)*

100. **(B)** The antipsychotic drug, haloperidol (Haldol), is available in several dosage forms including tablets, oral liquid, and parenteral. The injectable forms are designed for IV use with immediate activity and an elimination half-life of about 14 hours. The IM form has peak concentrations after 0.3 hours with an elimination half-life of 21 hours. Haloperidol decanoate in sesame oil is intended for sustained activity. It reaches peak concentrations in about 6 days with an elimination half-life of 3 weeks. Other drugs formulated as esters for slow (depot) release include fluphenazine decanoate (Prolixin). *(5; 17)*

101. **(D)** Targeted drug delivery or site-specific systems are intended to place a drug near or at its receptor site. This concept is especially useful when concentrating a drug in the cells of a tumor since lower concentrations of the drug are needed with less toxic effects throughout the body. One mechanism for drug targeting is the use of drugs enveloped in liposomes, which when injected, will concentrate at the tumor site. A second method is the administration of monoclonal antibodies (MAB), which are very receptor site specific, thus effective drug delivery carriers. Lyophilized powders are not classified as targeted drug delivery systems; instead they are powders, which have been dried to increase their stability. *(17; 24)*

102. **(E)** All of these drug characteristics are probably undesirable for a sustained-release dosage form. For a successful sustained-release product, the rate-limiting step must be drug release from the dosage form. If the drug has poor solubility, the dissolution rate may become the rate-limiting step. In this case, the patient may not absorb the quantity of drug needed for desired blood levels and therapeutic activity. Drugs with very long half-lives do not need to be formulated for sustained release because they will be biologically present for a long period of time. Intelligent dosing, such as every 12 or 24 hours (depending on the actual half-life), ensures sufficient blood levels. The release of drug from most sustained-release dosage forms is subject to individual biological variations. This patient-to-patient variability may result in the release of two or three times the normal dose in a particular patient. Therefore, a dangerous situation may develop if very large amounts of very potent drugs are formulated as sustained-release products. Thus, drugs that possess high therapeutic indexes are desired. Conversely, a drug with a very short half-life is also a poor candidate for sustained release. A very large amount of drug would have to be included in the dosage form, and rapid release of the drug would be necessary. *(17; 24)*

103. **(C)** The lag time is the time delay between drug administration and the beginning of absorption, usually reflected in the appearance of drug in the plasma. Enteric-coated tablets are intended for disintegration in the small intestine, which could slow absorption for several hours. Both delayed-release and sustained-release tablets are usually designed to begin some drug release shortly after administration. *(15)*

104. **(D)** The metabolic pathways of newborn infants are incompletely developed at birth; most notably, the oxidative and conjugative mechanisms that are known to metabolize many drugs. The reduced capacity to metabolize certain drugs will therefore result in prolonged biological half-lives of these drugs in newborn infants. Because of inadequate metabolic inactivation, the plasma concentration of chloramphenicol is higher in infants younger than 2 weeks of age than in older

infants. Kidney function also varies. Many drugs such as penicillin and gentamicin have longer half-lives in neonates than in adults (3.2 hours versus 0.5 hours for penicillin and 5 hours versus 2–3 hours for gentamicin). *(17)*

105. **(E)** Decreased efficiency in renal function occurs in approximately 70% of the geriatric population. Also, both blood circulation and hepatic function decrease in many of the elderly. Because both extracellular and other body fluids may decrease in volume, reported volume of distributions in some geriatric patients may be lower than expected. *(15; 17)*

106. **(B)** Since the volume of distribution is given as 100 mL/kg body weight, convert this to liter.

$$100 \text{ mL/kg} \times 70 \text{ kg} = 7,000 \text{ mL or } 7 \text{ L}$$

$$t_{0.5} = \frac{0.693 \times V_d}{CL}$$

$$3 \text{ h} = \frac{0.693 \times 7 \text{ L}}{CL} \qquad (17)$$

$$CL = 1.6 \text{ L/h}$$

107. **(B)** Drugs must be in solution for significant absorption from the GI tract to occur. Thus, drugs with poor water solubility may have their dissolution rate as the rate-limiting factor. However, making a drug dissolve faster (eg, by particle size reduction) will not increase the rate of its absorption if the absorption process itself is the rate-limiting step in the overall transport of the drug from its intact dosage form to the blood. The classical example of a drug formulated as a micronized powder is griseofulvin (Fulvicin U/F). This poorly water-soluble drug will dissolve faster in the GI tract due to an increase in surface area. Thus, larger quantities are available for absorption. *(1; 17)*

108. **(D)** Whenever extra information is included in a question, one must decide which equation to use and what values may be needed. An important concept is the interrelationship between dose or infusion rate and two factors: what blood concentration may be reached (C_{ss}) while the drug is constantly being removed (CL). The simplest equation will be

Dose = $[C_{ss}]$ [CL] (NOTE: where the dose is an infusion rate)

1 mg/min = $[C_{ss}]$ [0.5 L/min] (NOTE: cancel mins)

$$C_{ss} = \frac{1 \text{ mg}}{0.5 \text{ L}}$$

C_{ss} = 2 mg/L, Ans *(15; 17; 29)*

109. **(C)** The easiest equation to use will be

$$\text{Half-life} = \frac{(0.69)(V_d)}{CL}$$

$$\text{Half-life} = \frac{(0.69)(80 \text{ L})}{4 \text{ L/h}}$$

$$\text{Half-life} = 14 \text{ hours } (1; 15; 17)$$

110. **(B)** Based on the antibiotic's molecular weight, the active portion is 220 (mol. wt. active portion) ÷ 300 (mol. wt. of total molecule) = 0.73 (the *F* value). The dosing rate equals 300 mg ÷ 6 h. Some references use the symbol tau (τ) to represent the dosing time. Substituting into the equation:

$$\frac{(F)(\text{Dose})}{\tau} = (C_{ss})(CL)(V_d)$$

First, convert 20 μg/mL to 2 mg/dL and 20 L to 200 dL, then

(0.73) (300 mg/6 hours) = (2 mg/dL) (CL) (200 dL)

(NOTE: cancel all the units except h.)

36.5 = (2) CL (200)
CL = 0.09/h *(15; 17; 29)*

CHAPTER 6

Health Care Equipment and Supplies

The pharmacist should be cognizant of the patient's needs for durable medical equipment (DME) and other items necessary for maintaining a reasonable quality of life (QOL). Skills in fitting items such as walkers, wheelchairs, and neck braces are required. Also, counseling patients in their selection and proper use of supplies such as bandages and dressings, ostomy pouches, insulin administering, and other ambulatory infusion devices are competencies expected of the pharmacist. This chapter presents 60 questions to analyze the reader's knowledge in the above areas.

Questions

1. Criteria for DME include all of the following EXCEPT which of the following?

   (A) can withstand repeated use
   (B) are primarily used for a medical purpose
   (C) generally not useful to a patient in the absence of illness or injury
   (D) appropriate for use in the home
   (E) have wholesale price of at least $100

2. When a home health care pharmacy rents DME such as wheelchairs, it is best to sanitize the returned item. Which of the following solutions is probably the most appropriate for cleaning the equipment?

   (A) ammonia water
   (B) 6% acetic acid solution
   (C) household bleach 1:100
   (D) sterile normal saline
   (E) 3% sodium chloride solution

3. Which one of the following most closely describes a basal thermometer?

   (A) used to detect neuroleptic malignant syndrome
   (B) used to estimate time of ovulation
   (C) may determine patient's basal metabolic rate
   (D) graduated only in Celsius degrees
   (E) inserted into vagina

4. In what respect does the rectal clinical thermometers differ from oral thermometers?

   (A) bulb shaped
   (B) stem length

   (C) distance between graduation marks on the stem
   (D) standards for accuracy
   (E) stem shape

5. Which of the following is (are) true of a healthy ostomy stoma?

   I. bright red or pink in color
   II. no nerve feelings
   III. good muscle control by patient

   (A) I only
   (B) III only
   (C) I and II only
   (D) II and III only
   (E) I, II, and III

6. A nursing home aide calls to order ostomy pouches for one of her clients. Which of the following bits of information are needed to select an appropriate pouch?

   I. whether the unit is intended for a male versus a female
   II. whether an open or closed system is being used
   III. which size flange is required

   (A) I only
   (B) III only
   (C) I and II only
   (D) II and III only
   (E) I, II, and III

7. The effluent from which one of the following ostomies is most irritating to the skin?

   (A) ascending colostomy
   (B) descending colostomy
   (C) ileostomy
   (D) sigmoid colostomy
   (E) urostomy

8. In which type of ostomy is the patient in the greatest danger of dehydration?

   (A) ascending colostomy
   (B) descending colostomy
   (C) ileostomy
   (D) sigmoid colostomy
   (E) urostomy

9. Which of the following statements correctly describe(s) the Convatec Sur-Fit Natura ostomy system?

   I. a two-piece system
   II. can be used by patients with urostomies
   III. only suited for use with a drainable pouch

   (A) I only
   (B) III only
   (C) I and II only
   (D) II and III only
   (E) I, II, and III

10. Urostomy pouches differ from colostomy pouches in which of the following characteristics?

   I. only available as one piece units
   II. constructed of a different plastic
   III. have a flexible bottom tap or valve

   (A) I only
   (B) III only
   (C) I and II only
   (D) II and III only
   (E) I, II, and III

11. A patient has been told to use a tube of paste such as Convatec Stomahesive Paste. How should the pharmacist instruct the patient to use this paste with his two-piece ostomy system?

   (A) bind the pouch to the wafer
   (B) bind the wafer to the skin
   (C) place directly on the stoma
   (D) place around the stoma
   (E) place on the pouch flange to bind to the wafer flange

12. When a customer asks how his father should use the recently purchased product, Nullo, what does the pharmacist explain to do with the tablets?

   (A) place in the ostomy pouch
   (B) place in the urinary leg bag
   (C) swallow orally
   (D) dissolve in warm water and placed on the skin
   (E) dissolve in warm water and swallowed

13. A customer who is being taught to care for her elderly father recently purchased an ostomy irrigation kit. These kits or irrigation sets usually contain all of the following items except which of the following?

   (A) drain bag
   (B) reservoir bag
   (C) 1 L sterile normal saline solution
   (D) stoma cone
   (E) tubing with a clamp

14. Indwelling urinary catheters are suitable for use in which of the following populations?

   I. males
   II. females
   III. geriatrics

   (A) I only
   (B) III only
   (C) I and II only
   (D) II and III only
   (E) I, II, and III

15. What is a common name associated with the indwelling catheter?

    (A) Broviac
    (B) Foley
    (C) Henderson
    (D) Hickman
    (E) Texas

16. Which one of the following is the best description for a Texas catheter?

    (A) external catheter intended for children of either sex
    (B) external catheter suitable only for males
    (C) indwelling catheter suitable for either males or females
    (D) indwelling catheter suitable only for males
    (E) indwelling catheter suitable only for females

17. Which one of the following solutions would a pharmacist likely suggest to a client wishing to disinfect his urinary catheter?

    (A) 0.25% acetic acid
    (B) 3% sodium chloride
    (C) 0.9% sodium chloride solution
    (D) 1% sodium hypochlorite
    (E) 1% Betadine solution

18. A customer requests advice concerning an abdominal bulge below his belly button that has become progressively larger over the past few months. What should the pharmacist suggest?

    (A) a fitment of a hernia truss
    (B) contact his physician to schedule an in-hospital surgical procedure
    (C) contact his physician to schedule an outpatient surgical procedure
    (D) immediate visit to the emergency room for treatment
    (E) pushing the bulge back into place and cover with duct tape

19. What is pushing a hernia back into place referred to as?

    (A) contracting
    (B) reducing

    (C) strangulation
    (D) shrinking
    (E) shriveling

20. When fitting a pair of crutches to a patient, how should the underarm support fit?

    (A) loosely but firmly into the armpit
    (B) clears the armpit by 1 in
    (C) clears the armpit by 2 in
    (D) clears the armpit by 3 in
    (E) clears the armpit by 4 to 5 in

21. When properly fitted, which of the following parts of a forearm crutch will point forward in respect to the patient's body?

    (A) forearm cuff only
    (B) handgrip only
    (C) both the cuff and handgrip
    (D) neither the cuff or handgrip
    (E) fitment is optional for patient comfort

22. Which type of crutches is most appropriate for a patient with limited hand strength for lifting?

    (A) axillary
    (B) forearm
    (C) Lofstrand
    (D) platform
    (E) quad

23. Which of the following measurements are appropriate when fitting a wheelchair to a client?

    I. Determine width of patient directly across the hips then add 2 in
    II. Determine chair depth by measuring patient's distance from knee to hip and then subtracting 2 to 3 in
    III. When seated, the patient's knees should be approximately 2 in lower than the height of the seat.

    (A) I only
    (B) III only
    (C) I and II only
    (D) II and III only
    (E) I, II, and III

24. A customer requests information concerning the purchase of a hemi-wheelchair. Which one of the following is a basic characteristic of this chair?

  (A) seat height lower than that of a standard wheelchair
  (B) tipping levers
  (C) a reclining back
  (D) a headrest
  (E) large set-back wheels

25. A customer has purchased a monopod cane for support since he has a cast on his left leg. Which of the following should be communicated to the customer?

  I. the cane should be carried on the affected left side
  II. the cane handle should be approximately 2 in above the hip joint
  III. the cane should be moved forward at the same time as the affected leg

  (A) I only
  (B) III only
  (C) I and II only
  (D) II and III only
  (E) I, II, and III

26. Mrs. Wilson has been advised to purchase a "resting" splint. What is another name for this brace?

  (A) Air cushion
  (B) Carpel tunnel syndrome (CTS)
  (C) Knight
  (D) Philadelphia
  (E) Wrap-around

27. At what angle from the horizontal plane is the wrist usually supported with the above splint?

  (A) 30 degree angle rise
  (B) 45 degree angle rise
  (C) 90 degree angle rise
  (D) 30 degree depression
  (E) 90 degree depression

28. Mrs. Woodruff's elderly mother has some difficulty in walking because of her weak left leg. She is ambulatory and enjoys walking outdoors. Which one of the following support devices is probably most appropriate for her?

  (A) pair of forearm crutches
  (B) single forearm crutch
  (C) quad cane
  (D) offset monopod cane
  (E) axillary crutch

29. Fitment of a quad cane to a patient should include which of the following?

  I. The top of the handle should be level with the patient's trochanter.
  II. The longer two legs should point away from the patient's leg.
  III. The handle should be curved rather than flat.

  (A) I only
  (B) III only
  (C) I and II only
  (D) II and III only
  (E) I, II, and III

30. A home health care aide suggests that a family purchase a trapeze bar for their father who has been bedridden. What is the main purpose of this device?

  (A) assist in balancing
  (B) ease the pressure of bedcovers from the legs
  (C) exercise for the legs
  (D) exercise for the arms
  (E) as a positioning aid

31. In which of the following characteristics do abdominal binders differ from rib belts?

  I. wider in height
  II. available in both male and female designs
  III. intended to be worn 24 h a day

  (A) I only
  (B) III only
  (C) I and II only
  (D) II and III only
  (E) I, II, and III

32. Which one of the following devices is often employed by emergency rescue teams?

    (A) foam cervical brace
    (B) Philadelphia collar
    (C) figure-eight straps
    (D) Taylor brace
    (E) four-post neck brace

33. Which one of the following therapies is most appropriate for a patient with a diagnosis of chronic obstructive pulmonary disease (COPD)?

    (A) antibiotic for an anaerobic infection
    (B) antiglycemic drug therapy
    (C) cholesterol-reducing drug
    (D) heparin
    (E) oxygen

34. What is the usual flow rate established for oxygen in a home patient for relief of arterial hypoxemia?

    (A) 1 L/min
    (B) 5 L/min
    (C) 1 L/h
    (D) 2 L/h
    (E) 5 L/min

35. An ambulatory patient is receiving oxygen at a low flow rate but is annoyed with the nasal cannula. During which of the following activities may the caregiver safely reduce the flow rate?

    I. watching TV for a long period of time
    II. sleeping
    III. eating

    (A) I only
    (B) III only
    (C) I and II only
    (D) II and III only
    (E) I, II, and III

36. Which one of the following observations is an indication of patient oxygen depletion?

    (A) dry skin
    (B) fever
    (C) sputum with a greenish color

    (D) pedal edema
    (E) colorless, thick sputum

37. When discussing sources of home oxygen for an elderly patient, which one of the following is a disadvantage of an oxygen concentrator?

    (A) equipment is rather unsightly
    (B) need a constant source of electricity
    (C) not suitable for long-term use
    (D) oxygen tanks need replenishment
    (E) very expensive source of oxygen

38. A patient's family contacts your pharmacy to provide liquid oxygen for an 80-year-old man in his own home. Which of the following is (are) potential disadvantages of this type of oxygen?

    I. cannot obtain high flow rates
    II. not suitable for high-volume oxygen use
    III. danger of overmedication

    (A) I only
    (B) III only
    (C) I and II only
    (D) II and III only
    (E) I, II, and III

39. Which of the following is (are) potential disadvantages of providing gaseous oxygen to a frail 80-year-old man living alone?

    I. Home will need electricity.
    II. Patient will not be able to leave his home.
    III. The units are heavy and hard to turn on.

    (A) I only
    (B) III only
    (C) I and II only
    (D) II and III only
    (E) I, II, and III

40. A hospital order for a patient recovering from recent surgery is for a Respirex. What is the purpose of this type of unit?

    (A) exercise the lungs to improve breathing capacity

(B) measure peak air-flow volume

(C) measure absolute lung capacity

(D) provide antibiotic respiratory therapy

(E) provide liquid oxygen to the lungs

41. When visiting a nursing home, a consultant pharmacist checks the calculations of the nurse who has added 2 mL of 0.5% albuterol solution for inhalation into 8 mL of sterile water for nebulization. How many milligrams of albuterol is being inhaled in the 20-minute treatment if the residual volume of the nebulizer is 1.5 mL?

(A) 7.5 mg

(B) 8.5 mg

(C) 10 mg

(D) 42.5 mg

(E) 50 mg

42. Which one of the following factors is most conducive for wound healing?

(A) a dark environment

(B) exposure to air

(C) dry environment

(D) moist environment

(E) coverage with absorption-type dressing

43. Which of the following conditions is (are) desirable when discussing wound dressings?

I. puddling

II. windowing

III. wicking

(A) I only

(B) III only

(C) I and II only

(D) II and III only

(E) I, II, and III

44. Mr. Johnston has suffered an extensive burn to his thigh from a car muffler. Which of the following is most suitable to cover this burn that has some exudate?

(A) Adaptic

(B) Bioclusive

(C) butter

(D) Tegaderm

(E) cotton gauze covered with a secondary dressing

45. Mrs. Cassidy brings her son into the pharmacy with an extensive turf abrasion from playing football. What would be the most appropriate wound cleansing agent?

(A) a sterile 0.9% sodium chloride solution

(B) hydrogen peroxide

(C) iodine solution

(D) povidone iodine solution

(E) sodium hypochlorite solution

46. Which one of the following represents the most serious stage of decubitus ulcers (pressure sores)?

(A) A

(B) X

(C) IV

(D) I

(E) XXX

47. Which one of the following is the most appropriate treatment for a deep-pressure sore?

(A) ABD pad

(B) Debrisan granules

(C) enzyme cream

(D) hydrocortisone cream

(E) stomahesive cream

48. Which one of the following does NOT refer to a type of cushioning suitable for the prevention of decubitus ulcers?

(A) ABD pad

(B) APP pad

(C) sheepskin

(D) egg crate

(E) ROHO

49. Which of the following are basic characteristics of "stress incontinence"?

    I. involves loss of small volumes of urine
    II. therapy usually involves prescriptions for oxybutynin or tolterodine
    III. more prevalent in males than in females

    (A) I only
    (B) III only
    (C) I and II only
    (D) II and III only
    (E) I, II, and III

50. A customer requests a package of drain dressings for her father. How is the dressing used?

    (A) placed around a tube inserted into the body
    (B) placed upon the top of a suppurating wound
    (C) used to cover a burn area
    (D) placed into a deep wound
    (E) used to clean a wound before bandaging

51. A customer asks a pharmacy clerk to see some thromboembolytic devices (TEDs). Which area of the pharmacy will such devices be found?

    (A) ambulatory aids
    (B) bandages and dressings
    (C) enteral supplements
    (D) respiratory and oxygen therapy
    (E) support stockings

52. Support stockings with which degree of pressure in millimeters of mercury would a pharmacist suggest to a pregnant woman with mild varicosities?

    (A) 20
    (B) 30
    (C) 40
    (D) 50
    (E) 76

53. What is the usual use for a Sitz Bath?

    (A) eye irrigation
    (B) irrigation of colostomies
    (C) soaking tired feet
    (D) treatment of hemorrhoids
    (E) treatment of arthritis

54. Mr. Jackson's wife asks the pharmacist what is the TENS device that his doctor is suggesting to help relieve his back pain. The TENS device can best be explained as which of the following?

    (A) device that provides low electro-current through the skin
    (B) device that provides constant intravenous doses of an analgesic
    (C) implantable device that releases constant, small amounts of an analgesic
    (D) type of transdermal patch containing a strong analgesic
    (E) transdermal patch containing both a local anesthetic and an analgesic

55. A client has had a minor surgical procedure and needs a bandage to hold the incision site together. Which of the following are appropriate bandages?

    I. Butterfly
    II. Proxistrip
    III. Elastikon

    (A) I only
    (B) III only
    (C) I and II only
    (D) II and III only
    (E) I, II, and III

56. Mr. Collins is taking his scout troop on a long hike through the woods. He is interested in an antibacterial product that might help if any of the boys suffer minor cuts. Which of the following may be appropriate?

    I. new skin liquid bandage
    II. triple antibiotic ointment
    III. hydrocortisone cream 1%

    (A) I only
    (B) III only
    (C) I and II only
    (D) II and III only
    (E) I, II, and III

57. Which one of the following types of blood-pressure monitoring devices is considered to be the most accurate?

(A) aneroid monitor with stethoscope
(B) electronic monitor with upper arm cuff
(C) electronic monitor with finger cuff
(D) electronic monitor with wrist cuff
(E) mercury manometer with stethoscope

58. As a community service, a pharmacist conducts blood pressure measurements twice a week. Which one of the following procedures is NOT appropriate?

(A) conduct the reading after the customer has been sitting at least 5 minutes
(B) instruct the customer not to consume caffeine within 1 hour of the reading
(C) position the arm to be measured at chest level for the reading
(D) suggest that the readings be taken at the same time each day
(E) test each arm to ensure identical readings

59. The "French" scale is commonly used in this country for denoting the diameters of

I.   urinary catheters
II. enteral feeding tubes
III. syringe needles

(A) I only
(B) III only
(C) I and II only
(D) II and III only
(E) I, II, and III

60. Johnson and Johnson's "Band-Aid plus Antibiotics" contains which of the following?

(A) hydrocortisone + bacitracin
(B) hydrocortisone + polymyxin
(C) neomycin + bacitracin
(D) polymyxin + bacitracin
(E) polymyxin + neomycin

Answers and Explanations

Numbers within parentheses at the end of the answers refer to the numbered references that are listed in the front matter.

1. **(E)** While all of the other question choices describe criteria of DME, there is no dollar amount requirement. *(1; 22)*

2. **(C)** After cleaning the surface area with a mild soap solution and rinsing with water, an appropriate disinfectant would be household bleach such as commercial Clorox. A 1:100 dilution with tap water will kill most bacteria and fungi. The solution should be prepared fresh every day since it is relatively unstable. If it is necessary to inactivate HIV viruses, more concentrated solutions such as 1:10 dilution may be used. *(1; 22)*

3. **(B)** Because fertilization can occur within only a few hours (usually 24 hours) after ovulation, accurate knowledge of this effect could permit timing of intercourse to either increase or decrease the possibility of conception. Basal temperature (the lowest temperature of the body during waking hours) typically passes through a biphasic cycle over the course of the menstrual cycle. From an initially low temperature, a mid-cycle thermal shift occurs to a high level, where it remains until it again becomes low premenstrually. The temperature rise roughly corresponds to the time of ovulation. The thermometer should be used orally or rectally once daily, immediately on awakening in the morning and before getting out of bed. *(1)*

   Answer (D) is incorrect because the scale may be either Fahrenheit or Celsius. Since the temperature rise is only about 0.5 degree Fahrenheit, it would be difficult to measure on the usual clinical thermometer. The basal thermometer scale ranges only from 96 to 100 degrees Fahrenheit and is graduated to 0.1 degree Fahrenheit.

4. **(A)** The rectal thermometer bulb has a strong, blunt shape that facilitates insertion into the rectum with retention by the sphincter muscles. The oral bun is cylindrically elongated and thin walled for quick registration of temperature. Rectal thermometers can be used orally. The oral bulb is too easily broken and is not suitable for rectal use. The short, sturdy security bulb represents a compromise intermediate shape. *(1)*

5. **(C)** Stomas are formed from the inside wall of the intestines and the opening has a bright red or pink color. There are no nerves present. Because there is no muscle control by the patient, there may be constant discharge of GI contents. The sizes of stomas vary, and protrusion may occur. Usually, the stoma shrinks after surgery with its final size occurring in a few months. The skin around the stoma should be gently cleansed with mild soap and rinsed with water. *(2; 22)*

6. **(D)** The two basic ostomy systems are one piece consisting of a single-use, closed-end pouch and a two-piece that consists of a pouch which is attached to a skin barrier with a flange. These drainable pouches may be emptied through a bottom opening. One must also learn the size of the flange, expressed in inches, which attaches to the wafer previously attached to the skin

around the stoma. Pouches are intended for use on either sex. *(2; 22)*

7. **(C)** Ostomies are classified based on the location of the stoma from the surgery and the corresponding emptying body. Ileostomies are formed by bringing a portion of the small intestine (ileum) to the abdominal wall. The discharge is watery and contains stomach acid and digestive enzymes. Therefore, it is very irritating and odorous. Colostomies are created from a portion of the large intestine (colon). Further distinction is made as ascending, transverse, descending, and sigmoid colostomies with the discharge changing from semiliquid in the ascending colon to firm, solid stool in the sigmoid area. *(2; 22)*

8. **(C)** Patients that have had an ileostomy no longer have a working colon and are likely to lose large amounts of water and electrolytes. These patients must be instructed to drink large amounts of fluids to prevent dehydration. Diuretics may worsen the problem. *(1; 22)*

9. **(C)** Two-piece systems consist of a wafer that is placed directly onto the skin surrounding the stoma. The patient will either cut out an opening larger than the stoma or, more likely, purchase a commercial wafer with precut openings. The flange on the wafer can be easily fitted with the snap-on pouch. Although the drainable pouch is the most popular type, there are also closed-end pouches for one-time use and mini pouches intended for children or very active people. *(1; 22)*

10. **(B)** Pouches for the urostomate can be either one- or two-piece units. Each pouch has a flexible tap or valve at the bottom to allow emptying and an anti-reflux valve that prevents urine from pooling at the base of the stoma. *(1; 22)*

11. **(D)** Ostomy pastes such as Convatec Stomahesive protective paste are intended to prevent irritation of the skin around the stoma from the discharges entering the pouch. Usually the patient is directed to "caulk" or place a small amount of the paste into the area around the stoma and the opening in the wafer. Stomahesive

Paste and other similar products are pectin-based protective skin barriers or fillers. They do not possess adhesive properties. *(1; 2)*

12. **(A)** Nullo tablets are intended as a deodorant for ostomy patients. The tablets are placed directly into the ostomy pouch. *(1; 22)*

13. **(C)** Irrigation sets are intended for patients with either descending or sigmoid colostomies. By irrigating their ostomies, it may not be necessary to continuously wear a pouch. The stoma cone allows flow of the irrigating solution through the stoma into the intestines. Since the irrigated area is not sterile, there is no need for sterile normal saline solution; instead slightly warm tap water is used. *(1; 22)*

14. **(E)** The indwelling urinary catheter is inserted through the urethra into the bladder where it is intended to remain for several days. The small balloon at its tip in the bladder is inflated with 15 to 30 mL of water to ensure that the catheter remains in place without slippage. The indwelling catheter is appropriate for anyone especially patients that are ambulatory or senile. Usually a leg bag or other collection device is attached by tubing to collect the large volumes of urine. *(1; 22)*

15. **(B)** Indwelling retention catheters are commonly known as Foley catheters. They are sized based on their outside diameters using the French system in which the commonly used 18 French is larger than a 12 French. Most popular material of construction is silastic that does not readily adhere to the walls of the urethra. *(1; 22)*

16. **(B)** The Texas catheter has the appearance of a large condom. It is attached around the male penis to collect urine. *(1; 22)*

17. **(A)** Soaking a urinary catheter in a 0.25% acetic acid solution will disinfect the catheter without causing damage to the material. Soap and water would be a good cleansing solution but does not offer any antimicrobial activity. *(1; 22)*

18. **(C)** In modern practice, abdominal hernias are usually treated by minor surgery in an outpatient

setting. Under local anesthesia, the protrusion is pushed back into place, and a mesh is placed over the weakened area to prevent further protrusions. Thus, the patient avoids the need to permanently wear an uncomfortable truss. The customer may be advised to wear an abdominal binder to hold the protrusion in place until the surgery is performed. *(1; 22)*

19. **(B)** A patient may lay on his/her back and have the protruding hernia gently pushed back through the opening in the abdominal wall. The area can be covered temporarily with a bandage or more permanently with a truss. This reducing of the hernia can be performed by health professionals or the patient himself. *(1; 22)*

20. **(C)** A space of approximately 2 in between the axilla (armpit) and the top of the underarm supports will allow free movement without squeezing the armpit or damaging blood vessels. The height of the crutch handgrip is based on allowing a 25 to 30 degree bend at the elbow. *(1; 22)*

21. **(C)** Individuals needing more support than that provided by the standard pair of crutches may want to consider the forearm crutch, also known as Canadian or Lofstrand crutches. These crutches have a handgrip and a circular cuff that fits around the fleshy portion of the patient's forearm. This frees the patient's hand for other activities without the crutch falling to the ground. *(1; 22)*

22. **(D)** The platform crutch has a flat platform onto which the patient may rest his/her forearm. Either a handgrip or belt that can be attached to the arm aids the patient in moving the crutch. This type of crutch is especially useful for patients with partial body paralysis. The quad crutch is similar to a quad cane in having a base with four legs for additional support. *(1; 22)*

23. **(C)** A total of 2 in clearance between the chair seat and the client will allow easy transfer into and out of the chair. The chair depth must be less than the length between the knee and the hip to prevent the back of the knee (popliteal) touching the front edge of the seat. Otherwise blood flow may be impeded. Most wheelchair

fitters have the client sit in the chair and adjust the footrests so that the knee is even or slightly higher than the seat. This prevents the client from sliding forward and down. Appropriate cushioning is essential for the comfort of the client. *(1; 22)*

24. **(A)** The hemi-chair or low-seat chair is intended for use by a person with paralysis on one side of the body. The patient can push and steer the chair with his/her functional hand and foot. Characteristics of the chair include a low seat to encourage ambulation by having the feet on the ground, 20 rather than 24 in wheels, and no footplates. *(2; 22)*

25. **(D)** The cane height should be approximately 2 in above the hip joint so that the elbow is slightly bent at a 25 to 30 degree angle. Unless the therapist or physician instructs otherwise, the pharmacist should counsel the patient to carry the cane on the side opposite the affected leg, that is, on the stronger side. This allows the transfer of body weight to the cane while moving the good foot forward then transfer the weight to the good leg while moving the weak leg and cane forward. *(1; 22)*

26. **(B)** The CTS splint or brace is intended to relieve symptoms of CTS. Other common names for this brace is "resting" or "cock-up" splint. *(1; 22)*

27. **(A)** Since the purpose of the splint or brace is to raise the wrist for pain relief, a rise of 30 degree from the level is usually most comfortable. *(1; 22)*

28. **(C)** The quad cane is a monopod with four tips to provide greater support than that from the standard cane with a single tip. The use of forearm crutches is probably too restrictive, more difficult to use, and imply a more serious handicap than actually present. Axillary crutches that fit into the armpit area are intended mainly for heavy duty use, for example, with injured athletes. *(22)*

29. **(C)** Many fitters have patients stand with arms hanging loosely at their sides. The top of the handgrip should be at the same level as the

crease on the inside of the wrist that is also level with the trochanter. Two of the quad cane legs or tips are longer than the other two. The longer tip pair should face away from the patient's leg to provide additional support and also to lessen the possibility of tripping on the cane. Better-designed canes have a flat offset handle for more comfort and stability than that provided by the curved handle. *(1; 22)*

30. **(E)** A trapeze bar is attached to the bed's headboard or may be freestanding with its own floor stand. The patient may reach to grip the trapeze thereby repositioning himself in the bed. *(1; 22)*

31. **(C)** Usual widths of abdominal binders are 9 and 12 in with several ranges of waist sizes while most rib belts are only a few inches wide. The abdominal binder intended for females have a cutout for the breasts. Patients are advised to wear the rib belt 24 hours a day since rib support is necessary while sleeping. Abdominal binders are usually worn only during the day. *(1; 22)*

32. **(B)** The Philadelphia or extrication collar is a plastic unit that is easily fitted around the neck of a patient suspected of suffering a neck injury with possible paralysis. A soft foam collar offers only minimal physical support but does remind the wearer not to attempt much neck rotation. The figure-eight strap is a clavicle support used by ambulatory patients needing stabilization of their collar bone. The four-post neck brace is intended for patients requiring maximum immobilization usually in a hospital setting after neck or head surgery. The Taylor is a type of back brace worn over a long period of time. *(1; 22)*

33. **(E)** The acronym COPD designates a chronic obstructive pulmonary disease. While drugs including respiratory therapy are appropriate, the use of oxygen is often necessary to reduce energy expenditure and prevent hypoxemia. *(14; 22)*

34. **(A)** A flow rate of 1 L/min is usually ordered by the physician or respiratory therapist. *(22)*

35. **(A)** While the patient is sleeping, he/she cannot adequately control his/her breathing. Nocturnal hypoxemia may occur due to hypoventilation and abnormal oxygen transport. This may lead to nocturnal pulmonary hypertension and cardiac arrhythmias. Just before and during eating, the patient is expending a significant amount of energy. Usually watching TV requires little, if any, expenditure of energy, so intake of oxygen will be low. *(22)*

36. **(D)** Edema in the area of the ankles is often an indication of oxygen depletion in a patient. To evaluate the patient, the caregiver or the health professional will press and release the swollen ankle area. If the edema does not clear in less than 15 seconds (Class II pitting edema), the physician should be informed. Class III edema that does not clear in 15 seconds may require hospitalization. *(22)*

37. **(B)** Concentrators remove nitrogen from air thus leaving a concentrate of 80% to 98% pure oxygen. Oxygen flow rates of up to 6 L/min are possible. Since the concentrator is powered by electricity, power outages will present a problem. The concentrators are not unsightly; instead they look like a piece of furniture. After the initial purchase of the unit, its maintenance cost is fairly reasonable. *(1; 22)*

38. **(B)** Compressed liquid oxygen at temperatures of $-290°F$ is stored in canisters. By the use of a valve and tubing system, constant flow of oxygen is obtained over a long period of time. Since the patient may change the flow rate on the canister, there is some danger of overmedication. If the patient is ambulatory, he may have a small portable bottle of liquid oxygen that can be carried outside the home. *(1; 22)*

39. **(B)** Gaseous oxygen is supplied in large green cylinders of different sizes and internal pressures about 2,200 lb/in^2 A valve is used to release the gas and regulate flow rates. The duration of the largest unit is only about 50 hours. A small canister containing only 400 L will last 3 hours but can be carried outside the home. *(1; 22)*

40. **(A)** Postsurgical patients are instructed to either breathe deeply into a Respirex or similar devices to encourage and strengthen their inhalation and exhalation of air. This will likely increase their lung capacity and reduce the possibility of infections. Another popular volumetric exerciser is the Voldyne 5000. *(1; 22)*

41. **(B)** Two milliliters of 0.5% albuterol solution will contain 0.01 g or 10 mg of albuterol. The final dilution volume will be 2 mL active drug solution + 8 mL water = 10 mL, but only 8.5 mL of the solution is inhaled because the residual volume was 1.5 mL.

$$\frac{10 \text{ mg drug}}{10 \text{ mL}} = \frac{x \text{ mg}}{8.5 \text{ mL}}$$

$$\therefore x = 8.5 \text{ mg.}$$

42. **(D)** Today's health practice encourages maintaining a moist environment of endogenous fluids. The natural moisture in a wound bed allows the cells and natural chemicals to migrate for the healing process. *(2)*

43. **(D)** Wicking refers to the physical uptake of wound exudates by the covering dressing. This prevents the accumulation (puddling) of liquid exudates in the wound that may result in microbial growth. Windowing is a bandaging technique where the health provider places tape around the edges of all four sides of the dressing. This technique provides maximum physical support for the dressing. *(1; 2)*

44. **(A)** Burns should be covered with a dressing that will absorb some of the exudates but not stick to the wound. Adaptic, which has a petroleum emulsion coating, will serve both purposes. However, the dressing will need a covering bandage such as a dressing sponge (Johnson & Johnson Topper) or an all-purpose gauze (Nu Gauze). Adaptic is suitable for covering burns, pressure sores, and draining wounds. Most pharmacies now carry J & J's Soothing Non-Stick Dressing in place of Adaptic. The two products are virtually identical.

Bioclusive and Tegaderm are transparent dressings suitable for use over sutures since they are waterproof, and permeable to air. Other uses for Bioclusive include minor abrasions, ostomy sites, pressure sores, and even prevention of blistering due to new shoes. *(1; 2)*

45. **(A)** Sterile normal saline solution will cleanse the area with minimum pain, provide a moist environment, and promote granulation tissue formation. The popularity of hydrogen peroxide solution on topical abrasions has decreased since it provides minimal advantages. Iodine, povidone iodine, and sodium hypochlorite solutions are not favored as they are irritating and may damage tissue. *(1; 2; 22)*

46. **(C)** The assessment of pressure sores is by the stage or severity of the condition. In Stage I, the skin is intact but warm with induration or hardness. Stage II presents broken skin with the appearance of an abrasion often with blistering. Stage III has damage or necrosis of subcutaneous tissue. The most severe, Stage IV, shows extensive destruction of skin with deep-tissue necrosis and damage to muscle, tendons, and possible bone. Some sources subdivide Stage I into two observations—presence of erythema only versus blistering with erythema lasting over 30 minutes after pressure has been relieved. When either are observed, immediate action must be taken, for example, removing causative agents and rotating the patient to relieve contact points. *(2; 22)*

47. **(B)** Debrisan beads or Duoderm is sprinkled into a decubitus ulcer for absorption of large amounts of exudate and dead tissue thus stimulating wound healing (a chemotactic factor). The wound is then rinsed with sterile normal saline to remove the granules. Painful debridement is avoided. *(2; 22)*

48. **(A)** An ABD pad (abdominal pad) is a large dressing placed over wounds. APP or alternating pressure pad is used as an air mattress with movement that is intended to prevent pressure points. The egg crate mattress or seat pad has the appearance of an egg crate and will also relieve pressure points. The ROHO pad is a commercial product consisting of series of inflatable balloons that prevent buildup of pressure points and improve air circulation, thus effectively preventing pressure sores. *(1)*

49. **(A)** Stress incontinence involves the involuntary loss of small volumes of urine and is more common in women than men. Therapy may include use of estrogens. Oxybutynin and tolterodine are drugs of choice for treatment of urge incontinence. Urge incontinence involves the loss of moderate to large volumes of urine. The designation of urge is used if the patient has a strong desire to void. *(2; 22)*

50. **(A)** Drain dressings have a cutout slit into the center of the bandage. They are fitted around an infusion or drainage tube to keep the area clean. *(2; 22)*

51. **(E)** TEDs or thromboembolytic devices are anti-embolism stockings. Anti-embolism or hospital stockings provide fairly low (20 mm Hg) pressure onto the legs and are intended to reduce venous pooling and stasis. Many of the stockings have gradient compression with greatest support at ankle and less to the thigh.

52. **(A)** Stockings with 20 mm of pressure offer moderate support, which will be sufficient for pregnant women with mild varicosities. These stockings are also used for occupational stress (long standing such as experienced by pharmacists), mild swelling, and tired or aching legs. Stockings with 40 mm pressure or higher are intended for chronic venous insufficiency, orthostatic hypertension, and serious edema. Another popular brand of stockings is Sigvaris that have graduated pressures of 15 to 20 mm and 30 to 40 mm range. *(1)*

53. **(D)** The Sitz bath is a plastic unit that fits over the toilet rim. It is intended to soak the rectal area for the relief of hemorrhoids. *(2)*

54. **(A)** The acronym TENS refers to a transcutaneous electrical nerve stimulation or transdermal electro neurostimulation device. The small electric pulse generator or "black box" has two or more electrodes attached to the skin surface and electric pulses are produced to relieve pain. For some patients the device will relieve lower back, arthritis especially in the knees, and some other pains not entirely relieved by analgesics alone. *(1; 24)*

55. **(C)** Both the Butterfly and Proxistrip bandages are intended to be placed across an incision or suture area to hold the skin together. Neither is likely to adhere to healing tissue. Elastikon is an elastic tape similar to an ACE bandage but with adhesive. It will stretch thus is used as an adhering bandage. *(1; 2)*

56. **(C)** New skin liquid bandage contains 1% hydroxyquinoline and can be sprayed directly onto a minor cut. It will form a tough protective cover that is flexible and allows the skin to breathe. In recent years, several similar products have been developed including bandaids containing an antibiotic. Triple antibiotic ointment is still a major antibacterial topical for minor injuries. It contains bacitracin, neomycin, and polymyxin, a combination that will counteract virtually with all skin microorganisms. Hydrocortisone has good anti-inflammatory activity but not antibacterial action. *(1; 2)*

57. **(E)** The old-fashion mercury sphygmomanometer with a stethoscope allows the health professional to accurately detect the five phases of Korotkoff sounds. The resulting blood pressure values are the most accurate of all monitoring devices. However, the instrument is bulky and not suitable for home use. The next best choice will be the aneroid monitor with the pressure cuff placed on the upper arm and readings observed on a gauge. Most ambulatory patients prefer the electronic monitors. Placing the appropriate cuff on the upper arm usually results in more accurate readings than on the finger or wrist. *(1; 22)*

58. **(E)** Blood pressure reading between each arm may vary, usually with higher readings in the left arm. It is best that one arm be used each time so that day-by-day comparisons may be made. It is good technique to take a reading, have the patient rest for 1 minute, and then take a second reading. If the values differ by more than 5 mm of mercury, repeat the process. *(1; 22)*

59. **(C)** The French system is used for designating sizes of both urinary catheters and enteral

feeding tubing. One French unit equals 1 mm of outside circumference. Thus, a catheter with an outside circumference of 20 mm is identified as a 20 F or 20 Fr size. Syringe needles are sized by another system—the Stubbs number in which the number designation increases as the diameter of the needle shaft decreases. *(1; 2)*

60. **(D)** Several companies have marketed bandaid-type products that contain antibiotics. For example, J & J's "Band-Aid plus Antibiotics" contains two effective agents—polymyxin 10,000 units plus bacitracin zinc 500 units per gram. Patients may still prefer to use triple antibiotic ointment. *(1; 2)*

CHAPTER 7

Pharmaceutical Care

Pharmaceutical care is a term many have found difficult to define. A U.S. Supreme Court Justice, when challenged to define pornography, is said to have replied that although he could not define it, he was sure he could recognize it if he saw it. One could define pharmacy practice as the health science discipline in which pharmacists provide patient care that optimizes medication therapy and promotes health, wellness, and disease prevention. With this definition in mind, we have assembled a series of questions for this chapter that we believe fall under the category of pharmaceutical care—that is, they relate to patients, optimized medication therapy and the promotion of health, wellness, and disease prevention.

Questions

1. What is the primary advantage of piroxicam over most other nonsteroidal anti-inflammatory drugs (NSAIDs)?

    (A) It does not interact with warfarin.
    (B) It may be used concomitantly with aspirin.
    (C) It may be given on a once-a-day schedule.
    (D) It has a cytoprotective effect.
    (E) It has essentially no adverse GI effects.

2. Which of the following is (are) true of adalimumab (Humira)?

    I. It is a monoclonal antibody.
    II. It is indicated for the treatment of rheumatoid arthritis.
    III. It is a leukotriene inhibitor.

    (A) I only
    (B) III only
    (C) I and II only
    (D) II and III only
    (E) I, II, and III

3. A patient complains of GI intolerance when using ibuprofen for muscle aches. What should the pharmacist recommend?

    (A) celecoxib
    (B) oxaprozin
    (C) naproxen
    (D) acetaminophen
    (E) ketoprofen

4. When dispensing isotretinoin (Accutane) capsules to a 19-year-old female college student with acne, what should the pharmacist advise the patient?

    I. avoid pregnancy while using the drug
    II. the acne lesions may get worse before they get better
    III. increase her exposure to sunlight to help eliminate lesions

    (A) I only
    (B) III only
    (C) I and II only
    (D) II and III only
    (E) I, II, and III

5. Which of the following best describes the condition known as hypoprothrombinemia?

    (A) it is also called thrombocythemia
    (B) the development of deep vein thromboses (DVTs)
    (C) a low level of iron in the blood
    (D) a decrease in the production of red blood cells by the bone marrow
    (E) a reduced capability for blood to clot

6. A patient is brought to the emergency department (ED) with extensive hemorrhaging caused by the excessive use of warfarin. Which of the following could be used to reverse the patient's hemorrhaging?

I. dihydrotachysterol

II. ergocalciferol

III. phytonadione

(A) I only

(B) III only

(C) I and II only

(D) II and III only

(E) I, II, and III

7. A female patient complains of a reddish-orange discoloration of her urine. The pharmacist examines her drug profile. Which of the following drugs would most likely produce such an effect?

(A) cilostazol (Pletal)

(B) naratriptan

(C) sulfamethoxazole

(D) rifampin

(E) clonazepam

8. Which of the following is (are) true of menotropins?

I. It is only administered parenterally.

II. It is a gonadotropin.

III. It may be administered to pregnant women to reduce spontaneous abortion.

(A) I only

(B) III only

(C) I and II only

(D) II and III only

(E) I, II, and III

9. In counseling a patient about to begin using eplerenone tablets, what should the pharmacist advise the patient?

I. avoid large quantities of potassium-rich foods

II. avoid alcohol while using this drug

III. discontinue the use of all antihypertensive medication

(A) I only

(B) III only

(C) I and II only

(D) II and III only

(E) I, II, and III

10. The clinical investigation of a new drug consists of four phases. To whom is drug administered during Phase II of clinical testing?

(A) animals for toxicity studies

(B) patients suffering from the disease, administered by select clinicians

(C) animals to determine the effectiveness of the drug

(D) healthy volunteers, administered by select clinicians

(E) patients suffering from the disease, administered by general practitioners

11. Which of the following best describes the common clinical manifestations of hypoparathyroidism?

(A) hypocalcemia and hyperphosphatemia

(B) hypocalcemia and hypophosphatemia

(C) hypercalcemia and hypochlorhydria

(D) hypercalcemia and hypophosphatemia

(E) hypercalcemia and hyperphosphatemia

12. David Smith, a 42-year old musician, visits the ED of a large urban hospital with complaints of fever and severe chest congestion. He is diagnosed with *Legionella* pneumonia. Which of the following would be MOST appropriate to administer to Mr. Smith?

(A) vancomycin

(B) gentamicin

(C) imipenem

(D) levofloxacin

(E) fluoconazole

13. What may an adult patient who is hypothyroid have?

I. a goiter

II. Hashimoto's disease

III. low levels of TSH

(A) I only

(B) III only

(C) I and II only

(D) II and III only

(E) I, II, and III

14. Which of the following would be appropriate to use in treating a 10-year-old child with nocturnal enuresis?

    I. atomoxetine

    II. imipramine

    III. DDAVP

(A) I only

(B) III only

(C) I and II only

(D) II and III only

(E) I, II, and III

15. Which of the following should be avoided in patients who are hypersensitive to aspirin?

    I. Anacin

    II. Alka-Seltzer Blue

    III. Tylenol

(A) I only

(B) III only

(C) I and II only

(D) II and III only

(E) I, II, and III

16. Which of the following phrases best defines the clinical disorder known as hemochromatosis?

(A) absence of pigmentation in circulating red blood cells

(B) excessive storage of iron by the body

(C) a lack of circulating antibodies

(D) abnormally shaped red blood cells

(E) spontaneous hemolysis of red blood cells

17. Tendon rupture is a potential adverse effect in the use of which drug?

(A) ciprofloxacin

(B) clarithromycin

(C) vancomycin

(D) amphotericin B

(E) clindamycin

18. A patient who has been diagnosed with cystic fibrosis is likely to benefit from the use of which of the following?

    I. TOBI

    II. dornase alfa

    III. pancrelipase

(A) I only

(B) III only

(C) I and II only

(D) II and III only

(E) I, II, and III

19. Metoclopramide acts primarily as which of the following?

(A) H_2-receptor antagonist

(B) prokinetic agent

(C) proton pump inhibitor

(D) inhibitor of the amine pump

(E) *Helicobacter pylori* inhibitor

20. A patient with chronic inflammatory bowel disease claims to be allergic to sulfonamides. Which of the following products would be suitable for this patient?

    I. Dipentum

    II. Lialda

    III. Azulfidine

(A) I only

(B) III only

(C) I and II only

(D) II and III only

(E) I, II, and III

21. Which of the following is (are) true of ezetimibe?

    I. It should not be administered to diabetic patients.

    II. It inhibits the intestinal absorption of cholesterol.

    III. It may be used in combination with a "statin" drug.

(A) I only

(B) III only

(C) I and II only

(D) II and III only

(E) I, II, and III

22. Which of the following products is (are) indicated for the treatment of the human immunodeficiency virus (HIV) infection?

   I. Epzicom
   II. Trizivir
   III. Relenza

(A) I only
(B) III only
(C) I and II only
(D) II and III only
(E) I, II, and III

23. A patient complains about a headache that is localized in the periorbital area and seems to be worse in the morning than the afternoon. Which of the following would be the best way to characterize the headache?

(A) eye strain
(B) vascular migraine
(C) muscle contraction
(D) sinus
(E) tumorigenic

24. A patient wishes to know why combination drug treatment is used in treating his tuberculosis rather than using just one drug. Which of the following are acceptable explanations?

   I. shorten the duration of therapy
   II. delay the emergence of drug resistance
   III. enhance the antitubercular effects of treatment

(A) I only
(B) III only
(C) I and II only
(D) II and III only
(E) I, II, and III

25. What should patients taking the antitubercular drug rifampin (Rifadin) be told about the drug?

(A) it may cause diarrhea
(B) it may cause them to sunburn more easily

(C) it may impart an orange color to their urine and sweat
(D) it may produce nausea and vomiting if used with alcoholic beverages
(E) it should be swallowed whole (ie, not chewed) to prevent staining of the teeth

26. A patient using ticlopidine (Ticlid) should be monitored for the development of which of the following?

(A) pseudomembranous enterocolitis
(B) nephrotoxicity
(C) respiratory impairment
(D) agranulocytosis
(E) thrombotic thrombocytopenic purpura

27. Which of the following penicillin derivatives has significantly GREATER activity against *Pseudomonas* than amoxicillin?

(A) amoxicillin
(B) cloxacillin
(C) nafcillin
(D) piperacillin
(E) oxacillin

28. With what is antimicrobial-induced pseudomembranous colitis most commonly treated?

(A) sulfasalazine
(B) pentamidine
(C) mesalamine
(D) amphotericin B
(E) metronidazole (Flagyl)

29. A patient with Cushing's syndrome would likely exhibit which of the following?

(A) hemosiderosis
(B) adrenal hyperplasia
(C) hyperthyroidism
(D) polyuria
(E) excessive accumulation of copper in the body

30. Which of the following is (are) a characteristic of the aminoglycoside antibiotics?

    I.   may be used orally for serious systemic pseudomonas infections
    II. primarily eliminated renally
    III. bactericidal for a wide range of gram-positive and gram-negative micro-organisms

    (A) I only
    (B) III only
    (C) I and II only
    (D) II and III only
    (E) I, II, and III

31. Which of the following is (are) an infectious complication associated with HIV?

    I.   PCP
    II. MAC
    III. SARS

    (A) I only
    (B) III only
    (C) I and II only
    (D) II and III only
    (E) I, II, and III

32. What is a disadvantage of using Serevent in the treatment of asthma?

    (A) its nephrotoxicity
    (B) its brief duration of action
    (C) it may cause tachyphylaxis
    (D) it is ineffective in treating acute attacks
    (E) its instability at room temperature

33. Which of the following would be an appropriate drug for treating a patient with relapsing multiple sclerosis?

    I.   interferon beta-1a
    II. interferon beta-1b
    III. interferon alfa-2a

    (A) I only
    (B) III only
    (C) I and II only

(D) II and III only
(E) I, II, and III

34. What is the common name for the antidiuretic hormone elaborated by the posterior pituitary gland?

    (A) aldosterone
    (B) renin
    (C) oxytocin
    (D) vasopressin
    (E) secretin

35. Which of the following is (are) true of lithium carbonate (Eskalith, Lithane)?

    I.   Baseline liver function tests must be performed prior to initiating lithium therapy.
    II. Patients using it should be advised to limit their sodium intake.
    III. Its use may cause hypothyroidism.

    (A) I only
    (B) III only
    (C) I and II only
    (D) II and III only
    (E) I, II, and III

36. What should patients using alendronate be advised to do?

    I.   lie down for 60 minutes after taking each dose
    II. take each dose with a calcium supplement
    III. take each dose first thing in the morning

    (A) I only
    (B) III only
    (C) I and II only
    (D) II and III only
    (E) I, II, and III

37. How does insulin detemir provide a long-acting response?

    (A) precipitating at the injection site
    (B) binding to plasma proteins
    (C) being released from a liposomal dispersion

(D) partitioning into fatty tissue

(E) being slowly converted to its active metabolite

38. A patient who has been heparinized should be monitored by the use of which of the following parameters?

(A) international normalization ratio (INR)

(B) hematocrit

(C) prothrombin time (PT)

(D) activated partial thromboplastin time (APTT)

(E) complete blood count (CBC)

39. Two hours after receiving the last dose of heparin (9,000 units IV), a male patient begins bleeding from the gums after brushing his teeth. What is the most appropriate clinical action?

(A) discontinue heparin administration and wait for the anticoagulant effect to subside

(B) inject 10 mg of phytonadione intramuscularly (IM)

(C) inject 10 mg of phytonadione IV

(D) swab a small amount of epinephrine 1:100 onto the gum tissue to produce local vasoconstriction

(E) inject 30 mg of protamine sulfate IM

40. A 40-year-old woman with a history of DVT is stabilized on 5 mg of warfarin daily. The administration of which of the following medications to this patient would increase the risk of hemorrhage?

(A) acetaminophen (Tylenol) 650 mg q 4 h

(B) Avapro 300 mg daily

(C) pravastatin 20 mg hs

(D) zolpidem 5 mg hs

(E) itraconazole 200 mg daily

41. A pharmacist wishes to dispense lubiprostone (Amitiza) for use by a patient. What is this product usually used to treat?

(A) vernal keratoconjunctivitis

(B) herpes simplex keratitis

(C) open-angle glaucoma

(D) chronic idiopathic constipation

(E) shingles

42. Which of the following is (are) TRUE of etanercept (Enbrel)?

I. used to treat psoriasis

II. used to treat rheumatoid arthritis

III. it is a TNF inhibitor

(A) I only

(B) III only

(C) I and II only

(D) II and III only

(E) I, II, and III

43. What aspect of dopamine is an important advantage of using dopamine (Intropin) in cardiogenic shock?

(A) dopamine will not cross the blood–brain barrier and cause CNS effects

(B) dopamine will not increase blood pressure

(C) dopamine can be given orally

(D) dopamine produces dose-dependent increases in cardiac output and renal perfusion

(E) dopamine has no effects on alpha and beta receptors

44. A patient is experiencing signs of acute lorazepam (Serax) toxicity after having consumed approximately 15 times the normal dose in a suicide attempt. What is the appropriate agent to administer?

(A) flumazenil (Romazicon)

(B) naloxone (Narcan)

(C) EDTA

(D) naltrexone (ReVia)

(E) physostigmine (Antilirium)

45. A male patient who has been stabilized on 300 mg of Dilantin Kapseals once daily is having difficulty in swallowing capsules. His physician writes a new prescription for Dilantin suspension 300 mg once daily. What is this change likely to do?

    (A) reduce the phenytoin level because of decreased bioavailability from the suspension
    (B) increase the phenytoin level because of increased bioavailability from the suspension
    (C) have no impact on the phenytoin level
    (D) increase the phenytoin level because the 300 mg dose of suspension contains more of the active form of the drug
    (E) decrease the phenytoin level because the 300 mg dose of suspension contains less of the active form of the drug

46. A terminally ill hospice patient is experiencing severe pain associated with metastatic colon cancer. Which of the following would be the appropriate regimen to treat his pain?

    (A) Duragesic-50 applied q 72 h
    (B) codeine sulfate 30 mg PO qid
    (C) meperidine 50 mg PO qid
    (D) morphine sulfate PO, 15 mg prn pain
    (E) acetaminophen 500 mg PO q 4 h

47. Which of the following would be LEAST effective in the treatment of benign prostatic hyperplasia (BPH)?

    (A) tamulosin
    (B) pregabalin
    (C) dutasteride
    (D) saw palmetto
    (E) doxazosin

48. Respiratory distress is MOST likely to occur with the use of which of the following?

    (A) cisplatin
    (B) bleomycin
    (C) vincristine
    (D) daunorubicin
    (E) mitoxantrone

49. A male diabetic patient reports that he is planning a 4-week trip to Europe and will not have continuous access to a refrigerator to store insulin. What information would you give him?

    (A) Store the insulin in a small styrofoam box that can be kept cold with several ice cubes.
    (B) Be sure that insulin is available wherever you travel and purchase a fresh vial at least every third day.
    (C) The insulin will remain stable at room temperature during the time period in which a single vial will be used.
    (D) Increase your insulin dose by 10% to compensate for any deterioration.
    (E) See your doctor to prescribe a mixture of insulins that will be more stable.

50. Which of the following is (are) true of isotretinoin (Accutane)?

    I. may cause hyperlipidemia
    II. likely to cause cheilitis
    III. pregnancy category X

    (A) I only
    (B) III only
    (C) I and II only
    (D) II and III only
    (E) I, II, and III

51. Why are peripheral veins seldom used for the administration of total parenteral nutrition (TPN) fluids?

    (A) TPN fluids tend to infiltrate into surrounding tissue
    (B) the vessels are easily occluded
    (C) large-bore needles must be used
    (D) the hypotonic solution causes local hemolysis
    (E) the blood flow in peripheral vessels is not great enough to protect the peripheral vessels from irritation

52. A patient is diagnosed with a beta-lactamase–producing streptococcal infection. Which of the following would be suitable for treating this patient?

   I.   Amikin
   II. Timentin
   III. Augmentin

   (A) I only
   (B) III only
   (C) I and II only
   (D) II and III only
   (E) I, II, and III

53. A patient who began using Procardia XL a week ago calls to complain of the appearance of the tablet in his stool. What should you tell the patient?

   (A) he should crush or chew the tablet before swallowing
   (B) if he takes the medication with an alkaline food such as milk, the problem will not occur
   (C) he should return the remaining tablets to the pharmacy for replacement
   (D) if he takes the medication with an acidic food such as orange juice, the problem will not occur
   (E) he should not be concerned because this is a normal occurrence

54. Which of the following complications associated with the administration of TPN solutions is MOST likely to occur after the infusions have been discontinued?

   (A) pulmonary edema
   (B) hypoglycemia
   (C) hyperosmotic nonketotic hyperglycemia
   (D) respiratory alkalosis
   (E) hyperchloremic metabolic acidosis

55. Which one of the following provides the greatest number of cal/g?

   (A) ethanol
   (B) proteins
   (C) anhydrous dextrose
   (D) long-chain triglycerides
   (E) hydrous dextrose

56. A patient requires several administrations of high-dose cisplatin (Platinol) therapy for the treatment of advanced bladder cancer. During the first cisplatin administration, the patient develops severe nausea and vomiting. Which of the following drugs would be appropriate to administer to control these symptoms for future administrations?

   (A) escitalopram (Lexapro)
   (B) buspirone (BuSpar)
   (C) adalimumab (Humira)
   (D) formoterol (Foradil)
   (E) dolasetron (Anzemet)

57. Which drug has a similar mechanism of action to amiloride (Midamor)?

   (A) spironolactone (Aldactone)
   (B) hydrochlorothiazide (HydroDIURIL)
   (C) metolazone (Zaroxolyn)
   (D) chlorthalidone (Hygroton)
   (E) triamterene (Dyrenium)

58. A 50-year-old hypertensive patient has been maintained on spironolactone with hydrochlorothiazide (Aldactazide), methyldopa, and potassium (K-Tabs). The patient is admitted to the hospital for elective surgery and is found to be hyperkalemic (serum K of 6.4 mEq/L; normal range is 3.5–5.5 mEq/L) with no symptoms and a normal electrocardiogram. With what should this patient be treated?

   (A) IV sodium nitrite
   (B) oral EDTA
   (C) oral cholestyramine resin
   (D) IV normal saline
   (E) rectal sodium polystyrene sulfonate

59. A 55-year-old patient is to receive fonda-parinux (Arixtra). Which of the following is (are) TRUE of this drug product?

    I. It is administered by IV infusion.
    II. The patient's APTT must be monitored.
    III. It is used to prevent DVT.

    (A) I only
    (B) III only
    (C) I and II only
    (D) II and III only
    (E) I, II, and III

60. Which of the following drug products is (are) indicated for use in type 2 diabetes mellitus patients?

    I. miglitol (Glyset)
    II. saxagliptin (Onglyza)
    III. pioglitazone (Actos)

    (A) I only
    (B) III only
    (C) I and II only
    (D) II and III only
    (E) I, II, and III

61. Which of the following drugs is considered to be a drug of choice in treating status epilepticus?

    (A) carbamazepine (Tegretol)
    (B) lorazepam (Ativan)
    (C) buspirone (Buspar)
    (D) ethosuximide (Zarontin)
    (E) phenytoin (Dilantin)

62. The use of which of the following drugs has resulted in the development of a syndrome strongly resembling systemic lupus erythematosus (SLE)?

    (A) haloperidol
    (B) lamotrigine
    (C) amiodarone
    (D) procainamide
    (E) olanzapine

63. What may inhibit the antiparkinson effect of levodopa?

    (A) nicotinic acid
    (B) d-alpha tocopherol
    (C) pyridoxine HCl
    (D) dihydrotachysterol
    (E) cyanocobalamin

64. In terms of its major pharmacological effect, what is atenolol (Tenormin) most similar to?

    (A) formoterol
    (B) metaproterenol
    (C) fenoldopam
    (D) pindolol
    (E) albuterol

65. The pharmacist should advise a patient that he or she may experience dizziness and syncope after taking the first dose of which drug?

    (A) trandolapril
    (B) benazepril
    (C) prazosin
    (D) clonidine
    (E) labetalol

66. What is commonly measured to assess the degree of immunodeficiency in acquired immunodeficiency syndrome (AIDS) patients?

    (A) *Pneumocystis carinii* organisms
    (B) neutrophils
    (C) granulocytes
    (D) erythrocyte sedimentation rate (ESR)
    (E) CD4 cells

67. In the treatment of acute hypertensive crisis, how is nitroprusside (Nitropress) administered?

    (A) intrathecally
    (B) subcutaneously
    (C) as an IV bolus
    (D) as an IV infusion
    (E) sublingually

68. Which of the following drug products would be MOST appropriate for the treatment of schizophrenia?

    (A) paroxetine
    (B) aripiprazole
    (C) amitriptyline
    (D) atomoxetine
    (E) rasagiline

69. An IV admixture should NOT be prepared with tobramycin sulfate and which of the following?

    I. phenytoin sodium
    II. ticarcillin sodium
    III. sodium bicarbonate

    (A) I only
    (B) III only
    (C) I and II only
    (D) II and III only
    (E) I, II, and III

70. Which of the following agents would be LEAST effective in eradicating *H. pylori* from the GI tract?

    (A) clarithromycin
    (B) bismuth subsalicylate
    (C) metronidazole
    (D) metoclopramide
    (E) tetracycline

71. Cholestyramine (Questran) probably interferes with the GI absorption of which of the following?

    I. warfarin sodium
    II. levothyroxine sodium
    III. phenytoin sodium

    (A) I only
    (B) III only
    (C) I and II only
    (D) II and III only
    (E) I, II, and III

72. A clinically noticeable drug interaction resulting from the displacement of drug A by drug B from common plasma protein-binding sites is most often seen when which of the following occurs?

    (A) drug A has a high association constant (*K*) for binding the protein
    (B) drug B has a high association constant (*K*) for binding the protein and is given in large doses
    (C) drug B has a low association constant (*K*) for binding the protein and is given in large doses
    (D) drug B is more toxic than drug A
    (E) drug B is rapidly absorbed

73. A 5-year-old boy is brought to the ED after having ingested approximately 10 to 15 325 mg Tylenol tablets 2 hours ago. What is the appropriate agent to use in treating this boy?

    (A) EDTA
    (B) flumazenil
    (C) vitamin K
    (D) *N*-acetylcysteine
    (E) pralidoxime

74. Which of the following agents would likely affect the platelet aggregation of an adult?

    I. anagrelide
    II. clopidogrel
    III. dipyridamole

    (A) I only
    (B) III only
    (C) I and II only
    (D) II and III only
    (E) I, II, and III

75. Which of the following is a microorganism that is particularly dangerous to the eye?

    (A) *Streptococcus thermophilus*
    (B) *Bacillus subtilis*
    (C) *Pseudomonas aeruginosa*
    (D) *Aspergillus niger*
    (E) *Escherichia coli*

76. A patient has a purulent boil on his outer ear. Such lesions are usually caused by which genus species?

    (A) *Streptococcus*
    (B) *Candida*
    (C) *Pseudomonas*
    (D) *Staphylococcus*
    (E) *Tinea*

77. What is the treatment of choice for *Herpes simplex* infection of the eyelids and conjunctiva?

    (A) idoxuridine
    (B) oseltamivir
    (C) amphotericin B
    (D) metronidazole
    (E) valacyclovir

78. Which of the following antifungal agents is NOT effective against *Candida* organisms?

    (A) tolnaftate
    (B) clotrimazole
    (C) miconazole
    (D) amphotericin
    (E) nystatin

79. Tolterodine has been shown to be of clinical use in the management of which of the following?

    (A) Crohn's disease
    (B) Chronic obstructive pulmonary disease (COPD)
    (C) multiple sclerosis
    (D) rheumatoid arthritis
    (E) overactive bladder

80. Important potential complications of systemic corticosteroid therapy include(s)

    I. sodium depletion
    II. increased chance of developing cataracts
    III. dissemination of local infection

    (A) I only
    (B) III only
    (C) I and II only
    (D) II and III only
    (E) I, II, and III

81. Which of the following is a blood sugar concentration within normal limits for a fasting adult?

    (A) 500 mg/dL
    (B) 400 mg/dL
    (C) 300 mg/dL
    (D) 200 mg/dL
    (E) 100 mg/dL

82. Which of the following drugs can interfere with the diagnosis of pernicious anemia?

    (A) ascorbic acid
    (B) phytonadione
    (C) thiamine
    (D) pyridoxine
    (E) folic acid

83. Which of the following is (are) true of clomiphene citrate (Clomid)?

    I. It is used to treat polycystic ovarian disease.
    II. It has antiestrogenic effects.
    III. It promotes the secretion of follicle-stimulating hormone.

    (A) I only
    (B) III only
    (C) I and II only
    (D) II and III only
    (E) I, II, and III

84. A product insert indicates that a drug may cause glossitis. This means that the drug may cause inflammation of which of the following?

    (A) conjunctiva
    (B) urethra
    (C) eye
    (D) ear
    (E) tongue

85. The use of which of the following drugs is MOST likely to result in elevations of serum creatinine levels?

    (A) nifedipine
    (B) bisoprolol
    (C) valsartan

(D) fosinopril

(E) clonidine

86. What does hematocrit (HCT) measure?

(A) percentage of red blood cells per volume of blood

(B) weight of red blood cells per volume of blood

(C) number of red blood cells per volume of blood

(D) weight of hemoglobin per volume of blood

(E) total number of blood cells per volume of blood

87. Which of the following is NOT a white blood cell (or leukocyte)?

(A) basophil

(B) reticulocyte

(C) monocyte

(D) eosinophil

(E) lymphocyte

88. What is the BEST product to use in a 7-year-old child with otitis media (and no history of drug allergies)?

(A) amoxicillin

(B) mupirocin

(C) tetracycline HCl

(D) ciprofloxacin

(E) metronidazole

89. Which of the following agents is (are) capable of producing an antipyretic action in humans?

I. ibuprofen

II. acetylsalicylic acid

III. acetaminophen

(A) I only

(B) III only

(C) I and II only

(D) II and III only

(E) I, II, and III

90. What should patients receiving clozapine (Clozaril) be monitored for the development of?

(A) agranulocytosis

(B) heptatocellular necrosis

(C) Lupus-like effects

(D) thrombocytopenia

(E) Stevens–Johnson syndrome

91. Zollinger–Ellison syndrome can be best treated with which of the following agents?

(A) lithium carbonate

(B) pantoprazole

(C) zolmitriptan

(D) raloxifene

(E) betaserone

92. Intermittent IV therapy is used to

I. promote better diffusion of some drugs into the tissues because of a greater concentration gradient

II. reduce the potential of thrombophlebitis

III. avoid anticipated or potential stability or compatibility problems

(A) I only

(B) III only

(C) I and II only

(D) II and III only

(E) I, II, and III

93. Which of the following drugs is (are) classified as a mitotic inhibitor?

I. carboplatin

II. paclitaxel

III. vinblastine

(A) I only

(B) III only

(C) I and II only

(D) II and III only

(E) I, II, and III

94. Which of the following statements is (are) true of aspirin?

    I. High doses of aspirin may decrease plasma uric acid levels.
    II. Low doses of aspirin may increase plasma uric acid levels.
    III. Aspirin should not be used during the last trimester of pregnancy.

    (A) I only
    (B) III only
    (C) I and II only
    (D) II and III only
    (E) I, II, and III

95. Which of the following reference sources would be appropriate to use to find an American equivalent of a British drug?

    (A) *Martindale's Extra Pharmacopoeia*
    (B) *The Orange Book*
    (C) *Remington—The Science and Practice of Pharmacy*
    (D) *AHFS Drug Information*
    (E) *Facts and Comparisons*

96. Which of the following is (are) classified as a debriding agent?

    I. tenecteplase
    II. reteplase
    III. collagenase

    (A) I only
    (B) III only
    (C) I and II only
    (D) II and III only
    (E) I, II, and III

97. Which of the following cephalosporins would be appropriate to use in treating bacterial meningitis?

    I. cefprozil (Cefzil)
    II. ceftriaxone (Rocephin)
    III. cefotaxime (Claforan)

    (A) I only
    (B) III only

(C) I and II only
(D) II and III only
(E) I, II, and III

98. A patient has been diagnosed with herpes labialis. Which of the following agents would be MOST appropriate to recommend for treatment of this condition?

    (A) indinavir
    (B) penciclovir
    (C) oseltamivir
    (D) zalcitabine
    (E) saquinavir

99. With what should a patient with fungal blepharitis be treated?

    (A) natamycin
    (B) ketoconazole
    (C) caspofungin
    (D) micafungin
    (E) terbinafine

100. What should patients receiving doses of plantago (psyllium) be advised to do?

    (A) avoid dairy products
    (B) take the product with lots of water
    (C) mix the product with water and let stand for 30 minutes before administering
    (D) not lie down for at least 30 minutes after administration
    (E) take the medication with food

101. Which cation is MOST prevalent in the extracellular fluid of the human body?

    (A) sodium
    (B) chloride
    (C) calcium
    (D) potassium
    (E) magnesium

102. Systemic toxic effects of atropine sulfate may be treated by administering which of the following antidotes?

    (A) acetylcysteine
    (B) lactulase

(C) polyethylene glycol

(D) flumazenil

(E) physostigmine

103. The blood concentration of which of the following cations would normally rise if a patient became hypophosphatemic?

    I. calcium
    II. magnesium
    III. iron

(A) I only

(B) III only

(C) I and II only

(D) II and III only

(E) I, II, and III

104. In whom should products containing nicotine polacrilex be avoided?

    I. type 1 diabetic patients
    II. patients with severe angina
    III. pregnant women

(A) I only

(B) III only

(C) I and II only

(D) II and III only

(E) I, II, and III

105. What is a large overdose of acetaminophen likely to cause?

(A) hepatic necrosis

(B) seizures

(C) renal tubular necrosis

(D) respiratory alkalosis

(E) metabolic acidosis

106. With what should an adult patient who ingested 30 MS Contin 60 mg tablets 3 hours ago be treated?

(A) EDTA infusion

(B) *N*-acetylcysteine

(C) naloxone

(D) ipecac syrup

(E) sodium bicarbonate

107. Which of the following statements is (are) correct descriptions of sulfasalazine (Azulfidine)?

    I. used in treating ulcerative colitis and regional enteritis
    II. converted to mesalamine in the body
    III. poorly absorbed from the GI tract

(A) I only

(B) III only

(C) I and II only

(D) II and III only

(E) I, II, and III

108. Which of the following is the MOST potent enzyme inhibitor?

(A) acyclovir

(B) emtricitabine

(C) zalcitabine

(D) ritonavir

(E) didanosine

109. Nonselective beta-adrenergic blocking agents should be avoided in patients with

    I. supraventricular tachyarrhythmias
    II. insulin-dependent diabetes mellitus (IDDM)
    III. asthma

(A) I only

(B) III only

(C) I and II only

(D) II and III only

(E) I, II, and III

110. Which of the following agents would be most dangerous to use in a patient already receiving high doses of gentamicin?

(A) doxycycline

(B) bumetanide

(C) irbesartan

(D) ticarcillin sodium

(E) tamulosin

111. With what would a patient arriving in a hospital ED suffering from severe pulmonary hypertension most likely be treated?

(A) treprostinil
(B) methyldopa
(C) nitroprusside sodium
(D) minoxidil
(E) nesiritide

112. A patient with left ventricular failure is likely to exhibit which of the following signs or symptoms?

I. orthopnea
II. dyspnea
III. peripheral edema

(A) I only
(B) III only
(C) I and II only
(D) II and III only
(E) I, II, and III

113. Which of the following would be considered a level within normal range for a healthy adult?

I. LDL cholesterol 180 mg/dL
II. triglycerides 245 mg/dL
III. total cholesterol 175 mg/dL

(A) I only
(B) III only
(C) I and II only
(D) II and III only
(E) I, II, and III

114. Food containing tyramine should NOT be part of the diet of patients taking which of the following agents?

(A) eplerenone
(B) hydralazine
(C) selegeline
(D) methyldopa
(E) clonidine

115. Which of the following symptoms would be LEAST likely to be exhibited by a patient suffering from type 1 diabetes mellitus?

(A) weight loss
(B) excessive thirst
(C) glycosuria
(D) urinary retention
(E) weakness

116. A patient has been diagnosed as having impetigo. Which of the following drug products would be most useful in treating this condition?

(A) Primaxin
(B) Azactam
(C) Synercid
(D) Bactroban
(E) Trobicin

117. A pharmacy student reads a patient's chart and notes that the patient has blepharitis. Where is the patient's inflammation?

(A) colon
(B) eyelid
(C) throat
(D) tongue
(E) ear

118. Which of the following are uses for bupropion HCl?

I. antidepressant
II. smoking deterrent
III. seasonal affective disorder

(A) I only
(B) III only
(C) I and II only
(D) II and III only
(E) I, II, and III

119. Which of the following potential adverse effects of the phenothiazines is thought to be irreversible?

(A) akathisia

(B) orthostatic hypotension

(C) muscular rigidity

(D) tardive dyskinesia

(E) anticholinergic effects

120. Which of the following agents can be classified as an antagonist of angiotensin II receptors?

I. irbesartan

II. trandolapril

III. labetalol

(A) I only

(B) III only

(C) I and II only

(D) II and III only

(E) I, II, and III

121. What is the cause of Lyme disease?

(A) tick

(B) virus

(C) spirochete

(D) fungus

(E) lack of vitamin C

122. The use of olsalazine (Dipentum) is contraindicated in patients with a history of hypersensitivity to which of the following?

(A) sulfonamides

(B) imidazolines

(C) beta-adrenergic blocking agents

(D) phenothiazines

(E) salicylates

123. A patient has been receiving 50 mg of hydrocortisone IV every 6 hours for an acute exacerbation of ulcerative colitis. After several days of IV therapy, the physician wishes to switch the patient to an equivalent dose of oral prednisone. What is the equivalent total daily dose of prednisone?

(A) 50 mg

(B) 100 mg

(C) 200 mg

(D) 400 mg

(E) 600 mg

124. A 50-year-old patient with congestive heart failure is stabilized on digoxin 0.25 mg daily, hydrochlorothiazide 50 mg daily, and a low-sodium, potassium-rich diet. The patient then develops polyarteritis, which requires corticosteroid therapy. Which of the following glucocorticoids would be most appropriate for this patient?

(A) hydrocortisone

(B) cortisone

(C) prednisolone

(D) dexamethasone

(E) prednisone

125. A patient receiving chemotherapy develops blue-colored urine. Which of the following drugs is MOST likely to be responsible for this action?

(A) doxorubicin

(B) mitoxantrone

(C) cyclophosphamide

(D) cisplatin

(E) flutamide

126. A 20-year-old asthmatic patient has been treated with zileuton (Zyflo) 600 mg q.i.d. While the patient seems to tolerate the drug well, she has brief episodes of bronchospasm several times a week. Which of the following drugs would NOT be appropriate to recommend for the treatment of acute bronchospasm in this patient?

I. omalizumab (Xolair)

II. salmeterol (Serevent)

III. zafirlukast (Accolate)

(A) I only

(B) III only

(C) I and II only

(D) II and III only

(E) I, II, and III

127. A patient with rheumatoid arthritis cannot swallow tablets or capsules. Which of the following anti-inflammatory drugs is available in an oral liquid dosage form?

   I. ketoprofen
   II. Ibuprofen
   III. Naproxen

   (A) I only
   (B) III only
   (C) I and II only
   (D) II and III only
   (E) I, II, and III

128. A prescriber wishes to prescribe Lanoxicaps for a patient who has been receiving Lanoxin 0.25 mg tablets. Which strength of Lanoxicaps should the pharmacist recommend?

   (A) 0.05 mg
   (B) 0.1 mg
   (C) 0.3 mg
   (D) 0.5 mg
   (E) 0.2 mg

129. A secondary means of contraception should be recommended to patients using oral contraceptives when which of the following drugs is (are) also to be taken?

   I. rifampin
   II. cetirizine
   III. acetaminophen

   (A) I only
   (B) III only
   (C) I and II only
   (D) II and III only
   (E) I, II, and III

130. In addition to its anticonvulsant activity, what is carbamazepine also indicated for the treatment of?

   I. Kaposi's sarcoma
   II. bipolar disorder
   III. trigeminal neuralgia

   (A) I only
   (B) III only
   (C) I and II only
   (D) II and III only
   (E) I, II, and III

131. What is the advantage of naltrexone over naloxone?

   (A) its more rapid onset of action
   (B) that it is not addictive
   (C) its availability as sublingual tablets
   (D) that it does not have to be reconstituted immediately before use
   (E) its longer duration of action

132. Which of the following would be appropriate for the treatment of candidal vulvovaginitis?

   I. nystatin
   II. clotrimazole
   III. miconazole

   (A) I only
   (B) III only
   (C) I and II only
   (D) II and III only
   (E) I, II, and III

133. Polycythemia refers to an elevated number of which of the following?

   (A) platelets
   (B) leukocytes
   (C) erythrocytes
   (D) reticulocytes
   (E) granulocytes

134. In treating heparin overdose with protamine sulfate, why must caution be exercised to avoid using more protamine than is necessary?

   (A) protamine sulfate is toxic in small amounts
   (B) protamine sulfate is a cardiotoxic agent
   (C) the production of endogenous heparin will be stimulated

(D) protamine sulfate is also an anticoagulant

(E) the strongly basic protamine will produce alkalosis

135. Which of the following agents has the LONGEST duration of effect as a bronchodilator?

(A) salmeterol

(B) isoetharine

(C) levalbuterol

(D) terbutaline

(E) bitolterol

136. Which of the following would be the best choice for use in providing anticoagulant therapy for a pregnant patient near the anticipated time of delivery?

(A) heparin

(B) dipyridamole

(C) aspirin

(D) warfarin

(E) ticlopidine

137. The use of rizatriptan is contraindicated in which patients?

   I. patients with angina pectoris

   II. patients using MAO inhibitors

   III. patients who have received an ergotamine derivative within the past 24 hours

(A) I only

(B) III only

(C) I and II only

(D) II and III only

(E) I, II, and III

138. What is the most likely organism to cause an acute uncomplicated urinary tract infection?

(A) *Staphylococcus epidermidis*

(B) *Staphylococcus aureus*

(C) *Candida albicans*

(D) *E. coli*

(E) *Haemophilus influenza*

139. The Schilling test is useful for the detection of pernicious anemia. This test utilizes which of the following in its orally administered, radiolabeled form?

(A) folic acid

(B) cyanocobalamin

(C) iron

(D) intrinsic factor

(E) hemoglobin

140. Lipodystrophy experienced by patients using insulin can be avoided by recommending which of the following?

(A) use of longer-acting insulin

(B) use of shorter-acting insulin

(C) rotation of injection sites

(D) addition of a 2nd generation sulfonylurea to therapy

(E) addition of an alpha-glucosidase inhibitor to therapy

141. How is insulin aspart generally administered?

(A) one hour after the morning meal

(B) 15 minutes before a meal

(C) at bedtime

(D) one hour after dinner

(E) intravenously

142. Which of the following is (are) TRUE of liraglutide (Victoza)?

   I. For treatment of type 1 or type 2 diabetes mellitus.

   II. Should only be administered with the morning meal.

   III. It is only given subcutaneously.

(A) I only

(B) III only

(C) I and II only

(D) II and III only

(E) I, II, and III

143. A patient has been told by his physician to consume foods that are high in lycopene because it may decrease his chance of developing prostate cancer. Which of the following foods would be the BEST dietary source of lycopene?

    (A) cabbage
    (B) walnuts
    (C) tomato sauce
    (D) aged cheeses
    (E) cold-water fish

144. Patients receiving analgesic doses of morphine should be monitored for the development of

    I. respiratory depression
    II. nausea
    III. diarrhea

    (A) I only
    (B) III only
    (C) I and II only
    (D) II and III only
    (E) I, II, and III

145. Which of the following is true of combination oral contraceptive product?

    I. They suppress follicle-stimulating hormone (FSH) and luteinizing hormone (LH).
    II. They decrease viscosity of cervical mucus.
    III. Most contain medroxyprogesterone and ethinyl estradiol.

    (A) I only
    (B) III only
    (C) I and II only
    (D) II and III only
    (E) I, II, and III

146. A 28-year-old female visits a neighborhood clinic complaining of flu-like symptoms that began about 24 hours ago. She is diagnosed as having uncomplicated influenza A. Which of the following would be appropriate to prescribe for this patient?

    I. valacyclovir
    II. zanamivir
    III. oseltamivir

    (A) I only
    (B) III only
    (C) I and II only
    (D) II and III only
    (E) I, II, and III

147. Which of the following drugs is particularly useful for the treatment of acute hypoglycemic reactions when oral or IV administration of glucose is not possible?

    (A) insulin lispro
    (B) glucocorticoids
    (C) glucagon
    (D) pancreatin
    (E) glimepiride (Amaryl)

148. Which of the following would be the BEST drug to use in treating a pregnant patient who is HIV-positive in order to reduce the likelihood of transmission of HIV to the newborn child?

    (A) zidovudine
    (B) nevirapine
    (C) didanosine
    (D) ritonavir
    (E) enfurvitide

149. A patient is admitted to the ED with marked hypotension and appears to be in shock. What is the drug of choice to treat this condition?

    (A) dobutamine
    (B) milrinone
    (C) epinephrine HCl
    (D) nitroprusside
    (E) dopamine HCl

150. Which of the following oral contraceptive products could be prescribed for a woman who does not wish to use an estrogen-containing contraceptive product?

    I. Yaz
    II. Ovrette
    III. Nor-QD

(A) I only

(B) III only

(C) I and II only

(D) II and III only

(E) I, II, and III

151. How would the erythrocytes of an iron-deficient patient be described?

(A) microcytic and hypochromic

(B) microcytic and hyperchromic

(C) normocytic and hyperchromic

(D) macrocytic and hyperchromic

(E) macrocytic and hypochromic

152. A postmenopausal female patient has a prescription filled for one Estring. At what interval should she be expected to return for her refills?

(A) 30 days

(B) 60 days

(C) 90 days

(D) 180 days

(E) 1 year

153. Which of the following is (are) TRUE of calcitonin salmon?

I. it is administered by inhalation

II. it should not be refrigerated

III. it is administered daily

(A) I only

(B) III only

(C) I and II only

(D) II and III only

(E) I, II, and III

154. Why should loperamide NOT be given to patients taking oral clindamycin?

(A) the antimicrobial action of clindamycin will be impaired

(B) aplastic anemia may be more likely to occur

(C) toxic effects of clindamycin may be enhanced

(D) the rate of hydrolytic destruction of clindamycin in the GI tract will increase

(E) an insoluble complex will be formed

155. What is an advantage of loperamide (Imodium) over diphenoxylate (Lomotil) as an antidiarrheal?

(A) loperamide does not cause drowsiness or dizziness

(B) loperamide has a direct effect on the CNS and therefore works more rapidly than does diphenoxylate

(C) loperamide is available in a parenteral form

(D) loperamide does not appear to have opiate-like effects

(E) loperamide has significant adsorbent action

156. A woman has had two unplanned pregnancies. Each pregnancy was associated with failure to correctly use the oral contraceptive prescribed for her. Which of the following would be a reasonable alternative for this patient to reduce the likelihood of future pregnancies?

I. Mirena

II. Natazia

III. Clomid

(A) I only

(B) III only

(C) I and II only

(D) II and III only

(E) I, II, and III

157. A patient using felodipine should be advised to do which of the following?

(A) take the product on an empty stomach

(B) avoid aspirin while taking the product

(C) take the product at bedtime

(D) take each dose with a fatty food

(E) avoid the use of grapefruit juice while using the product

158. A patient under the influence of crack cocaine is brought to an acute-care facility. To which drug are the symptoms of cocaine intoxication most similar?

(A) heroin
(B) tetrahydrocannabinol (THC)
(C) ethanol
(D) dextroamphetamine
(E) morphine

159. The initiation of therapy with which one of the following agents would be LEAST likely to cause therapeutic problems in a patient already taking warfarin (Coumadin)?

(A) acetaminophen
(B) colestipol
(C) phenytoin
(D) aspirin
(E) cimetidine

160. A patient's physician changes his medication from captopril to valsartan. Which of the following is (are) TRUE of valsartan (Diovan)?

  I. It is angiotensin II receptor blocker.
  II. It is less likely to cause angioedema than captopril.
  III. It is less likely than captopril to cause a nonproductive cough.

(A) I only
(B) III only
(C) I and II only
(D) II and III only
(E) I, II, and III

161. A nutritional product is said to contain 11 g of protein, 22 g of carbohydrate, and 5 g of fat in each 100-mL serving. What is the caloric content of one serving?

(A) 238 kcal
(B) 198 kcal
(C) 218 kcal
(D) 177 kcal
(E) 378 kcal

162. Patients experiencing toxicity as a result of methotrexate administration should be given which of the following?

(A) potassium citrate
(B) sodium bicarbonate
(C) bioflavinoids
(D) leucovorin calcium
(E) misoprostol

163. A 19-year-old college student visited Mexico during her spring break and acquired an acute GI disorder characterized by severe diarrhea. Over the past week, she has lost 5 lb and feels weak and run down. Which of the following would be most appropriate to administer to this patient?

(A) Nulytely
(B) K-Lyte
(C) Isomil
(D) Pedialyte
(E) Lypressin

164. Parenteral administration of 1 L of 5% dextrose in water provides the patient with approximately how many kilocalories of energy?

(A) 150–200 kcal
(B) 350–400 kcal
(C) 450–500 kcal
(D) 800–850 kcal
(E) 1,000 kcal

165. Which of the following is (are) true of Hepatitis B vaccine?

  I. must be stored in a refrigerator
  II. will also protect against hepatitis A
  III. administered intradermally

(A) I only
(B) III only
(C) I and II only
(D) II and III only
(E) I, II, and III

166. A patient is said to have a significantly elevated PSA level. What is this indicative of?

(A) BPH

(B) tuberculosis

(C) an underlying *Pseudomonas* infection

(D) cystic fibrosis

(E) cholestatic hepatitis

167. Which of the following would be (a) good alternative(s) to penicillin V in a pregnant patient allergic to penicillins?

I. erythromycin

II. trimethoprim

III. demeclocycline

(A) I only

(B) III only

(C) I and II only

(D) II and III only

(E) I, II, and III

168. Which one of the following sulfonamide-containing products is best suited for the topical treatment of serious burns?

(A) sulfacetamide

(B) sulfamethoxazole/trimethoprim

(C) sulfisoxazole

(D) silver sulfadiazine

(E) sulfasalazine

169. Which of the following drugs would be MOST appropriate to use for the treatment of an uncomplicated gonorrhea infection in a poorly compliant patient?

(A) ceftriaxone

(B) pipericillin

(C) tetracycline

(D) clindamycin

(E) itraconazole

170. Which of the following drugs used in the treatment of acute gouty arthritis does (do) NOT affect urate metabolism or excretion?

I. indomethacin

II. probenecid

III. allopurinol

(A) I only

(B) III only

(C) I and II only

(D) II and III only

(E) I, II, and III

171. The antiemetic effect of which of the following drugs is the result of increased rate of gastric emptying?

(A) promethazine

(B) granisetron

(C) olsalazine

(D) baclofen

(E) metoclopramide

172. Which of the following agents is (are) indicated for the treatment of Parkinson's disease?

I. amantadine

II. selegiline

III. entacapone

(A) I only

(B) III only

(C) I and II only

(D) II and III only

(E) I, II, and III

173. Patients diagnosed with Alzheimer's disease may be treated with which of the following agents?

I. galantamine

II. memantine

III. clomipramine

(A) I only

(B) III only

(C) I and II only

(D) II and III only

(E) I, II, and III

174. Patients receiving metformin for the treatment of diabetes mellitus should be monitored for the development of

(A) photosensitivity

(B) tendon rupture

(C) lactic acidosis

(D) respiratory alkalosis

(E) agranulocytosis

175. A pharmacist tells a young mother about clinical (fever) thermometers and advises her to report to the pediatrician both the degrees of temperature and whether the temperature was taken rectally or orally. Why is this good advice?

    (A) oral temperature is about 1° Fahrenheit (1°F) higher than rectal temperature
    (B) oral thermometers have degree calibrations that differ from rectal thermometers
    (C) the normal temperature (marked with an arrow) is 99.6°F on the rectal thermometer and 98.6°F on the oral one
    (D) rectal temperature is about 1°F higher than oral temperature
    (E) the bulb on the rectal thermometer is round and contains more mercury than in the thin cylindrical bulb of the oral thermometer

176. What is the BEST emergency advice that a pharmacist could give an individual who has just suffered a minor burn?

    (A) apply bacitracin cream onto the burn site
    (B) immerse the burned area in warm water followed by cold water
    (C) apply petrolatum to the burn
    (D) contact a physician immediately
    (E) immerse the burned area in cold water

177. What should a patient who is planning to use montelukast sodium be advised to do?

    I. take the drug daily as prescribed even when they are asymptomatic
    II. stop using bronchodilator drugs
    III. use one inhalation at the onset of an asthma attack

    (A) I only
    (B) III only
    (C) I and II only
    (D) II and III only
    (E) I, II, and III

178. Which of the following is (are) an effect associated with the use of pilocarpine ophthalmic products?

    I. miosis
    II. cholinergic agonism
    III. inhibition of carbonic anydrase

    (A) I only
    (B) III only
    (C) I and II only
    (D) II and III only
    (E) I, II, and III

179. For what should patients using amiodarone be monitored?

    I. pulmonary toxicity
    II. visual changes
    III. intestinal polyp formation

    (A) I only
    (B) III only
    (C) I and II only
    (D) II and III only
    (E) I, II, and III

180. Which of the following should NOT be administered to a patient being treated for narrow-angle glaucoma?

    (A) tropicamide
    (B) dorzolamide
    (C) latanoprost
    (D) carteolol
    (E) levobunolol

181. A patient tells a pharmacist that his physician has recommended that he purchase tocopherol OTC. With what should the pharmacist provide this patient?

    (A) vitamin E capsules
    (B) vitamin A capsules
    (C) pyridoxine tablets
    (D) thiamine tablets
    (E) benzoyl peroxide lotion

182. Which of the following is (are) true of GoLYTELY?

    I. must be reconstituted before use
    II. ingredients are enzymatically converted to active form in colon
    III. contains loperamide

(A) I only

(B) III only

(C) I and II only

(D) II and III only

(E) I, II, and III

183. Which of the following is (are) true of orlistat (Xenical, Alli)?

    I. inhibits absorption of dietary fats

    II. patient should consume diet that contains at least 30% of calories from fat

    III. not more than one dose should be taken in any 24-hour period

(A) I only

(B) III only

(C) I and II only

(D) II and III only

(E) I, II, and III

184. Scabies is a contagious skin disease, caused by a

(A) mite

(B) herpes virus

(C) flea

(D) spider

(E) tick

185. How is psoriasis characterized?

(A) granulomatous lesions

(B) small, water-filled blisters

(C) silvery gray scales

(D) small red vesicles

(E) pustules

186. A patient with a documented allergy to morphine should NOT receive which one of the following analgesics?

    I. codeine

    II. fentanyl

    III. pentazocine

(A) I only

(B) III only

(C) I and II only

(D) II and III only

(E) I, II, and III

187. Which of the following agents is (are) classified as an immunosuppressive agent?

    I. cyclosporine

    II. tacrolimus

    III. cilostazol

(A) I only

(B) III only

(C) I and II only

(D) II and III only

(E) I, II, and III

188. Which of the following is (are) TRUE of darbepoetin alfa?

    I. the pharmacist should store unopened containers in the refrigerator

    II. indicated for treatment of hemosiderosis

    III. may be used orally or intranasally

(A) I only

(B) III only

(C) I and II only

(D) II and III only

(E) I, II, and III

189. Which of the following antihypertensive agents is available in a transdermal patch dosage form?

(A) penbutolol

(B) clonidine

(C) aliskiren

(D) telmisartan

(E) terazosin

190. Ideally, what should be the approximate pH value of stomach contents after the use of an antacid?

(A) 3.5

(B) 5.5

(C) 6.5

(D) 7.5

(E) 9.5

191. Which of the following is (are) an indication for the use of epoetin alfa (Epogen, Procrit)?

    I. treatment of severe chronic neutropenia
    II. treatment of anemia associated with cancer chemotherapy
    III. treatment of anemia associated with chronic renal failure

    (A) I only
    (B) III only
    (C) I and II only
    (D) II and III only
    (E) I, II, and III

192. A patient with Parkinson's disease has been receiving levodopa (1 g four times daily) with fairly good response but with excessive adverse effects. The patient's physician wishes to switch him from levodopa to Sinemet. What would be the approximate starting dose of Sinemet?

    (A) one 10/100 tablet daily
    (B) one 10/100 tablet four times daily
    (C) one 25/250 tablet daily
    (D) one 25/250 tablet four times daily
    (E) four 25/250 tablets four times daily

193. A patient is being treated effectively for Parkinson's disease with levodopa. Suddenly, all therapeutic benefits of the levodopa are lost and the adverse effects also disappear. Which one of the following facts obtained from a medication history would most likely explain this phenomenon?

    (A) The patient has forgotten to take two doses of the medication.
    (B) The patient began using an OTC multivitamin product.
    (C) Selegiline was added to the drug regimen for 1 week.
    (D) The patient took occasional doses of an antacid.
    (E) The patient regularly consumed alcoholic beverages.

194. Patients receiving miglitol should

    I. expect some flatulence and diarrhea to occur

    II. take each dose on an empty stomach
    III. expect to use a higher insulin dose while on the medication

    (A) I only
    (B) III only
    (C) I and II only
    (D) II and III only
    (E) I, II, and III

195. Which of the following drugs is associated with the "Gray Baby Syndrome" in infants?

    (A) kanamycin
    (B) ciprofloxacin
    (C) demeclocycline
    (D) amphotericin B
    (E) chloramphenicol

196. A nursing student asks a pharmacist about the use of nitroprusside sodium. Which of the following is (are) correct about this drug?

    I. It is used in treating hypertensive emergencies.
    II. Solutions of the drug should be discarded if they turn pink.
    III. It is administered by IV infusion.

    (A) I only
    (B) III only
    (C) I and II only
    (D) II and III only
    (E) I, II, and III

197. What is an obese individual most likely suffering from?

    (A) polydipsia
    (B) hypotonia
    (C) polyphagia
    (D) polyhydrosis
    (E) polymorphism

198. A headache is a commonly experienced side effect of which drug?

    (A) clonidine
    (B) nitroglycerin

(C) doxazosin

(D) diltiazem

(E) captopril

199. Which of the following is (are) true of misoprostol?

  I. It is used in the treatment of psoriasis.

  II. It is a prostaglandin analog.

  III. It is in pregnancy category X

(A) I only

(B) III only

(C) I and II only

(D) II and III only

(E) I, II, and III

200. All of the following terms relate directly to body muscles EXCEPT which of the following?

(A) myalgia

(B) myositis

(C) myoclonus

(D) myocardia

(E) myopia

201. What should patients taking lithium products be advised to do?

  I. stop taking the medication if tremors or diarrhea occur

  II. consume 2–3 L of fluid each day

  III. reduce their salt intake

(A) I only

(B) III only

(C) I and II only

(D) II and III only

(E) I, II, and III

202. Which of the following drug products would be MOST useful in treating a patient with a diagnosis of irritable bowel syndrome (IBS) whose primary bowel symptom is constipation?

(A) alosetron

(B) tegaserod

(C) granisetron

(D) pantoprazole

(E) dicyclomine

203. When dispensing Adderal, what should the patient be told about the drug?

  I. that it may cause palpitations

  II. that it may cause weight gain

  III. to take the medication at bedtime

(A) I only

(B) III only

(C) I and II only

(D) II and III only

(E) I, II, and III

204. A 60-year-old patient with congestive heart failure who has been stabilized for 3 months on digoxin, furosemide, and potassium chloride is gradually placed on the following additional medicines. Which of these drugs is most likely to cause a problem?

(A) aspirin

(B) temazepam

(C) meperidine HCl

(D) quinidine sulfate

(E) nitroglycerin

205. Which of the following diuretics would be LEAST likely to produce a hypokalemic effect in a patient?

(A) ethacrynic acid

(B) torsemide

(C) chlorthalidone

(D) furosemide

(E) eplerenone

206. Mannitol is used therapeutically primarily as a (an)

(A) cardiac stimulant

(B) sucrose substitute

(C) antianginal agent

(D) osmotic diuretic

(E) plasma expander

207. Which of the following drugs is (are) indicated for the treatment of enuresis?

   I. defasirox
   II. imipramine
   III. desmopressin

(A) I only
(B) III only
(C) I and II only
(D) II and III only
(E) I, II, and III

208. In monitoring acute MI patients who are using warfarin sodium (Coumadin), what should their INR ideally be between?

(A) 0.1–0.2
(B) 2–3
(C) 4–5.5
(D) 9–14
(E) 80–120

209. What should patients using phenytoin be monitored for the development of?

   I. gingival hyperplasia
   II. nystagmus
   III. pseudomembranous enterocolitis

(A) I only
(B) III only
(C) I and II only
(D) II and III only
(E) I, II, and III

210. What is the potential problem of using butorphanol in a patient who is dependent on codeine?

(A) additive respiratory depression
(B) increased tolerance to codeine
(C) precipitation of narcotic withdrawal symptoms
(D) impaired renal excretion of codeine
(E) excessive CNS stimulation

Answers and Explanations

Numbers within parentheses at the end of the answers refer to the numbered references that are listed in the front matter.

1. **(C)** Although the NSAIDs are structurally different, they all possess similar pharmacological properties and all inhibit prostaglandin synthesis. Furthermore, these drugs produce similar adverse effects, including GI intolerance. Piroxicam (Feldene) and oxaprozin (Daypro) have the longest half-life of the group (approximately 42–80 hours) and may be given on a once-a-day basis. *(3)*

2. **(C)** Adalimumab (Humira) is a monoclonal antibody that is directed against tumor necrosis factor-alpha (TNF-α). It is indicated for reducing the signs and symptoms and inhibiting the progression of structural damage in adults with moderate-to-severe active rheumatoid arthritis who have failed previous treatment with disease-modifying antirheumatic drugs. *(3)*

3. **(D)** Acetaminophen (Tylenol) is a useful alternative to NSAIDS when used in the treatment of mild–moderate muscle pain. Alternatively, the pharmacist could encourage the patient to take their ibuprofen with food or milk. *(11)*

4. **(C)** When dispensing isotretinoin (Accutane) to a woman of childbearing potential, the pharmacist should advise the patient of the dangers of becoming pregnant during therapy. In addition, the patient should be advised that the lesions will initially appear worse but then improve and that prolonged exposure to sunlight or sunlamps should be avoided while using the drug. *(3)*

5. **(E)** In the condition known as hypoprothrombinemia, there is a reduction in the levels of prothrombin in the blood. This substance is essential in the blood-clotting mechanism. *(14)*

6. **(B)** Rapid reversal of warfarin-induced hypoprothrombinemia can be accomplished by discontinuing warfarin therapy and, if necessary, the administration of phytonadione (vitamin K_1). Phytonadione, when used for this purpose, is best administered IM or SC in a single dose. The dose may be repeated if the patient does not adequately respond within 6 to 8 hours. *(6)*

7. **(D)** Rifampin (Rifadin, Rimactane) is a highly colored red substance that commonly causes discoloration of the urine and other body fluids. It is used primarily for the treatment of tuberculosis. *(6)*

8. **(C)** Menotropins (Repronex) is a product that has moderate FSH and LH activity. The product is administered parenterally to induce ovulation in patients with amenorrhea or in other conditions that cause anovulatory cycles. It may also be used in males to enhance spermatogenesis. It is classified in pregnancy category X. *(6)*

9. **(A)** Eplerenone (Inspra) is a potassium-sparing diuretic. Patients should be advised to avoid large quantities of potassium-rich foods because their use with this drug product could cause serious hyperkalemia. *(3)*

10. **(B)** Animal testing of a new drug is completed before the investigational new drug (IND) status is obtained for clinical testing. In Phase I of the study, healthy volunteers are tested to determine drug tolerance, dosing schedules, side effects, and pharmacokinetic data. This is followed by Phase II, in which actual patients suffering from the disease are tested with the drug. Drug efficacy is observed, and side effects not evident in healthy volunteers may occur. Phase III involves administration of the drug to large numbers of patients by private practitioners. Phase IV is the continuous investigation or monitoring of the drug after marketing. *(1)*

11. **(A)** Hypoparathyroidism usually presents itself as a disorder of calcium metabolism in which serum calcium levels of the patient decrease while levels of phosphate increase in an inversely proportional manner. Low serum calcium levels may precipitate a potentially serious condition known as tetany. To prevent the development of this disorder and to treat the hypoparathyroidism, calcium supplements, such as calcium gluconate, calcium carbonate, or calcium lactate may be prescribed. *(14)*

12. **(D)** *Legionella* organisms are aerobic, gram-negative rods. Typical drugs used to treat this organism in adults are fluoroquinolones such as ciprofloxacin and levofloxacin and macrolides such as erythromycin. Azithromycin (Zithromax) is often recommended for use in children with the disease. *(3)*

13. **(C)** The hypothyroid state is characterized by marked retardation of mental and physical activity; hoarseness; dry sparse hair; thickening of the skin and subcutaneous tissues; constipation; cold intolerance; anemia; and dry, pale, coarse skin. However, because of the nature of the general symptoms, hypothyroidism is usually recognized and treated before all of the previously mentioned symptoms develop. Patients with hypothyroidism frequently develop enlargement of the thyroid glands (goiter) and may have elevated TSH levels. Hashimoto's disease (autoimmune thyroiditis) is a common cause of hypothyroidism in adults. *(14)*

14. **(D)** Nocturnal enuresis is also called bed-wetting. While fairly common in children, it may also continue in some through the teen years and adulthood. A variety of possible causes exist, including psychological, diabetes insipidus, weakness of the bladder sphincter, and others. It is often treated with antidiuretic hormones such as DDAVP or imipramine, which exerts anticholinergic effects. *(14)*

15. **(C)** Anacin and Alka-Seltzer Blue each contain aspirin the only agent listed that contains aspirin. *(3)*

16. **(B)** Hemochromatosis is an iron storage disorder characterized by excessive amounts of iron in parenchymal tissues with resultant tissue damage. Such a condition may be caused by a number of factors, one of which is the prolonged use of excessive doses of iron preparations. *(14)*

17. **(A)** Tendon rupture is more likely to occur in patients using fluoroquinolone drugs such as ciprofloxacin.

18. **(E)** Dornase alfa (Pulmozyme) is a mucolytic agent that liquefies the tenacious respiratory mucus that is often a characteristic of cystic fibrosis. Pancrelipase (Ultrase) is a pancreatic enzyme product indicated for patients with cystic fibrosis. Such a product is useful in this disease because of the common presence of thick mucus plugs in the pancreatic duct, which may block the passage of pancreatic enzymes into the GI tract. TOBI is an aminoglycoside antimicrobial agent called Tobramycin. It is used by inhalation in patients with cystic fibrosis. *(3)*

19. **(B)** Metoclopramide is a prokinetic agent that promotes gastric emptying. It is most commonly used in treating diabetic gastroparesis and peptic ulcer disease. *(3)*

20. **(C)** Patients with chronic inflammatory bowel disease may use olsalazine sodium (Dipentum) or mesalamine (Asacol, Pentasa, Rowasa, Lialda) if they are allergic to sulfa drugs, because these drugs do not contain a sulfa

component. Sulfasalazine (Azulfidine) contains a sulfa component. *(3)*

21. **(D)** Ezetimibe (Zetia) is a lipid-lowering compound that selectively inhibits the intestinal absorption of cholestrol. It may be administered alone or it may be administered in combination with an HMG-CoA reductase inhibitor (ie, a statin drug), such as is seen with Vytorin. *(3)*

22. **(C)** Epzicom is combination product containing abacavir and lamivudine, both NRTIs. Trizivir is a product containing abacavir, lamivudine, and zidovudine. All are NRTIs. Relenza is an antiviral product containing zanamavir. It is used in the treatment and prevention of influenza A and B. *(3)*

23. **(D)** Patients with sinus headaches generally experience pain in the periorbital area. Pain is usually greatest on awakening because of the accumulation of fluid in the sinus cavities. *(14)*

24. **(D)** Combined drug treatment is usually required because of the rapid development of resistant organisms when a single agent is used. It has also been demonstrated that combined drug therapy enhances the antitubercular effects of the individual drugs. *(14)*

25. **(C)** The color change imparted to urine and sweat is a predictable and harmless side effect. Patients should be told to expect this effect so that they are not alarmed by it. *(3)*

26. **(D)** Ticlopidine (Ticlid) is a platelet aggregation inhibitor used to reduce the risk of thrombotic stroke. While using this drug the patient may be at higher risk of abnormal bleeding and the development of a serious condition known as thrombotic thrombocytopenic purpura (TTP). *(3)*

27. **(D)** Piperacillin (pipracil) is an extended-spectrum penicillin that is active against both gram-positive and many gram-negative microorganisms. It is particularly useful in treating serious gram-negative infections caused by *Pseudomonas* or *Proteus*. *(3)*

28. **(E)** Pseudomembranous colitis is a severe and occasionally fatal complication of antibiotic therapy. One etiology appears to be the presence of an exotoxin produced by overgrowth of *Clostridium difficile* in the bowel. Clindamycin, lincomycin, and ampicillin have been the most commonly implicated antibiotics, although other antibiotics have also been implicated. Treatment is directed against the offending organism and its exotoxin. Oral metronidazole (Flagyl) 250 to 500 mg three to four times daily for 10 days is most commonly used. *(3)*

29. **(B)** Cushing's syndrome is a condition characterized by adrenal hyperplasia caused by overproduction of ACTH by the pituitary gland. Patients with this disease often have obesity, hypertension, and gonadal dysfunction. *(14)*

30. **(D)** The aminoglycosides have activity against a wide range of microorganisms particularly serious gram negative organisms such as pseudomonas and proteus. After parenteral administration, they are excreted unchanged in the urine. Because of their well-established nephrotoxicity and ototoxicity, they are not suitable for long-term treatment of chronic urinary tract infections. *(3)*

31. **(C)** Mycobacterium avium complex (MAC) and *P. carinii* pneumonia (PCP) are both infectious complications of HIV. Sudden acute respiratory syndrome (SARS) is a highly transmissible viral disorder that is not specifically related to the presence of HIV. *(14)*

32. **(D)** Serevent is a long-acting bronchodilator that is not suitable for the treatment of acute attacks. *(3)*

33. **(C)** Interferon beta-1a (Avonex) and beta-1b (Betaseron) are used to treat multiple sclerosis. Interferon alfa-2a (Roferon-A) is used to treat leukemia and AIDS-related Kaposi's Sarcoma. *(6)*

34. **(D)** Vasopressin, which is a purified preparation of the antidiuretic hormone, is used therapeutically in the treatment of diabetes insipidus, a disease of pituitary origin. When

administered in any one of a number of available dosage forms [IM, IV, subcutaneous (SC), and nasal insufflation or spray], vasopressin usually reverses the symptom of excessive urination (polyuria), which is the primary symptom of patients suffering from this disease. The initially observed action of the hormone was vasoconstriction, which led to the name vasopressin; this is still the official USP designation. *(3)*

35. **(B)** Lithium carbonate (Lithane, Eskalith) is primarily indicated for treating manic episodes in patients with manic–depressive illness. It is administered orally in daily divided doses of 600 mg to 1.8 g. Lithium users may experience hypothyroidism because of the affinity of the thyroid for lithium. Patients on lithium should be advised not to reduce their sodium intake, as this may increase the likelihood of lithium toxicity. *(3)*

36. **(B)** Alendronate is a biphosphonate compound that inhibits normal and abnormal bone resorption. It is used for the treatment and prevention of osteoporosis in postmenopausal women. Patients should be advised to take their daily dose first thing in the morning, at least 30 minutes before the first food, beverage, or medication of the day is consumed. The drug should be taken with a full glass of plain water. The patient should be advised not to lie down for at least 60 minutes following the administration of the drug, to reduce the possibility of esophageal irritation. Ibandronate is available in a once-monthly regimen as well. *(3)*

37. **(A)** Glucose-6-phosphate dehydrogenase (G6PD) controls the initial step in the pentose-phosphate pathway, bringing about the oxidation of glucose-6-phosphate to 6-phosphogluconate, which reduces NADP to NADPH. Many oxidizing drugs (eg, primaquine, sulfisoxazole, probenecid) increase the rate of oxidation of glutathione. This increases the intracellular demand for NADPH to maintain glutathione in the reduced form. In patients with a deficiency in erythrocyte G6PD, oxidized glutathione accumulates and, by some unknown mechanism, disrupts erythrocyte

membrane integrity with subsequent hemolysis. *(6)*

38. **(D)** The anticoagulant effect of heparin is quantified by measuring the APTT. The usual therapeutic goal is to prolong the APTT to 2 to 2.5 times that of the laboratory control. *(6)*

39. **(E)** Because of heparin's brief duration of action, mild hemorrhaging is usually treated by simply withdrawing the drug. In the presence of severe hemorrhage, the use of a specific heparin antagonist (eg, protamine sulfate) is imperative. If protamine sulfate is required, generally 1 mg of protamine sulfate IV is utilized to neutralize 100 units of heparin. After the IV administration of heparin, the quantity of protamine required decreases rapidly with time. Only 0.5 mg of protamine is required to neutralize 100 units of heparin 30 minutes after IV administration of heparin. *(6)*

40. **(E)** Itraconazole potentiates the effects of oral anticoagulants by decreasing the rate of hepatic metabolism of warfarin. Itraconazole causes a reversible but significant increase in plasma warfarin concentration and, consequently, in the PT. In this case, it is necessary to recognize this interaction and decrease the dose of warfarin or use a safer alternative to itraconazole. *(3)*

41. **(A)** Cromolyn sodium 4% ophthalmic solution (Crolom) is used to treat ocular allergic disorders such as vernal keratoconjunctivitis. It is effective only if it is used at regular intervals. Cromolyn acts to inhibit degranulation of sensitized mast cells that occurs after exposure to specific antigens. *(3)*

42. **(E)** Etanercept (Enbrel) is a drug that acts as a TNF antagonist. It is indicated for the treatment of plague psoriasis and moderate to severe rheumatoid arthritis in patients who have not responded to more conservative forms of therapy (eg, NSAIDs). This drug must be used with great caution in patients who have a preexisting infection. Treatment with this drug should be discontinued if the patient develops a serious infection while on

the drug. The drug is administered subcutaneously every week. *(3)*

43. **(D)** Dopamine (Intropin) is a sympathomimetic drug that acts directly on alpha and beta-receptors and produces indirect effects due to release of norepinephrine. Dopamine also dilates renal and mesenteric vessels through a dopamine receptor effect. The hemodynamic effects of dopamine are dose related. At low infusion rates (1–5 mg/kg/min), dopamine increases renal blood flow without much change in cardiac output or total peripheral resistance. In higher doses (5–20 mg/kg/min), cardiac output and heart rate increase, the increase in renal perfusion persists, and total peripheral resistance is variable. At higher infusion rates, renal vasoconstriction occurs, total peripheral resistance rises, and blood pressure increases. Consequently, the infusion rate must be adjusted and monitored carefully to achieve the desired response. *(3)*

44. **(A)** Flumazenil (Romazicon) is a specific benzodiazepine antagonist used to reverse the toxic effects of benzodiazepine intoxication. It should not be used in patients also using tricyclic antidepressants because it may increase the risk of seizures in such patients. *(6)*

45. **(D)** Although there are no reported differences in bioavailability between phenytoin capsules and suspension, this patient's phenytoin level is likely to increase because the milligram-for-milligram conversion is equivalent to an increase in dose. The capsule form of Dilantin is the sodium salt and contains only 92% phenytoin. The suspension is the free acid and contains 100% phenytoin. In this situation, the patient would be going from a daily dose of 276 mg phenytoin (as 300-mg phenytoin sodium) to 300 mg phenytoin. *(3)*

46. **(A)** Fentanyl (Duragesic) patches are effective in treating chronic severe pain. They are applied every 72 hours and provide a continuous release of analgesic during that period. PRN treatment is not advisable in treating severe pain because it may cause patient anxiety. Codeine, oral meperidine, and aceta-

minophen are generally not effective enough to control chronic severe pain. *(3)*

47. **(B)** Pregabalin is an anticholinergic drug that would likely cause urinary retention. All of the other choices will tend to increase urine flow by reducing prostatic size. *(3)*

48. **(B)** Respiratory distress is a serious adverse effect associated with the use of bleomycin (Blenoxane). It is most likely to occur in elderly patients and in those receiving a total dose of 400 units or more. *(3)*

49. **(C)** In general, all insulin products currently available are reasonably stable at room temperature (ie, 59–85°F). Traveling diabetic patients should be advised to avoid prolonged exposure of their insulin to very high temperatures, and told that it is not necessary to refrigerate the vial in use. Insulin vials stored in pharmacies are required to be refrigerated because they may be kept in stock for a long period of time. *(3)*

50. **(E)** Isotretinoin (Accutane) is a vitamin A derivative indicated for the treatment of recalcitrant cystic acne in patients who do not respond to more conservative therapy. Approximately 90% of patients using this product experience cheilitis, a cracking around the margin of the lips. Elevation of lipid levels may also occur. Isotretinoin is a category X drug and it, therefore, should not be used in pregnant women. *(3)*

51. **(E)** Fluids employed in TPN are generally very hypertonic and hyperosmotic. Until the technique of subclavian vein catheterization was perfected, it was too irritating and inflammatory to use the usual sites of IV administration. Peripheral veins are seldom used in the administration of hypertonic nutrient solutions because blood flow is insufficient to provide the necessary dilution of the fluid to protect the intima of the vessel. The exception occurs when the slightly hypertonic amino acid solutions containing limited amounts of dextrose are administered. *(1)*

52. **(D)** Timentin, is a combination of ticarcillin and clavulanate potassium (a beta-lactamase inhibitor). Augmentin contains amoxacillin and clavulanate. Since clavulanate is a beta-lactamase inhibitor, these products would be suitable for this patient. Amikin, which contains amikacin (an aminoglycoside), is primarily effective against serious gram-negative infections. *(3)*

53. **(E)** Use of sustained-release nifedipine products, as well as some other sustained-release drug products, may cause what appears to be an intact, undissolved, tablet in the stool. This is the plastic matrix from which the drug diffused and it is devoid of the active drug. *(3)*

54. **(B)** Suddenly discontinuing the administration of dextrose solution may cause a rebound hypoglycemia in response to the sudden elimination of the sustained glucose load of the TPN solution. It is best to maintain the patient on a nominal amount of dextrose such as D_5W or to wean the patient slowly from the TPN solution.

    (E, incorrect)—Hyperchloremic metabolic acidosis may occur during TPN therapy when the total chloride ion content is high. The amino acids in the protein salts are usually chloride or hydrochloride salts. Additional amounts of chloride are obtained when sodium or potassium chlorides are added to the TPN solutions. It may be useful to supply either sodium or potassium as acetate salts.

    (C, incorrect)—Hyperosmotic nonketotic hyperglycemia is a result of infusing an overload of glucose. Causes include an overly rapid infusion rate, dextrose solutions that are too concentrated, and malfunction of pancreatic secretion of insulin. *(14)*

55. **(D)** Long-chain triglycerides are fats that provide approximately 9 kcal/g. Ethanol provides approximately 7 kcal/g, hydrous dextrose provides approximately 3.4 kcal/g and protein provides approximately 3 to 4 kcal/g. *(3)*

56. **(E)** Dolasetron (Anzemet) is an orally administered selective 5-HT$_3$ receptor antagonist used to prevent nausea and vomiting associated with cancer chemotherapy. The usual dosage regimen for this drug is 100 mg given 1 hour prior to initiating chemotherapy. *(3)*

57. **(E)** Amiloride is a potassium-sparing diuretic with a mechanism of action similar to that of triamterene. Both drugs exert a diuretic effect by promoting the exchange of sodium for potassium in the distal portion of the renal tubule. In contrast to spironolactone, neither of these drugs inhibits aldosterone. Metolazone and chlorthalidone are thiazide-like diuretics. *(3)*

58. **(E)** Treatment of hyperkalemia can be approached by three methods. First, in the presence of ECG changes, calcium should be given to counteract the effects of excess potassium on the heart. Second, bicarbonate or glucose plus insulin can be used to shift potassium rapidly from extracellular to intracellular fluid compartments. Third, exchange resins such as sodium polystyrene sulfonate (Kayexalate) or dialysis can be used to remove potassium from the body. In this case, because there are no symptoms of ECG changes, the rectal administration of sodium polystyrene sulfonate (enemas containing 50 g in 70% sorbitol solution) is the most appropriate option. *(14)*

59. **(B)** Fondaparinux (Arixtra) is a synthetic pentasaccharide. The five-sugar sequence that comprises this product is the same as the fraction of heparin that binds to antithrombin. Dalteparin sodium (Fragmin) and enoxaparin sodium (Lovenox) are low-molecular-weight heparin products prepared from porcine (pork) heparin. They are administered subcutaneously only to prevent DVTs. It is not necessary to monitor APTT when a patient is using any of these fractionated heparin products. *(3)*

60. **(E)** Miglitol (Glyset) is an alpha-glucosidase inhibitor. Saxagliptin (Onglyza) is a dipeptidyl peptidase-4 (DPP-4) inhibitor that increases insulin secretion after meals when glucose levels are elevated. Pioglitazone (Actos) enhances insulin receptor sensitivity. All are indicated for the treatment of type 2 diabetes mellitus. *(3)*

61. **(B)** When administered parenterally, lorazepam (Ativan) is a rapidly acting anticonvulsant

with fewer tendencies to produce respiratory depression than the barbiturates. It has become a common choice for initial therapy of status epilepticus. *(14)*

62. **(D)** Chronic administration of procainamide has been associated with the development of a syndrome clinically indistinguishable from disseminated lupus erythematosus. This lupus-like syndrome (fever, arthralgia, splenomegaly, edema, and the presence of lupus erythematosus cells in the peripheral blood) has also been associated with hydralazine use. *(6)*

63. **(C)** Vitamin B_6 (pyridoxine) use by patients using levodopa may decrease the effectiveness of levodopa by promoting the peripheral decarboxylation of levodopa by dopadecarboxylase. This is not a problem in patients using levodopa in combination with carbidopa (Sinemet). *(6)*

64. **(D)** Atenolol (Tenormin) blocks beta-adrenergic receptors. It differs from pindolol primarily in that it has some preferential effect on $beta_1$-adrenoreceptors, which are located chiefly in the cardiac muscle. This preferential effect is not absolute and, at higher doses, atenolol may also inhibit $beta_2$-adrenoreceptors, which are located chiefly in bronchial and vascular musculature. Although the mechanism of its antihypertensive effect is not known, the drug is indicated in the management of hypertension either alone or in combination with other antihypertensive drugs. *(6)*

65. **(C)** Prazosin (Minipress) is an $alpha_1$-adrenergic blocker that causes peripheral vasodilation. Side effects of therapy may include a precipitous fall in blood pressure, possibly accompanied by tachycardia and syncope following the first several doses. Other *"sin"* drugs, such as terazosin (Hytrin) and doxazosin (Cardura), may also produce this "first dose" effect. *(6)*

66. **(E)** CD4 cells are a type of T lymphocytes whose primary role is to stimulate other cells in the immune response. The lower the level of these cells in the patient's blood, the more susceptible the patient becomes to the development of opportunistic infections such as PCP. *(14)*

67. **(D)** Nitroprusside has marked antihypertensive activity when given by IV infusion. It appears to lower blood pressure by relaxing vascular smooth muscle, thereby dilating peripheral arteries and veins. Solutions of nitroprusside must be protected from light. Discolored solutions or those with visible particulate matter should be discarded. Excessive doses may produce symptoms of cyanide poisoning. *(6)*

68. **(B)** Aripiprazole (Abilify) is an atypical or second-generation antipsychotic agent used for the treatment of schizophrenia and bipolar disorder.

69. **(E)** Tobramycin sulfate is the salt of a weak base and a strong acid. Combining such a drug with alkaline drugs, such as those listed, will result in a chemical incompatibility. *(6)*

70. **(D)** All of the agents listed, except metoclopramide, are employed in the treatment of *H. pylori*-related peptic ulcer disease. Metoclopramide (Reglan) is an antiemetic and prokinetic agent used in treating GERD and diabetic gastroparesis. *(6)*

71. **(E)** Cholestyramine is a basic anion exchange resin. This quaternary ammonium chloride compound exchanges the chloride ion for the negatively charged bile acids, thereby preventing their reabsorption. Cholestyramine binds many organic acids, including warfarin, levothyroxine, and phenytoin. *(6)*

72. **(B)** If drug B has a greater affinity (ie, a higher association constant) for specific protein-binding sites than does drug A, it will have a tendency to displace drug A from these sites. Furthermore, if drug B is given in large doses, the degree of this displacement will increase because there will be a greater amount of drug B competing with drug A for the binding sites. *(6)*

73. **(D)** When large doses of acetaminophen are consumed and/or the metabolic capacity of the liver has been impaired by alcohol or by disease, there may be insufficient glutathione present to metabolize toxic metabolites that have formed. *N*-Acetylcysteine (Acetadote) is a specific acetaminophen antidote that prevents the accumulation of these toxic metabolites. *(6)*

74. **(E)** Anagrelide (Agrylin), dipyridamole (Persantine), and clopidogrel (Plavix) each exhibit antiplatelet action. *(6)*

75. **(C)** Penetration of the cornea by *P. aeruginosa* will often lead to destruction of the cornea and interior portions of the eye. Blindness may result. This organism is a common contaminant in water. The need for sterility of ophthalmic products is well recognized. *(6)*

76. **(D)** Boils caused by *Staphylococcus* organisms form in the anterior portion of the external auditory meatus. They are usually self-limiting, and treatment with antibiotic ointments prevents spreading. *(14)*

77. **(A)** Idoxuridine is an antimetabolite that inhibits the replication of viral DNA with greater selectivity than does that of the host cell. It is used primarily in the treatment of herpes simplex keratitis, a disease of viral origin that can cause blindness. *(6)*

78. **(A)** Although tolnaftate is effective against several types of fungi, it is ineffective against *Candida* organisms. Miconazole, clotrimazole, and amphotericin (Fungizone) are relatively broad-spectrum antifungal agents with activity against some species of *Candida*. *(3)*

79. **(E)** Tolterodine (Detrol) is muscarinic receptor antagonist (anticholinergic) that is used in treating symptoms of overactive bladder, including incontinence, urinary frequency, and urgency. *(3)*

80. **(D)** Complications of systemic corticosteroid therapy are usually related to the length of time that they have been administered and the dosage used. Corticosteroids suppress normal tissue responses to infection (increasing susceptibility to infection) and allow further dissemination of existing infections. Because tissue responses to infection are suppressed, the subjective, objective, and laboratory manifestations of infection may be masked. Corticosteroids may also cause sodium and water retention and increased likelihood of cataract development. *(6)*

81. **(E)** Normal fasting blood sugar values for adults range from 80 to 120 mg/dL (or 80–120 mg%). When the fasting blood sugar levels exceed 120 mg/dL, diabetes mellitus should be suspected. Levels below 60 mg/dL may suggest insulin overdosage, glucagon deficiencies, and/or hypoactivity of various endocrine glands. *(6)*

82. **(E)** The administration of pharmacological doses (0.4 mg/d or more) of folic acid can stimulate reticulocytosis and improve the anemia associated with vitamin B_{12} deficiency. However, folic acid administration does not prevent the development or progression of the neurologic manifestations of pernicious anemia. *(6)*

83. **(D)** Clomiphene citrate (Clomid) is a nonsteroidal estrogen agonist–antagonist that causes the hypothalamus to release gonadotropin-releasing hormone. This increases the peripheral concentrations of FSH and LH and promotes ovulation. *(6)*

84. **(E)** Glossitis may occur when the tongue is either acutely or chronically inflamed. This may be the result of infection, trauma, pernicious anemia, or chemical or thermal injury. *(14)*

85. **(D)** Angiotensin converting enzyme (ACE) inhibitors such as fosinopril and other *"pril"* drugs may increase serum creatinine levels. Serum creatinine concentration should be checked in all patients within 1 week of starting ACE inhibitor therapy, and rechecked if clinical conditions change or medications are changed. ACE inhibitor therapy should be

stopped if the serum creatinine concentrations increase by more than 1 mg/dL. *(6)*

86. **(A)** Whole blood treated with anticoagulant is centrifuged in a calibrated hematocrit tube. The volume ratio of the packed red blood cells to total blood volume is determined. The hematocrit is normally 39 to 49 for men and 33 to 43 for women. It gives some indication of both the number and the size of the red blood cells present in an individual. *(14)*

87. **(B)** A reticulocyte is an immature erythrocyte (red blood cell). *(14)*

88. **(A)** Amoxicillin is an effective drug for the treatment of otitis media. The other choices are either unlikely to be active against organisms that commonly cause otitis media or they are too toxic to use in young children. *(3)*

89. **(E)** Aspirin, ibuprofen, and acetaminophen are capable of reducing elevated body temperature by altering the hypothalamic set-point. *(11)*

90. **(A)** Clozapine (Clozaril) is an antipsychotic agent that is used to treat patients with severe schizophrenia, who do not respond to standard antipsychotic treatment. The drug is capable of causing agranulocytosis, a potentially life-threatening adverse drug reaction. Patients who are to receive the drug should have a baseline white blood cell and differential count performed before the initiation of treatment. Once therapy has begun, a white blood cell count should be performed weekly for the first 6 months. After 6 months of therapy, the patient should have testing done every 2 weeks. At the end of 1 year of continuous monitoring, the patient need only get bloodwork done every 4 weeks. *(3)*

91. **(B)** Zollinger–Ellison syndrome is a condition characterized by gastric acid hypersecretion and recurrent peptic ulceration. It is generally the result of a gastrin-producing tumor. The proton pump inhibitors such as pantoprazole (Protonix) are effective in managing the acid secretion in this condition. *(3)*

92. **(E)** The administration of a drug by intermittent (rather than continuous) IV injection is accomplished over a period of minutes (rather than hours). Stability and/or compatibility problems are less likely to occur because the drug does not remain in contact with a large-volume IV fluid for long periods of time. The potential for thrombophlebitis is reduced because the drug is not in constant contact with the blood vessel tissue at the site of the injection. Finally, the greater concentration gradient produced by a more rapid injection may promote better diffusion of some drugs into tissues. *(1)*

93. **(D)** Vinblastine, vinorelbine (Navelbine), and other vinca alkaloids such as vincristine are considered to be mitotic inhibitors. Paclitaxel (Taxol) and docetaxel (Taxotere) are taxanes. They are also antimitotic agents. *(3)*

94. **(E)** Aspirin should be avoided during the last trimester of pregnancy. Aspirin exerts a dose-dependent action on uric acid excretion. *(11)*

95. **(A)** *Martindale's Extra Pharmacopoeia* is probably one of the most comprehensive, international, single-volume references on drugs and drug products. *Martindale's* is divided into three parts: The first part consists of monographs on drugs and ancillary substances. (Although drugs that are manufactured in the United Kingdom are stressed, generic and proprietary products from many other countries are included.) The monographs include physiochemical data, storage, incompatibilities, uses, doses, and toxic effects. The second part contains a supplementary discussion of new drugs, obsolete drugs, and miscellaneous substances. The third part lists formulas of OTC products sold in the United Kingdom. There is also a directory of worldwide pharmaceutical manufacturers. *(1)*

96. **(B)** Collaginase (Santyl) is a debriding agent that helps to remove necrotic material from a wound. The other two choices are tissue plasminogen activators used as thrombolytic agents. *(14)*

97. **(D)** Ceftriaxone (Rocephin) and cefotaxime (Claforan) are third-generation cephalosporins while cefprozil (Cefzil) is a second-generation cephalosporin. Third-generation cephalosporins are more effective in treating CNS infections, such as meningitis, because they penetrate the CNS better than first- or second-generation agents. *(3)*

98. **(B)** Penciclovir (Denavir) is an antiviral drug that is indicated specifically for the treatment of herpes labialis or cold sores. It is applied topically at the earliest sign of a fever blister and should be applied every 2 hours, while awake, for 4 days. If applied appropriately, this agent will generally reduce the severity and duration of cold sore symptoms. *(3)*

99. **(A)** Natamycin (Natacyn) is an antibiotic that has antifungal activity. It is used as an intraocular suspension for the treatment of fungal blepharitis, conjunctivitis, and keratitis. *(3)*

100. **(B)** Plantago (psyllium) is a bulk-forming laxative agent. Patients using it should mix the dose with a glass of water or other fluid and drink it down quickly. This should be followed with more fluids. *(11)*

101. **(A)** The relative concentration of different anions and cations varies considerably between intracellular and extracellular fluids of the body. Intracellular body fluids contain high concentrations of potassium (a cation) and phosphate (an anion), whereas extracellular fluid contains high concentrations of sodium (a cation) and chloride (an anion). *(14)*

102. **(E)** Acute toxicity associated with an overdose of the anticholinergic drug atropine sulfate may be treated by the administration of the cholinergic compound physostigmine. *(6)*

103. **(A)** There is a reciprocal relationship between the concentration of calcium and phosphorus in the blood. For example, hypoparathyroidism is characterized by low serum calcium and high serum phosphorus, whereas hyperparathy-roidism is characterized by low serum phosphorus and high serum calcium. *(14)*

104. **(D)** Nicotine polacrilex contains nicotine bound to an ion exchange resin in a chewing gum base. It is used to assist smokers in their withdrawal from cigarette use. The drug may cause peripheral vasoconstriction, tachycardia, and high blood pressure, so it should be avoided in patients with severe angina. The drug is also classified in pregnancy category X, meaning that it should not be used in pregnant women. *(3)*

105. **(A)** Acetaminophen is metabolized in the liver primarily by conjugation to glucuronide or sulfate metabolites. A small percentage is metabolized by the hepatic cytochrome P450 mixed-function oxidase system to a toxic intermediate metabolite. Normally, this metabolite is preferentially conjugated to glutathione and excreted in the urine. When large doses of acetaminophen are ingested, the glucuronide and sulfate pathways become saturated, and stores of glutathione become inadequate to conjugate the amount of toxic metabolite that is produced. The metabolite binds covalently to hepatocytes and produces hepatic necrosis. *(6)*

106. **(C)** MS Contin is a potent analgesic product that contains morphine sulfate. Because the drug was ingested 3 hours ago, the likelihood of removing a large amount of drug from this patient's stomach with ipecac syrup is small. Activated charcoal could bind some of the drug if given soon after ingestion, but its use here is also unlikely to be of value because of the elapsed time. Naloxone is a pure narcotic antagonist that would be a specific antidote for the effects of systemic morphine toxicity. *(14)*

107. **(E)** Because of the poor absorption of sulfasalazine from the GI tract, its localized activity is valuable as one of the first-line treatments for various forms of colitis and enteritis. In the gut, sulfasalazine is broken down into sulfapyridine and mesalamine. The drug is available as an oral tablet (Azulfidine) and as a suspension. *(3)*

108. (D) Ritonavir (Norvir), a protease inhibitor, is a potent enzyme inhibitor. It is, therefore, often combined with other protease inhibitors in order to inhibit their metabolic rate and thereby "boost" their plasma concentration. *(11)*

109. (D) Nonselective beta-adrenergic blocking agents may cause bronchoconstriction. In addition, the drugs may mask the effects of hypoglycemia, thereby placing type 1 diabetic patients (IDDM) at risk. These drugs are often useful in treating patients with supraventricular tachyarrhythmias. *(3)*

110. (B) Bumetanide is a loop diuretic that is capable of producing ototoxicity, which would enhance the similar toxicity produced by gentamicin. *(3)*

111. (A) Treprostinil (Remodulin) is a prostaglandin used to treat the primary symptoms of pulmonary hypertension. Treprostinil relaxes blood vessels, thereby increasing blood flow to the lungs and reducing the workload on the heart. *(3)*

112. (C) Left ventricular failure is associated with bronchial edema, increased airway resistance, and dyspnea. In addition, orthopnea (dyspnea that occurs while the patient is in the supine position) also often occurs. Peripheral edema is more likely to occur with right ventricular failure. *(14)*

113. (B) For a healthy adult, values of <200 mg/dL are considered desirable levels of total cholesterol, <150 mg/dL for triglycerides, and a value of <130 mg/dL is a desirable level for low-density lipoproteins (LDL) cholesterol. Desirable levels may be considerably lower in patients with one or more risk factors such as hypertension and diabetes. *(14)*

114. (C) Selegeline (Eldepryl) is an MAO-B inhibitor used to treat Parkinson's disease. It may interact with pressor amines such as tyramine in some cheeses, wines, and beers to produce a hypertensive crisis that may be life threatening. *(6)*

115. (D) Frequent urination (polyuria) is a common symptom of diabetes mellitus. *(14)*

116. (D) Impetigo is a bacterial condition that may cause the formation of blisters or sores on the face and hands. It is one of the most common skin conditions of children. Most common causative organisms are Group A *Streptococcus* or *S. aureus*. Mupirocin (Bactroban) is specifically indicated for the topical treatment of impetigo. *(14)*

117. (B) Blepharitis is a condition characterized by chronic inflammation of the eyelids. This may result in redness, itching, and tearing of the eye. Often, antimicrobial and/or anti-inflammatory ophthalmic products are used to treat this condition. *(14)*

118. (E) Bupropion (Wellbutrin) is indicated for the treatment of depression. The product Zyban, which contains bupropion as its active ingredient, is used as a smoking deterrent in smoking cessation programs. Bupropion is also indicated for the treatment of seasonal affective disorder (SAD). *(3)*

119. (D) Tardive (late-occurring) dyskinesia (involuntary muscular movements) is a drug-induced neurologic disorder that appears to be irreversible and unresponsive to drug treatment. It is characterized by involuntary movements of the lips, tongue, or jaw and is commonly observed as a smacking of the lips, rhythmical movement of the tongue, or facial grimaces. This disorder may be due to hypersensitivity of dopaminergic receptors to endogenous dopamine after long-term blockade by antipsychotic drugs.

(A, incorrect)—Akathisia is a feeling of restlessness or a compelling need for movement. *(6)*

120. (A) Irbesartan (Avapro) is an angiotensin II-receptor antagonist. It is employed in the treatment of hypertension. *(3)*

121. (C) Lyme disease is caused by the bacterium *Borrelia burgdorferi*, a spirochete, and is transmitted to humans by the bite of infected blacklegged ticks. If not treated, infection can spread to joints, the heart, and the nervous system. *(14)*

122. **(E)** Olsalazine is a salicylate compound that is converted to 5-aminosalicylic acid (mesalamine) in the gut. This agent produces an anti-inflammatory effect in the gut. It is used to treat ulcerative colitis. *(3)*

123. **(A)** Prednisone is approximately four times more potent than hydrocortisone. Because this patient was receiving a total daily dose of 200 mg of hydrocortisone, an equivalent anti-inflammatory dose of prednisone would be 50 mg/d. *(3)*

124. **(D)** Glucocorticoids associated with a lesser degree of mineralocorticoid activity (eg, dexamethasone, triamcinolone, methylprednisolone, and betamethasone) should be used in patients with conditions such as congestive heart failure in which sodium retention can be an aggravating factor. Because all glucocorticoids can induce potassium loss, regardless of their mineralocorticoid activity, even dexamethasone should be used with caution in this patient. *(6)*

125. **(B)** Mitoxantrone (Novantrone) is available as a deep blue solution intended for parenteral use. Patients who receive this drug may experience a bluish tinge in the whites of their eyes and may have their urine turn into blue-green color for about 24 hours after the drug has been administered. Doxorubicin causes a red color change in patients who receive parenteral doses of it.

126. **(E)** None of these agents would be appropriate for the treatment of acute bronchospastic attacks because they are only indicated for asthma prophylaxis. *(3)*

127. **(D)** Ibuprofen and naproxen each come in both a solid and a liquid oral dosage form while ketoprofen does not. *(3)*

128. **(E)** Lanoxicaps contain digoxin in a more bioavailable form than in digoxin tablets. A 20% reduction in dosage is generally required to achieve a comparable therapeutic response with Lanoxin tablets. *(3)*

129. **(A)** Rifampin is a potent microsomal enzyme inducer and may reduce effectiveness of hormones supplied by oral contraceptive products. *(3)*

130. **(D)** Carbamazepine (Tegretol) is indicated for the treatment of trigeminal neuralgia, a painful disorder affecting the trigeminal nerve. It is also used for the treatment of acute mania as well as for prophylaxis of bipolar disorder. *(6)*

131. **(E)** Naltrexone (Revia) is a pure opioid antagonist that is used to reverse opioid effects. It has a longer duration of effect than naloxone (Narcan) and is, therefore, more effective in reversing the effects of long-acting opioid compounds. *(3)*

132. **(E)** Each of these agents exerts an antifungal action against *Candida* (yeast) organisms. *(3)*

133. **(C)** Mild polycythemia is normal in persons who exercise excessively and in persons who live at high altitudes. Polycythemia vera is a state in which the rate of red cell production is far greater than normal, even though there is no apparent physiologic need for the increased production. It is believed that this disease may result from a malignancy of the bone marrow stem cells. Phlebotomy whenever the hematocrit rises higher than 55% may suffice as the only treatment for patients who do not have severe thrombocytosis. Drugs used to treat polycythemia include busulfan (Myleran) and radioactive phosphorus ^{32}P. *(14)*

134. **(D)** Protamine is a strongly basic substance that combines with the strongly acidic heparin to produce a stable salt with loss of anticoagulant activity. Because protamine itself possesses anticoagulant properties, it is unwise to administer more than 50 mg of protamine over a short period of time unless it is known that there is a definite need for a larger amount. *(6)*

135. **(A)** Salmeterol (Serevent) is the longest acting of these beta$_2$-adrenergic agonists. Its duration

of action is greater than 12 hours. Isoetharine has the shortest duration (0.5–2.0 h), while the others have an intermediate duration of approximately 4 to 8 hours. *(3)*

136. **(A)** Although monitoring the PT of the mother closely can minimize the risk of hemorrhage in the fetus, it is probably best to use heparin if anticoagulant therapy is necessary. Because heparin is a high molecular weight mucopolysaccharide, it does not cross the placenta and enter the fetal circulation. *(6)*

137. **(E)** Rizatriptan (Maxalt) is a 5-HT$_1$ receptor agonist used to abort a migraine headache. It is contraindicated in patients with angina pectoris, previous myocardial infarction, and/or uncontrolled hypertension. It should also not be used if a patient has used an ergotamine derivative within the past 24 hours, or within 2 weeks after discontinuing use of the MAO inhibitor. *(3)*

138. **(D)** Acute uncomplicated urinary infections are most commonly caused by *E. coli*. Such infections are most common in women and are characterized by the presence of dysuria, urinary urgency, and suprapubic discomfort. *(14)*

139. **(B)** In normal individuals, more than 50% of an oral dose of cyanocobalamin (vitamin B$_{12}$) is absorbed from the GI tract. This absorption occurs only in the presence of the intrinsic factor of Castle, with which the vitamin must presumably combine in order to pass through the intestinal walls. By means of radioactive cobalt–labeled cyanocobalamin, it has been shown that more than one-half of an oral dose soon appears in the blood. Normally, only a small amount of radioactivity appears in the urine. However, if a large flushing dose (1,000 mg) of cyanocobalamin is given parenterally within an hour of the tagged oral dose, the renal threshold for cyanocobalamin is exceeded and radioactivity is observed in the urine. In patients with pernicious anemia, there is a deficiency in intrinsic factor that results in poor absorption of the radioactive cyanocobalamin. Most of the radioactivity in these patients will be detected in the feces. *(6)*

140. **(C)** Lipodystrophy is either the breakdown or the accumulation of subcutaneous fat at the insulin injection site. It can best be avoided by having the patient rotate the site of insulin injection so that the same site is not used more frequently than once every 30 days. *(14)*

141. **(B)** Insulin aspart (NovoLog) is a rapidly acting insulin. The onset of action takes about 15 minutes and its peak action occurs within 30 to 90 minutes. This form of insulin is generally given 15 minutes before a meal to permit effective utilization of the dietary glucose that is absorbed. *(3)*

142. **(B)** Liraglutide (Victoza) is a glucagon-like peptide (GLP-1) agonist that is used as an adjunct to diet and exercise to improve diabetic control in patients with type 2 diabetes. It works to increase insulin release in the presence of increased levels of glucose in the body. It is available in a pen device that contains multiple doses of the drug. One dose of the drug is administered subcutaneously daily at any time. Before the pen device is used for the first time, it should be stored in a refrigerator, but not frozen. Once the pen device begins to be used by the patient it may be stored at controlled room temperature for up to 30 days. When used with insulin secretagogues, liraglutide can increase the likelihood of hypoglycemia. *(10)*

143. **(C)** Lycopene is a carotenoid that contains 13 double bonds. This makes it a useful compound that is capable of neutralizing free radicals, substances that have been associated with the development of aging, cancers, and other degenerative diseases. Foods that have a deep red color, such as tomatoes, watermelon, guava, and pink grapefruit tend to have high levels of lycopene in the *trans* form. Processing these foods, particularly with heat, tends to convert the *trans* form of the lycopene into the *cis* form, which is more biologically active. (6)

144. **(C)** Morphine and its chemical derivatives commonly cause respiratory depression, nausea, and constipation. *(6)*

145. **(A)** Combination oral contraceptive products usually contain norethindrone (a progestin) and ethinyl estradiol (an estrogen). The estrogen component suppresses the production of FSH and LH and thereby prevents ovulation. The progestin component increases the viscosity of cervical mucus and makes the endometrial lining of the uterus less receptive to the implantation of a fertilized ovum. *(6)*

146. **(D)** Zanamivir (Relenza) and oseltamivir (Tamiflu) are antiviral drugs used for the treatment of uncomplicated influenza A or B. In order to be effective, therapy with these agents must begin within 2 days of symptom onset. Zanamivir is administered as a powder for inhalation using a Diskhaler device while oseltamivir is administered orally. For treatment of influenza A or B, these medications should be administered twice daily for 5 days. Valacyclovir (Valtrex) is used to treat *Herpes simplex* and *Herpes zoster* (shingles). *(3)*

147. **(C)** The usual method of treating an acute hypoglycemic reaction is to give glucose orally or, in unconscious patients, by IV in concentrated solutions. However, if these routes cannot be used, 0.5 to 1 mg of glucagon may be given SC or IM as well as IV. Glucagon is an endogenous hormone produced by the alpha cells of the pancreatic Islet of Langerhans. Glucagon increases blood glucose by stimulating hepatic gluconeogenesis and glycogenolysis. *(3)*

148. **(A)** Zidovudine (AZT, Retrovir) is a nucleoside reverse transcriptase inhibitor that is employed in treating pregnant women who are HIV-positive in order to reduce the likelihood of transmission of the virus to their offspring. When used in this manner, zidovudine is administered orally to the pregnant women during the second and third trimesters of pregnancy. During labor, an IV dose of zidovudine is administered. After delivery zidovudine is administered orally to the newborn for approximately 6 weeks. *(14)*

149. **(E)** Dopamine exerts a positive inotropic effect by direct action on beta-adrenergic receptors and causes a release of norepinephrine from storage sites. A major advantage of the drug is that controlling the infusion rate can vary its hemodynamic effects. *(6)*

150. **(D)** Ovrette and Nor-QD are oral contraceptive products that contain only progestin. Although they are not as effective as combination oral contraceptive products, they are useful for women who cannot take estrogen-containing products or who wish to use an oral contraceptive product while they are breastfeeding. Yaz is a combination oral contraceptive that contains drospirinone and ethinyl estradiol. *(3)*

151. **(A)** In the iron-deficient state, the iron storage compartment becomes depleted. This is followed by a reduction in plasma transferrin saturation. Subsequently, the number and size of the erythrocytes as well as their hemoglobin content will be decreased. The lack of hemoglobin causes the erythrocytes to become pale (hypochromic) in color. *(14)*

152. **(C)** Estring is an intravaginal ring that contains 2 mg of estradiol. When inserted into the vagina it releases a consistent amount of estrogen for 90 days. It is used to treat postmenopausal vaginal symptoms such as atrophy and dryness. *(3)*

153. **(B)** Calcitonin salmon (Miacalcin, Fortical) is used once daily as a nasal spray in women who are at least 5 years postmenopausal in order to retard the progressive loss of bone mass. It is used in conjunction with adequate calcium and vitamin D intake. The product should be stored in the refrigerator. *(10)*

154. **(C)** The development of inflammatory conditions of the colon (eg, nonspecific colitis or a more severe pseudomembranous colitis) has been associated with antibiotic therapy. Although many antibiotics have been implicated, there have been a disproportionate number of reports specifically involving clindamycin and lincomycin. Colitis has been associated with both oral and parenteral administration of these drugs, and no clear predisposing conditions have been identified.

Because antiperistaltic drugs (eg, loperamide, diphenoxalate) used to treat the resulting diarrhea seem to prolong the disease (probably by retaining the toxins produced by the *Clostridium* causative organism), they should not be used. *(3)*

155. **(D)** Loperamide (Imodium) inhibits peristaltic activity by a direct effect on the musculature of the intestinal wall. Loperamide appears to be devoid of opiate-like effects. *(3)*

156. **(A)** Mirena is an intrauterine contraceptive device (IUD) that releases levonorgestrel over a period of 5 years. It, therefore, does not require any conscious need to remember to take doses and could be an appropriate product for this patient. Natazia is a quadphasic oral contraceptive product that would also be a poor choice for a forgetful patient. Clomid is an antiestrogen product used to promote ovulation and pregnancy. *(3)*

157. **(E)** Felodipine (Plendil) is a calcium channel blocking agent used in treating angina and hypertension. When taken with grapefruit juice, there is evidence that the AUC of felodipine will be increased. Therefore, grapefruit juice should be avoided when using this product. *(3)*

158. **(D)** Cocaine, like the amphetamines, is a potent CNS stimulant. The other agents listed are CNS depressants. *(6)*

159. **(A)** Acetaminophen will not displace warfarin from its protein-binding sites or interfere with warfarin metabolism. It is less likely therefore to cause a therapeutic problem in this patient. All of the other choices either have a high affinity for plasma proteins or may alter warfarin absorption or metabolism. *(6)*

160. **(E)** Valsartan (Diovan) is an angiotensin II receptor blocker (ARB) that is used to treat hypertension. ARB drugs, unlike ACE inhibitors, are not as likely to cause angioedema or nonproductive cough. *(3)*

161. **(D)** Each gram of protein supplies about 4 kcal, each gram of carbohydrate supplies about

4 kcal, and each gram of fat supplies about 9 kcal. It is obvious, therefore, that strictly on a weight basis, fats are better caloric sources than are other nutrients. *(14)*

162. **(D)** Leucovorin calcium is a derivative of folic acid used as an antidote for drugs used as folic acid antagonists such as methotrexate. *(6)*

163. **(D)** Pedialyte is an orally administered electrolyte solution containing dextrose; potassium chloride; and sodium, calcium, and magnesium salts. It is used to supply water and electrolytes in a balanced proportion in order to prevent serious deficits from occurring in patients suffering from mild to moderate fluid loss. The product does not contain protein or fat. *(3)*

164. **(A)** Each gram of dextrose supplies approximately 3.4 kcal of energy to a patient. Because a liter of dextrose 5% solution contains 50 g of dextrose, the administration of the liter will supply the patient with approximately 170 kcal. *(1)*

165. **(A)** Hepatitis B vaccine (Engerix-B) is used to immunize people of all ages against all known subtypes of hepatitis B virus. It must be stored in a refrigerator and is usually administered IM. *(3)*

166. **(A)** Prostate-specific antigen (PSA) is a glycoprotein produced only by prostate cells. Levels of PSA are determined for prostate cancer screening. PSA levels may also be elevated in men with acute prostatitis or BPH. *(14)*

167. **(A)** Of the drugs listed, erythromycin has the lowest degree of toxicity and the spectrum of action most similar to penicillin. Demeclocycline may inhibit skeletal growth in the fetus. Deposition of tetracyclines in the teeth of the fetus has been associated with enamel defects and staining of the teeth. Trimethoprim is a teratogenic drug. *(3)*

168. **(D)** Silver sulfadiazine (Silvadene) cream applied topically to burns has been found to be quite effective in inhibiting the invasion of the affected site by both gram-positive and gram-negative bacteria. The cream is usually

applied to a thickness of about 1/16 in twice daily over the entire burned surface. Mafenide (Sulfamylon) cream is also used topically for the same purpose. *(3)*

169. **(A)** The drug of choice in treating most forms of gonorrhea is ceftriaxone (Rocephin). The drug is generally given in a single 125 mg IM dose. In patients who cannot tolerate a beta-lactam antimicrobial agent, ciprofloxacin (Cipro) 500 mg PO once or Ofloxacin (Floxin) 400 mg PO once may be given instead. *(14)*

170. **(A)** Indomethacin (Indocin) and other NSAIDs are effective agents in the treatment of acute gouty arthritis. They act by reducing the joint inflammation responsible for the excruciating pain associated with the disease. *(6)*

171. **(E)** Metoclopramide exerts a potent antiemetic effect by inhibiting dopamine receptors in the chemoreceptor trigger zone of the brain. It also stimulates GI motility and increases the rate of gastric emptying. This enhances the antiemetic activity by eliminating stasis that precedes vomiting. All of the other drugs listed, decrease the rate of gastric emptying. *(6)*

172. **(E)** Most antiparkinson agents act by increasing dopaminergic activity. *(6)*

173. **(C)** Galantamine (Razadyne) is an acetylcholinesterase inhibitor and memantine (Namenda) is a NMDA receptor used in treating Alzheimer's disease. Clomipramine is a tricyclic antidepressant used for obsessive–compulsive disorder. *(3)*

174. **(C)** Metformin is a biguanide that, in rare cases, may cause lactic acidosis. This is a condition that may be fatal in 50% of cases. *(6)*

175. **(D)** Inserting a clinical thermometer into either the mouth or rectum can make a satisfactory approximation of the temperature of the internal organs. Both of these are closed cavities with good blood supply. The accepted average oral temperature is 98.6°F, with the recognition that both individual and diurnal

variations occur regularly. The rectum is about 1°F warmer. Rectal and oral thermometers have the same temperature scales and markings, differing only in the shape of the bulb. To avoid the potential confusion and errors in subtracting or adding degrees from readings, physicians prefer that the actual temperature and the method be reported; for instance, 102.5°F taken rectally. *(1)*

176. **(E)** Immediate treatment of the burn is recommended. Application of cold water will often reduce the severity of the burn. The burn area should be kept in cold water until no further pain is experienced whether in or out of the water. If necessary, a physician may then be contacted. *(14)*

177. **(A)** Montelukast sodium (Singulair) is an orally active leukotriene receptor antagonist used to provide prophylaxis and chronic treatment of asthma. It should be taken daily to prevent asthma attacks, even when the patient is asymptomatic. If required, rapid-acting bronchodilator drugs may be used to control acute attacks. *(6)*

178. **(C)** Pilocarpine is a cholinergic drug that produces a miotic effect (pupillary constriction). It does not affect carbonic anhydrase. *(6)*

179. **(C)** Amiodarone (Cordarone) is a Class III antiarrhythmic agent that can produce a number of serious adverse effects including visual impairment, pulmonary toxicity, and proarrhythmic effects. *(6)*

180. **(A)** Tropicamide is parasympatholytic agent used ophthalmically as a mydriatic, particularly to facilitate eye examinations. Mydriatic drugs may exascerbate narrow-angle glaucoma. Dorzolamide is a carbonic anhydrase inhibitor and latanoprost is prostaglandin derivative. Both of these agents are useful in glaucoma treatment. *(3)*

181. **(A)** Vitamin E has a number of synonyms. They include tocopherol, alpha-tocopherol, tocotrienol, etc *(11)*

182. **(A)** GoLYTELY is a bowel evacuant product that is used to cleanse the bowel prior to GI examination. It contains polyethylene glycol and a mixture of electrolytes that must be reconstituted with water before it is administered. The usual dose is 4 L of reconstituted solution consumed in doses of 240 mL every 10 minutes, until the contents of the container have been consumed or the rectal effluent is clear. *(3)*

183. **(A)** Xenical (Orlistat, Alli) is a lipase inhibitor that inhibits the absorption of dietary fats. It is used in the management of obesity by having patients to take one 120 mg capsule of the drug three times daily with each main meal containing fat. A dose may be skipped if a meal is low in fat or if a meal is skipped. Patients using xenical are often advised to limit their intake of fats to not more than 30% of their total calories. *(3)*

184. **(A)** Scabies is a disorder caused by the mite *Sarcoptes scabeii*. The mite burrows into the skin. Its droppings cause a hypersensitivity reaction characterized by intense itching. *(14)*

185. **(C)** The distinctive lesion is a vivid red macule, papule, or plaque covered by silvery lamellated scales. Usually the scalp, elbows, knees, and shins are affected first. *(14)*

186. **(A)** If morphine allergy is present, codeine (methyl morphine) should also be avoided because both codeine and morphine are structurally similar phenanthrene derivatives. Also, codeine is partially (10%) demethylated to morphine. *(6)*

187. **(C)** Tacrolimus (Prograf) and cyclosporine (Sandimmune, Neoral) are immunosuppressive drugs that are used to reduce organ rejection in patients who receive an organ transplant. Cilostazol (Pletal) is a drug used for the treatment of intermittent claudication. *(3)*

188. **(A)** Darbepoetin (Arenesp) is a synthetic form of erythropoetin. It is used to increase red blood cell growth in the bone marrow. It must be kept refrigerated. It is administered either subcutaneously or intravenously. *(3)*

189. **(B)** Clonidine is a central alpha-adrenergic stimulant that reduces peripheral vascular resistance and heart rate. Patients who use oral clonidine are susceptible to rebound hypertension if they discontinue their use of the tablets. The transdermal dosage form (Catapres TTS) releases clonidine at a constant rate for about 7 days, thereby improving compliance and reducing the likelihood of rebound hypertension. *(3)*

190. **(A)** Raising the intragastric pH from 1.5 to 3.5 neutralizes 99% of the acid and greatly reduces the proteolytic activity of pepsin. Buffering to a higher pH serves no useful purpose and may actually trigger further release of hydrochloric acid. *(11)*

191. **(D)** Epoetin alfa (Epogen, Procrit) is a glycoprotein that stimulates red blood cell production. It is generally used to treat anemia in patients on cancer chemotherapy or in those with chronic renal failure. It is not effective in treating patients with neutropenia (inadequate white blood cells). *(3)*

192. **(D)** Sinemet is a combination product containing carbidopa and levodopa in a ratio of 1:4 or 1:10. Because carbidopa inhibits the peripheral decarboxylation of levodopa, much smaller doses of levodopa can be used. This in turn generally reduces the peripheral side effects associated with high doses of levodopa. Dosage levels of levodopa can be decreased by approximately 75%. *(3)*

193. **(B)** The administraton of pyridoxine, even in small doses (5 mg or more) contained in ordinary vitamin preparations, is equivalent to a reduction in dosage of levodopa. Pyridoxine is believed to be a cofactor for the enzyme dopa decarboxylase, which is responsible for the peripheral metabolism of levodopa. The decarboxylated metabolic product cannot enter the brain, which is the intended site of action. *(6)*

194. **(A)** Miglitol (Glyset) is an alpha-glucosidase inhibitor that delays the digestion of ingested carbohydrates. This results in a smaller increase

in blood glucose concentration after meals and permits better control of type 2 diabetic patients who cannot control their hyperglycemia with diet alone. *(6)*

195. **(E)** Gray baby syndrome occurs in premature and full-term newborn infants when chloramphenicol is administered during the first few days of life. The syndrome results from the inability of the infant to metabolize the drug because of a deficient enzyme, glucuronyl transferase, which is required to detoxify the drug by changing it to the glucuronide. Symptoms consist of cyanosis, vascular collapse, and elevated chloramphenicol levels in the blood. *(6)*

196. **(E)** Nitroprusside sodium (Nitropress) is a vascular smooth muscle relaxant that is used to treat hypertensive emergencies. Solutions of nitroprusside develop colored decomposition products. Any discolored nitroprusside solution should, therefore, be discarded. Light may increase the likelihood of decomposition. Therefore, nitroprusside solutions should be protected from light by using an opaque covering on administration containers. The solution is administered by IV infusion. *(3)*

197. **(C)** Polyphagia is defined as an excessive craving for food. *(14)*

198. **(B)** Nitroglycerin is a dilator of peripheral vascular tissue, thereby causing a drop in blood pressure. It also is a coronary vasodilator and increases blood flow to the heart muscle. Nitroglycerin almost always causes cranial vasodilation, which causes headache to occur. *(6)*

199. **(D)** Misoprostol is a synthetic prostaglandin E1 analog that inhibits gastric acid secretion. It is used orally to prevent NSAID-induced gastric ulcers. The drug is in pregnancy category X. *(6)*

200. **(E)** Myopia is the condition of nearsightedness.
(A, incorrect)—Myalgia is pain in a muscle.
(B, incorrect)—Myositis is inflammation of a voluntary muscle.

(C, incorrect)—Myoclonus is muscular twitching or contraction.
(D, incorrect)—Myocardia pertains to the heart muscle. *(14)*

201. **(C)** Lithium products are used for the maintenance treatment of manic episodes of manic-depressive illness. Since lithium decreases renal sodium reabsorption, patients should be advised to maintain a normal salt and fluid intake. Anything that depletes the patient of sodium (eg, sweating, diarrhea, and use of diuretics) may increase lithium toxicity. Signs of lithium toxicity include the development of diarrhea and/or tremors. *(6)*

202. **(B)** Tegaserod (Zelnorm), a partial 5-HT4 agonist, is indicated for IBS that is constipation predominant. Alosetron (Lotronex) is a selective 5-HT3 receptor antagonist that is indicated for diarrhea-predominant IBS. *(3)*

203. **(A)** Amphetamines (Adderal) are CNS stimulants. Patients should be advised to take the medication early in the day to avoid insomnia and warned that the drug may cause palpitations. With prolonged use, amphetamine products are likely to cause weight loss. *(3)*

204. **(D)** Although digoxin and quinidine may be used together, administering quinidine to a patient previously stabilized on digoxin will cause serum digoxin levels to rise to an average of 2- to 2.5-fold. The mechanism of this interaction may involve both a displacement of digoxin from tissue-binding sites and a reduction in renal clearance of digoxin. Even though the significance of this interaction remains controversial, many clinicians suggest reducing the dose of digoxin by 50% when adding quinidine. In any case, the patient should be monitored carefully for signs of digoxin toxicity. *(3)*

205. **(E)** Eplerenone (Inspra) is an aldosterone blocking agent that, like spironolactone (Aldactone), triamterene (Dyrenium), and amiloride (Midamor) may exert a potassium-sparing action. Potassium supplements should not be used with these drugs because of the possibility of causing hyperkalemia. *(3)*

206. **(D)** Mannitol is usually administered IV as a hypertonic 10% to 25% solution (an isotonic solution is about 5.5%). The introduction of a hypertonic solution promotes urine flow. Mannitol solutions are used in prophylaxis of acute renal failure, in the evaluation of acute oliguria, and for the reduction of the pressure and volume of the intraocular and cerebrospinal fluids. *(6)*

207. **(D)** Imipramine (Tofranil) is a tricyclic antidepressant that is indicated for the treatment of nocturnal enuresis. It is not recommended for children younger than 6 years of age. Doses of imipramine range from 25 to 75 mg, lower than those used for treatment of depression. Desmopressin (DDAVP) is a posterior pituitary hormone that has an antidiuretic effect. It is administered once daily either orally or as a nasal spray. *(3)*

208. **(B)** The INR is used to monitor anticoagulant efficacy for patients using warfarin sodium (Coumadin). For patients who have had an acute MI, the INR should ideally be between 2 and 3. *(14)*

209. **(C)** Use of phenytoin (Dilantin) is associated with a number of adverse effects, including nystagmus (oscillation of the eyeball) and gingival hyperplasia (excessive gum growth). *(6)*

210. **(C)** Butorphanol tartrate (Stadol) is a mixed narcotic agonist–antagonist capable of relieving moderate to severe pain. In subjects dependent on such narcotics as morphine and codeine, nalbuphine precipitates a withdrawal syndrome. Although it is capable of producing euphoria similar to morphine, its effect on respiration seems to exhibit a ceiling effect, such that doses higher than 30 mg produce no further respiratory depression. *(3)*

CHAPTER 8

Patient Profiles

The pharmacist, whether practicing in a community or an institutional setting, must constantly refer to patient profiles for information regarding the medical and pharmaceutical history of a specific patient. Analysis of profile data requires a strong knowledge base in the pharmacy disciplines already reviewed in this book.

In this section, there are 30 patient medication profiles. Some are related to community pharmacy practice and some to institutional practice.

Questions

Community Pharmacy Medication Record

Patient Name: Henry Wallace
Address: 649 Terrace Avenue
Age: 64   Race: African American   Height: 5'10"
Sex: M   Weight: 263 lb
History: Mother died of stroke at age 63; father died of MI at age 51

DIAGNOSIS

Primary	Secondary
1. Hypertension	1.
2. BPH	2.
3.	3.

MEDICATION RECORD

Date	Rx No.	Physician	Drug and Strength	Quantity	Sig	Refills
1. 7/21	37325	Castro	hydrochlorothiazide 25 mg	30	1 daily	1
2. 8/20	37325	Castro	refill	30	1 daily	0
3. 9/18	39334	Castro	hydrochlorothiazide 25 mg	30	1 daily	2
4. 9/18	39335	Castro	Candesartan 8 mg	30	1 daily	2
5. 10/14	39334	Castro	refill	30	1 daily	1
6. 11/05	50478	McCullum	Avodart 0.5 mg	30	1 daily	2

PHARMACIST'S NOTES AND OTHER PATIENT INFORMATION

Date	Comment
9/24	Claritin-D # 5 OTC

DIRECTIONS (Questions 1a through 1l): Each of the numbered items or incomplete statements in this section is followed by answers or completions of the statement. Select the ONE lettered answer or completion that is BEST in each case.

1a. A drug product that is most similar in action to hydrochlorothiazide is

(A) torsemide

(B) acetazolamide

(C) ethacrynic acid

(D) hydroxyurea

(E) metolazone

1b. Which of the following lab tests would be useful in determining the presence of BPH?

(A) HbA_{1c}

(B) TSH

(C) PUD

(D) PSA

(E) CPK

1c. Candesartan can best be described as a (an)

(A) alpha$_2$-receptor agonist

(B) ACE inhibitor

(C) angiotensin II receptor blocker

(D) alpha$_1$-receptor blocker

(E) direct renin antagonist

1d. When using hydrochlorothiazide the patient should be advised to

  I. take the dose with food or milk

  II. restrict the intake of fluids while using the medication

  III. take the dose at bedtime

(A) I only

(B) III only

(C) I and II only

(D) II and III only

(E) I, II, and III

1e. Avodart can best be described as a (an)

(A) prostaglandin antagonist

(B) alpha$_1$-adrenergic blocker

(C) prostaglandin analog

(D) androgen

(E) antiandrogen

1f. Which of the following is (are) an adverse effect of Avodart?

  I. reflex tachycardia

  II. hirsutism

  III. fetal damage

(A) I only

(B) III only

(C) I and II only

(D) II and III only

(E) I, II, and III

1g. The chronic use of hydrochlorothiazide may result in the development of

  I. hypercalcemia

  II. hypomagnesemia

  III. hypokalemia

(A) I only

(B) III only

(C) I and II only

(D) II and III only

(E) I, II, and III

1h. Patients who exhibit hypersensitivity to hydrochlorothiazide should avoid the use of

(A) acetaminophen

(B) COMT antagonists

(C) aspirin

(D) monoamine oxidase (MAO) inhibitors

(E) sulfa drugs

1i. The pharmacist should advise Mr. Wallace to

(A) take Claritin-D three times a day

(B) avoid the concomitant use of hydrochlorothiazide and candesartan

(C) avoid the use of potassium-rich foods

(D) avoid the use of Claritin-D

(E) avoid vigorous exercise

1j. Which of the following drug products is (are) indicated for the treatment of BPH?

  I. Cardura

  II. Uroxatral

  III. Inspra

(A) I only

(B) III only

(C) I and II only

(D) II and III only

(E) I, II, and III

1k. A patient is brought to the emergency department (ED) and diagnosed as having hypertensive emergency. Which of the following drugs is (are) appropriate for the treatment of this condition?

  I. treprostinil
  II. febuxostat
  III. nitroprusside

(A) I only
(B) III only
(C) I and II only
(D) II and III only
(E) I, II, and III

1l. The best choice for a pregnant woman who needs to be treated for essential hypertension is

(A) propranolol
(B) hydrochlorothiazide
(C) epoprostenol
(D) methyldopa
(E) telmisartan

■ PROFILE NO. 2

Community Pharmacy Medication Record

Patient Name: Paula Mitogrand
Address: Bellafiore Nursing Home
Age: 89   Height: 5'3"
Sex: F   Weight: 154 lb
Allergies: Codeine

DIAGNOSIS

Primary	Secondary
1. Osteoarthritis	1.
2. Angina	2.
3.	3.

MEDICATION RECORD

Date	Rx No.	Physician	Drug and Strength	Quantity	Sig	Refills
1. 4/12	34094	Mouseau	Nitroglycerin 0.4 mg	100	p.r.n.	5
2. 4/12	34095	Mouseau	Celebrex 100 mg	60	b.i.d.	3

PHARMACIST'S NOTES AND OTHER PATIENT INFORMATION

Date	Comment
1. 4/21	Senokot Tablets (OTC)
	Cosamin DS (OTC)

DIRECTIONS (Questions 2a through 2l): Each of the numbered items or incomplete statements in this section is followed by answers or completions of the statement. Select the ONE lettered answer or completion that is BEST in each case.

2a. Celebrex is an example of a (an)

    I. nonsteroidal anti-inflammatory drug (NSAID)

    II. cyclooxygenase-2 (COX-2) inhibitor

    III. coronary vasodilator

    (A) I only

    (B) III only

    (C) I and II only

    (D) II and III only

    (E) I, II, and III

2b. Celecoxib should NOT be prescribed for a patient with a

    (A) BP < 100

    (B) HR < 60

    (C) $CL_{Cr} < 25$

    (D) FPG < 65

    (E) HDL < 40

2c. Nitroglycerin sublingual tablets must be

    I. discarded within 30 days after opening the container

    II. refrigerated

    III. packaged in a glass container

    (A) I only

    (B) III only

    (C) I and II only

    (D) II and III only

    (E) I, II, and III

2d. Another name for vasospastic angina is

(A) thrombotic thrombocytopenic purpura
(B) Prinzmetal's angina
(C) Babinski's angina
(D) Carlton's angina
(E) Pauling's angina

2e. Cosamin DS is a (an)

(A) cartilage enhancer
(B) anti-inflammatory
(C) vasodilator
(D) treatment for hypoglycemia
(E) treatment for hyperglycemia

2f. After using Celebrex for several weeks, Ms. Mitogrand develops GI upset. Which of the following would be helpful in reducing this problem?

(A) administer Cytoxan
(B) recommend that Feldene be used instead of Celebrex
(C) take the Celebrex on an empty stomach
(D) administer Cytotec
(E) recommend that Celebrex doses be taken at bedtime

2g. Which of the following is (are) an effect associated with the use of nitroglycerin sublingual tablets?

I. a burning sensation under the tongue
II. headache
III. paresthesia

(A) I only
(B) III only
(C) I and II only
(D) II and III only
(E) I, II, and III

2h. Which of the following is NOT a dosage form of nitroglycerin?

(A) oral suspension
(B) ointment

(C) IV
(D) transdermal patch
(E) sustained-release capsule

2i. Ms. Mitogrand's physician wishes to replace the Celebrex with a different oral analgesic product. Which of the following would be a suitable analgesic for this patient?

(A) Restasis
(B) Humira
(C) Ultram
(D) Comtan
(E) Ativan

2j. The active ingredient of Senokot can best be described as a (an)

(A) amylase inhibitor
(B) intestinal lubricant
(C) anthraquinone glycoside
(D) pyrimidine analog
(E) lactase inhibitor

2k. An appropriate method for using Nitrolingual spray is

(A) spray one or two doses onto or under the tongue
(B) inhale once p.r.n.
(C) inhale one to two times p.r.n.
(D) inhale one to two times before each meal
(E) spray once into each nostril

2l. When using nitroglycerin sublingual tablets the patient should be advised to avoid the use of

I. alcohol
II. vardenafil
III. aspirin

(A) I only
(B) III only
(C) I and II only
(D) II and III only
(E) I, II, and III

■PROFILE NO. 3

Community Pharmacy Medication Record

Patient Name: Lydia Hernandez
Address: 210 Morris Avenue
Age: 38   Height: 5'7"
Sex: F   Weight: 144 lb
Allergies: Aspirin

DIAGNOSIS

Primary	Secondary
1. Generalized tonic–clonic seizures since age 7	1. Constipation
2.	2.
3.	3.

MEDICATION RECORD

Date	Rx No.	Physician	Drug and Strength	Quantity	Sig	Refills
1. 1/2	32601	Mazur	Plan B One Step	1	As directed	0
2. 2/2	34568	Mazur	Micronor	1	1 daily	3
3. 3/1	34568	Mazur	Refill			2
4. 3/21	35908	Wilson	Dilantin Kapseals. 0.1	90	3 daily	2

PHARMACIST'S NOTES AND OTHER PATIENT INFORMATION

Date	Comment
1. 4/2	Ortho Gynol II Extra Strength Vaginal Jelly 2.85 oz (OTC)
2. 4/2	Centrum Ultra Women's Tablets # 100 (OTC)
3. 4/9	Colace 100 mg #100 (OTC)

DIRECTIONS (Questions 3a through 3q): Each of the numbered items or incomplete statements in this section is followed by answers or completions of the statement. Select the ONE lettered answer or completion that is BEST in each case.

3a. Micronor can best be described as a (an)

(A) vaginal deodorant product

(B) biphasic oral contraceptive

(C) triphasic oral contraceptive

(D) ovulation inducer

(E) progestin-only oral contraceptive

3b. Which of the following is (are) true of Ortho Gynol II Extra Strength Jelly?

I. is only used with a diaphragm

II. contraceptive

III. vaginal lubricant

(A) I only

(B) III only

(C) I and II only

(D) II and III only

(E) I, II, and III

3c. A synonym for generalized tonic–clonic seizures is

(A) Jacksonian seizures

(B) absence seizures

(C) grand mal seizures

(D) status epilepticus

(E) focal seizures

3d. Which of the following drugs are reasonable alternative drugs to phenytoin for the treatment of this patient's seizures?

    I. valproic acid
    II. carbamazepine
    III. lamotrigine

(A) I only
(B) III only
(C) I and II only
(D) II and III only
(E) I, II, and III

3e. The Dilantin product prescribed may be administered

    I. in three divided daily doses
    II. as a single daily dose
    III. on a p.r.n. basis

(A) I only
(B) III only
(C) I and II only
(D) II and III only
(E) I, II, and III

3f. In the course of receiving Dilantin the patient develops gingival hyperplasia. This is a disorder of the

(A) skin
(B) gums
(C) tongue
(D) hematological system
(E) cardiac rhythm

3g. Which of the following is associated with the use of phenytoin?

(A) Michaelis–Menten kinetics
(B) myelosuppression
(C) cheilosis
(D) first-pass effect
(E) pseudomembranous enterocolitis

3h. A plasma phenytoin determination is performed after the patient has been using phenytoin sodium for about 1 month. It reveals a concentration of 5 μg/mL. This indicates that

(A) hepatic impairment may exist
(B) the patient may have renal impairment
(C) the concentration is within the therapeutic range
(D) the patient may not be taking all prescribed doses
(E) the patient may be taking more doses than prescribed

3i. The prescriber should be called because of

(A) cross-sensitivity between Colace and Dilantin
(B) carcinogenicity with Dilantin
(C) reduction in Dilantin effectiveness
(D) reduction in Micronor effectiveness
(E) improper Dilantin dose prescribed

3j. Which of the following is a phenytoin prodrug?

(A) Mysoline
(B) Keppra
(C) Monurol
(D) Cerebyx
(E) Gabitril

3k. Which of the following is true of parenterally administered Dilantin?

    I. Dilantin parenteral solutions must be kept refrigerated until just prior to administration.
    II. IM administration should generally be avoided.
    III. Precipitation is likely to occur when Dilantin is combined with B-complex with C in an IV admixture.

(A) I only
(B) III only
(C) I and II only
(D) II and III only
(E) I, II, and III

3l. Patients receiving Dilantin may develop a morbilliform rash. Morbilliform refers to

(A) measles-like
(B) butterfly-shaped
(C) unilateral
(D) acne-like
(E) multicolored

3m. Which of the following drugs would be appropriate to use in the treatment of status epilepticus?

I. propofol
II. midazolam
III. lorazepam

(A) I only
(B) III only
(C) I and II only
(D) II and III only
(E) I, II, and III

3n. A patient on long-term phenytoin therapy should receive supplements of

(A) cyanocobalamin
(B) folic acid
(C) calcium
(D) iron
(E) inositol

3o. The active ingredient of Ortho Gynol II Extra Strength Jelly is

(A) misoprostol
(B) benzalkonium chloride
(C) buconazole
(D) sodium lauryl sulfate
(E) nonoxynol-9

3p. The active ingredient in Colace is a (an)

(A) nonionic surfactant
(B) coprecipitated laxative
(C) anionic surfactant
(D) osmotic laxative
(E) cationic surfactant

3q. An ingredient of some Centrum products is lycopene. The purpose of this ingredient is to

(A) prevent hemolysis
(B) reduce the likelihood of osteoporosis
(C) prevent urinary infection
(D) prevent cataract formation
(E) improve prostate health

■ PROFILE NO. 4

Community Pharmacy Medication Record

Patient Name: Timothy Bologna
Address: 64 West State Street
Age: 79   Height: 5'10"
Sex: M   Weight: 164 lb
Allergies:

DIAGNOSIS

Primary	Secondary
1. Parkinson's disease	1.
2.	2.
3.	3.

MEDICATION RECORD

Date	Rx No.	Physician	Drug and Strength	Quantity	Sig	Refills
1. 2/3	56445	Mosely	Sinemet 10/100	90	1 t.i.d.	2
2. 3/1	56445	Mosely	Refill			
3. 3/19	59008	Mosely	Sinemet 25/250	90	t.i.d.	2
4. 3/19	59009	Mosely	Akineton 2 mg	90	1 tid	2
5. 4/15	59008	Mosely	Refill			
6. 4/15	61122	Mosely	Comtan 200 mg	60	1 t.i.d.	3

DIRECTIONS (Questions 4a through 4m): Each of the numbered items or incomplete statements in this section is followed by answers or completions of the statement. Select the ONE lettered answer or completion that is BEST in each case.

4a. The function of carbidopa in the Sinemet formulation is to

(A) act as a prodrug for levodopa
(B) act as a COMT inhibitor
(C) act as an MAO inhibitor
(D) inhibit decarboxylation of levodopa in the CNS
(E) inhibit peripheral decarboxylation of levodopa

4b. Patients receiving levodopa should avoid using vitamin supplements that contain

(A) folic acid
(B) thiamine
(C) pyridoxine
(D) calcium
(E) cyanocobalamin

4c. A patient using Sinemet complains of an appreciable darkening of the urine beginning about 3 days after starting Sinemet therapy. The pharmacist should tell the patient to

(A) disregard the discoloration because it is not harmful

(B) check the expiration date on the Sinemet container to make sure it has not expired

(C) immediately stop taking the Sinemet and call the prescriber

(D) avoid the use of acidic foods while on Sinemet

(E) avoid the use of alkaline foods while on Sinemet

4d. Akineton has been prescribed because of its action as a (an)

(A) centrally acting skeletal muscle relaxant

(B) COMT inhibitor

(C) anticholinergic

(D) MAO-B inhibitor

(E) GABA-mimetic agent

4e. Which of the following is NOT employed in the treatment of Parkinson's disease?

(A) rasagiline (Azilect)

(B) tiagabine (Gabitril)

(C) ropinirole (Requip)

(D) bromocriptine (Parlodel)

(E) selegiline (Eldepryl)

4f. After several months of being well controlled on Sinemet, the patient experiences a relapse. This is likely due to

(A) neuroleptic malignant syndrome

(B) an interaction with Akineton

(C) the first-pass effect

(D) the on–off effect

(E) enterohepatic cycling

4g. Diplopia is an adverse effect related to the use of levodopa. This can best be described as

(A) double vision

(B) a facial tic

(C) hearing loss

(D) loss of taste sensation

(E) a cardiac tachyarrhythmia

4h. When a patient on levodopa is to be switched to Sinemet, which of the following is (are) true?

I. Permit at least 8 hours to elapse between the last dose of levodopa and the first dose of Sinemet.

II. The daily levodopa dose in the Sinemet should be 75% lower than when levodopa is used alone.

III. Plasma levodopa levels must be measured each day for the first 5 days of Sinemet therapy.

(A) I only

(B) III only

(C) I and II only

(D) II and III only

(E) I, II, and III

4i. The prolonged use of which of the following drugs is associated with Parkinson-like symptoms?

(A) citalopram

(B) loxapine

(C) raloxifene

(D) methylphenidate

(E) paroxetine

4j. Which one of the following products may be used to provide individual doses of carbidopa?

(A) Lodosyn

(B) Enablex

(C) Tegretol

(D) Dopar

(E) Zometa

4k. An adverse effect associated with the use of Akineton is

(A) aplastic anemia

(B) constipation

(C) the first-dose effect

(D) ptosis

(E) nyctalopia

41. A patient using selegiline (Eldepryl) for the treatment of Parkinson's disease should be advised to avoid

   I. cheese

   II. wine

   III. nasal decongestants

(A) I only

(B) III only

(C) I and II only

(D) II and III only

(E) I, II, and III

4m. The patient wishes to know more about a new product for depression she has read about called Emsam recently. Which of the following is true of Emsam?

   I. It is a COMT inhibitor

   II. It is a MAO inhibitor

   III. It is available as a transdermal product.

(A) I only

(B) III only

(C) I and II only

(D) II and III only

(E) I, II, and III

■ PROFILE NO. 5

Community Pharmacy Medication Record

Patient Name: Susan Wilson
Address: 425 Reading Way
Age: 69   Height: 5'7"
Sex: F   Weight: 186 lb
Allergies: Pollen, penicillin

DIAGNOSIS

Primary   Secondary
1. Open-angle glaucoma, primary   1.
2. Emphysema   2.
3.   3.

MEDICATION RECORD

Date	Rx No.	Physician	Drug and Strength	Quantity	Sig	Refill
1. 7/29	59083	Weber	Timoptic-XE 0.25%	5 mL	gtt 1 os daily	2
2. 8/20	59083	Weber	Refill			
3. 9/11	65002	Weber	Betagan 0.5%	10 mL	gtt 1 os b.i.d.	2
4. 10/21	65002	Weber	Lumigan 0.03%	2.5 mL	gtt 1 os daily	1

PHARMACIST'S NOTES AND OTHER PATIENT INFORMATION

Date	Comment
1. 9/14	Motrin IB
2. 10/7	Visine-A Allergy Relief (OTC)

DIRECTIONS (Questions 5a through 5l): Each of the numbered items or incomplete statements in this section is followed by answers or completions of the statement. Select the ONE lettered answer or completion that is BEST in each case.

5a. The PRIMARY action of Timoptic-XE in the treatment of glaucoma is as a (an)

(A) cycloplegic
(B) alpha blocker
(C) miotic
(D) 5HT blocker
(E) beta blocker

5b. Timoptic is most similar in pharmacologic action to

(A) carbachol
(B) acetazolamide
(C) dipivefrin
(D) propofol
(E) metipranolol

5c. Several weeks after using Timoptic-XE, the patient's intraocular pressure is measured as 14 mm Hg. This indicates that

(A) the patient's intraocular pressure is under control
(B) the patient has narrow-angle glaucoma
(C) an error in measurement must have occurred
(D) the dose of Timoptic-XE should be increased
(E) the dose of Timoptic-XE should be decreased

5d. The Timoptic-XE dosage form can best be described as a (an)

(A) suspension

(B) gel-forming solution

(C) liposome dispersion

(D) emulsion

(E) microsomal dispersion

5e. The use of Timoptic has been reported to produce urticaria in some patients. Another name for urticaria is

(A) hair loss

(B) dry eye

(C) tooth decay

(D) hives

(E) cold extremities

5f. Acetazolamide is sometimes indicated for the treatment of glaucoma. Which of the following best describes the mechanism of action of this drug?

(A) tocolytic

(B) miotic

(C) carbonic anhydrase inhibitor

(D) mydriatic

(E) cycloplegic

5g. Which of the following is likely to be an adverse effect associated with the use of bimatoprost (Lumigan)?

    I. nyctalopia

    II. cataracts

    III. conjunctival hyperemia

(A) I only

(B) III only

(C) I and II only

(D) II and III only

(E) I, II, and III

5h. Betagan ophthalmic solution contains edetate disodium. Which of the following best describes the function of this ingredient?

(A) buffer

(B) antibacterial

(C) metal scavenger

(D) viscosity builder

(E) antifungal

5i. The patient returns to the pharmacy to purchase more Motrin IB. If the pharmacy was out of Motrin IB which of the following products could the pharmacist recommend as the closest substitute?

(A) Datril

(B) Advil

(C) Excedrin

(D) Aleve

(E) Anacin

5j. The Visine-A Allergy Relief purchased OTC by this patient contains a (an)

(A) beta$_1$ blocker

(B) beta$_2$ agonist

(C) alpha$_2$ agonist

(D) alpha$_1$ agonist

(E) beta$_1$ antagonist

5k. The pharmacist should contact the prescriber to discuss the possibility of

(A) blood dyscrasias

(B) respiratory distress

(C) urinary retention

(D) interaction between Timoptic-XE and Betagan

(E) interaction between Timoptic-XE and Lumigan

5l. Patients with glaucoma should avoid drugs that are

(A) sympathomimetics

(B) broad-spectrum antimicrobial agents

(C) peripheral vasodilators

(D) potassium depleters

(E) anticholinergics

■ PROFILE NO. 6

Community Pharmacy Medication Record

Patient Name: Karl Schmidt
Address: 2204 North Street
Age: 17
Sex: M
Allergies: Penicillin

Height: 6'1"
Weight: 180 lb

DIAGNOSIS

Primary
1. Acne vulgaris—cystic
2.
3.

Secondary
1.
2.
3.

MEDICATION RECORD

Date	Rx No.	Physician	Drug and Strength	Quantity	Sig	Refills
1. 6/7	45023	Thomas	Benzac Ac Gel 10%	45 g	ut dict	3
2. 6/22	48399	Wilson	Retin-A Micro 0.1%	20 g	Apply p.r.n.	2
3. 7/13	45023	Thomas	Refill			2
4. 8/24	45023	Thomas	Refill			1
5. 9/17	57888	Wilson	Cleocin T Gel	30 g	Apply topically	3
6. 10/5	59778	Thomas	Claravis 10 mg	60	1 b.i.d.	5

PHARMACIST'S NOTES AND OTHER PATIENT INFORMATION

Date	Comment
1. 7/1	Brasivol Medium
2. 7/30	Pernox Scrub 60 mL

DIRECTIONS (Questions 6a through 6m): Each of the numbered items or incomplete statements in this section is followed by answers or completions of the statement. Select the ONE lettered answer or completion that is BEST in each case.

6a. The active ingredient in Benzac is

(A) budesonide
(B) benzoyl peroxide
(C) isotretinoin
(D) benzyl alcohol
(E) benzalkonium chloride

6b. Patients using Retin-A should avoid

I. excessive sunlight
II. having the product come in contact with their eyes
III. use of antimicrobial agents

(A) I only
(B) III only
(C) I and II only
(D) II and III only
(E) I, II, and III

6c. Retin-A liquid contains butylated hydroxytoluene. The function of this ingredient is as a (an)

(A) viscosity builder
(B) solvent
(C) abrasive
(D) chelating agent
(E) antioxidant

6d. Retin-A Micro is a product that is only available as a (an)

(A) water-soluble cream

(B) micronized powder

(C) water-insoluble cream

(D) gel

(E) ointment

6e. Which of the following adverse effects is associated with the systemic use of Cleocin?

(A) diarrhea

(B) crystalluria

(C) hemorrhagic cystitis

(D) photosensitivity

(E) aplastic anemia

6f. The Cleocin-T product contains 10 mg of clindamycin per milliliter and is available in a 30-mL package size. This means that the strength of clindamycin in the solution is

(A) 1%

(B) 3%

(C) 0.1%

(D) 10%

(E) 0.3%

6g. Claravis is most closely related to

(A) pantothenic acid

(B) ascorbic acid

(C) ergocalciferol

(D) beta-carotene

(E) cyanocobalamin

6h. Which of the following is (are) common adverse effects associated with the use of Claravis?

I. chelitis

II. conjunctivitis

III. hyperlipidemia

(A) I only

(B) III only

(C) I and II only

(D) II and III only

(E) I, II, and III

6i. Before receiving and using Claravis, the patient MUST have received a (an)

I. informed consent form

II. patient package insert

III. sunscreen with an SPF 30 or greater

(A) I only

(B) III only

(C) I and II only

(D) II and III only

(E) I, II, and III

6j. Acne can BEST be described as a (an)

(A) dermatological response to excessive intake of dietary fats

(B) allergic response

(C) infection

(D) autoimmune disease

(E) inflammatory response to free fatty acids

6k. Brasivol contains aluminum oxide. This ingredient is employed in this product as a (an)

(A) buffering agent

(B) abrasive

(C) oxidizing agent

(D) astringent

(E) desiccating agent

6l. Pernox scrub contains salicylic acid. This ingredient is employed in this product as a (an)

(A) buffer

(B) antiseptic

(C) antioxidant

(D) keratolytic

(E) astringent

6m. Patients with acne often secrete large amounts of

(A) lactic acid

(B) dihydrotachysterol

(C) pectin

(D) sebum

(E) cerumen

■PROFILE NO. 7

Community Pharmacy Medication Record

Patient Name: Lois Petrowski
Address: 422 Clarindon Court
Age: 25   Height: 5′4″
Sex: F   Weight: 136 lb
Allergies:

DIAGNOSIS

Primary	Secondary
1. Asthma	1.
2. IBS	2.
3.	3.

MEDICATION RECORD

Date	Rx No.	Physician	Drug and Strength	Quantity	Sig	Refills
1. 6/19	40098	Churchill	Singulair 10 mg	30	p.r.n.	2
2. 7/7	40098	Churchill	Refill			1
3. 8/1	46443	Churchill	Proventil-HFA Aero.	17 g	p.r.n.	2
4. 8/1	46444	Churchill	Flovent Diskus 100	1	p.r.n.	1
5. 9/22	48998	Churchill	Amitiza 8 mcg	60	b.i.d.	2

PHARMACIST'S NOTES AND OTHER PATIENT INFORMATION

Date	Comment
1.	Patient smokes 2 packs of cigarettes daily.
2. 9/1	Habitrol Film 7 mg/24 h also as—1 box OTC

DIRECTIONS (Questions 7a through 7k): Each of the numbered items or incomplete statements in this section is followed by answers or completions of the statement. Select the ONE lettered answer or completion that is BEST in each case.

7a. The active ingredient in Singulair is most similar to the active ingredient in

(A) Serevent
(B) Ventolin HFA
(C) Accolate
(D) Intal
(E) Pulmicort

7b. In an acute asthmatic attack, the patient uses one dose of Singulair and, after 5 minutes, still has not been relieved. The patient should be advised to

(A) go to the local emergency department immediately

(B) administer a second dose of Singulair if relief is not evident

(C) use the Proventil-HFA Aerosol product instead of the Singulair

(D) breathe into a brown bag for 6 minutes to increase the respiratory concentration of carbon dioxide

(E) use a corticosteroid inhalation immediately before the Singlulair

7c. In reviewing the patient's profile, it is evident that the prescriber needs to be contacted because of an error in prescribing which of the following products?

    I. Amitiza

    II. Singulair

    III. Flovent Diskus

  (A) I only

  (B) III only

  (C) I and II only

  (D) II and III only

  (E) I, II, and III

7d. The Proventil-HFA Aerosol product contains

  (A) bitolterol

  (B) zafirlukast

  (C) ipratropium bromide

  (D) terbutaline

  (E) albuterol

7e. When using Proventil-HFA Aerosol in an elderly patient, it may be necessary to use a

  (A) beta-adrenergic blocking agent with intrinsic sympathomimetic activity (ISA)

  (B) nasal cannula

  (C) Busher injector

  (D) nebulizer

  (E) spacer device

7f. The HFA in the product Proventil-HFA Aerosol refers to a(n)

  (A) propellant

  (B) preservative

  (C) type of nozzle

  (D) an inhalation containing a powder

  (E) a surfactant

7g. Rotacaps are

  (A) capsules that contain a powder for inhalation

  (B) oral capsules that must be emptied into food before use

  (C) sustained-release capsules

  (D) enteric-coated capsules

  (E) capsules containing ingredients separated by a semipermeable membrane

7h. The active ingredient in Flovent Diskus can best be described as a (an)

  (A) respiratory surfactant

  (B) leukotriene receptor antagonist

  (C) corticosteroid

  (D) bronchodilator

  (E) anticholinergic

7i. When Proventil-HFA Aerosol and Flovent Diskus are to be used at the same time

  (A) the Flovent Diskus should be used first

  (B) the patient should be advised to rinse her mouth with water immediately before administering the first drug product

  (C) the Proventil-HFA should be used first

  (D) a saline aerosol should be administered first

  (E) a spacer device should be used

7j. Which of the following is true of Habitrol Patches?

    I. They are applied for a 24-hour period.

    II. They contain the same active ingredient as Nicoderm.

    III. The area to which they are to be applied should be moistened before use.

  (A) I only

  (B) III only

  (C) I and II only

  (D) II and III only

  (E) I, II, and III

7k. Flovent Diskus contains the same active ingredient as

  (A) Atrovent HFA

  (B) Advair HFA

  (C) Maxair

  (D) Serevent

  (E) Dulera

■ PROFILE NO. 8

Community Pharmacy Medication Record

Patient Name: Helen Bayerwood

Address: 4 Woodline Court

Age: 77   Height: 5′4″

Sex: F   Weight: 164 lb

Allergies:

DIAGNOSIS

Primary	Secondary
1. Chronic stable angina	1.
2. Chronic alcoholism	2.
3.	3.

MEDICATION RECORD

Date	Rx No.	Physician	Drug and Strength	Quantity	Sig	Refills
1. 1/14	40952	Cohen	Nitrostat 0.4 mg	100	p.r.n.	3
2. 1/30	42772	Cohen	Nitro-Dur 0.1	30	Apply daily	5
3. 2/26	42772	Cohen	Refill			4
4. 3/16	42772	Cohen	Refill			3
5. 4/7	42772	Cohen	Refill			2
6. 4/28	50632	Cohen	Nitro-Dur 0.3 mg	30	1 daily	2
7. 4/28	50633	Cohen	Tranxene 7.5 mg	30	1 t.i.d.	2
8. 4/28	50634	Cohen	Persantine 25 mg	90	1 t.i.d.	3

PHARMACIST'S NOTES AND OTHER PATIENT INFORMATION

Date	Comment
1. 3/2	Dristan Tabs (OTC)

DIRECTIONS (Questions 8a through 8J): Each of the numbered items or incomplete statements in this section is followed by answers or completions of the statement. Select the ONE lettered answer or completion that is BEST in each case.

8a. An advantage of Nitrostat over many other sublingual nitroglycerin products is that it is

(A) available in color-coded tablets

(B) more rapidly absorbed

(C) less subject to potency loss

(D) effective when used orally as well as sublingually

(E) longer acting

8b. Nitrostat should be dispensed

   I. in its original container

  II. in quantities not greater than 25 tablets

 III. with a "Refrigerate" auxiliary label

(A) I only

(B) III only

(C) I and II only

(D) II and III only

(E) I, II, and III

8c. The patient should be advised to apply the Nitro-Dur transdermal system to

    I.   the distal parts of the extremities

    II. only onto the chest close to the heart

    III. a hairless site

(A) I only

(B) III only

(C) I and II only

(D) II and III only

(E) I, II, and III

8d. When discontinuing therapy with Nitro-Dur

(A) the number of hours per day that it is applied should be reduced gradually over 7 days

(B) the dosage and frequency of application should be reduced gradually over a 3-day period

(C) the dosage and frequency of application should be reduced gradually over a 4–6-week period

(D) severe nausea and vomiting may occur

(E) the patient should be advised to take prophylactic aspirin doses for 2 weeks prior to discontinuation

8e. In addition to being employed in the treatment of angina, dipyridamole (Persantine) is also used as a (an)

(A) antiviral

(B) antiplatelet

(C) antimalarial

(D) antihypertensive

(E) antiarrhythmic

8f. The reason why nitroglycerin products are generally NOT administered orally is because nitroglycerin

(A) rapidly decomposes in stomach acid

(B) it can cause GERD

(C) is decomposed rapidly by pepsin

(D) undergoes rapid first-pass deactivation

(E) is poorly absorbed from the GI tract

8g. Patients using nitroglycerin should be advised to AVOID the use of

    I.   antiplatelet drugs

    II. alcohol

    III. tadalafil

(A) I only

(B) III only

(C) I and II only

(D) II and III only

(E) I, II, and III

8h. Solutions of nitroglycerin intended for IV administration should be

(A) administered using the administration set provided by the manufacturer

(B) kept covered with an opaque shield to protect it from decomposition

(C) warmed for 15 minutes prior to infusion to dissolve crystalline material

(D) given only by rapid IV injection

(E) refrigerated until 30 minutes prior to administration

8i. When nitroglycerin topical ointment is administered

    I.   it should be rubbed into the skin until no further ointment is evident on the skin surface

    II. the area to which it is applied should not be occluded

    III. the dose is measured in inches

(A) I only

(B) III only

(C) I and II only

(D) II and III only

(E) I, II, and III

8j. One of the ingredients in Dristan is tablets phenylephrine. This drug's therapeutic action in this product can BEST be described as a (an)

(A) beta$_1$ blocker

(B) beta$_2$ agonist

(C) alpha$_1$ agonist

(D) alpha$_1$ blocker

(E) alpha$_2$ agonist

■ PROFILE NO. 9

Community Pharmacy Medication Record

Patient Name: Amelia Wasserman
Address: 1705 N. 16th St
Age: 64   Height: 5'5"
Sex: F   Weight: 178 lb
Allergies: Sulfas

DIAGNOSIS

Primary	Secondary
1. Type 1 diabetes mellitus	1.
2.	2.
3.	3.

MEDICATION RECORD

Date	Rx No.	Physician	Drug and Strength	Quantity	Sig	Refills
1. 9/11	29087	Madison	Humalog	10 mL	p.r.n.	5
2. 9/11	29088	Madison	Lantus Insulin	10 mL	24 U daily	5
3. 9/11	29089	Madison	B-D Micro-Fine+ Insulin Syringes	100		5
4. 9/11	29090	Madison	Ascensia Elite Meter	1	As directed	

PHARMACIST'S NOTES AND OTHER PATIENT INFORMATION

Date	Comment
1. 9/1	Theragran M #100
2. 9/11	Ascencia Elite Reagent Strips
3. 9/20	Sudafed PE Tablets 10 mg #72 (OTC)

DIRECTIONS (Questions 9a through 9o): Each of the numbered items or incomplete statements in this section is followed by answers or completions of the statement. Select the ONE lettered answer or completion that is BEST in each case.

9a. The term "type 1 diabetes mellitus" is also referred to as

(A) diabetes insipidus

(B) insulin-dependent diabetes mellitus

(C) adult-onset diabetes mellitus

(D) insulin-resistant diabetes mellitus

(E) brittle diabetes mellitus

9b. Which of the following is (are) true of Humalog?

I. It should be administered first thing in the morning.

II. It is a clear solution.

III. It is prepared by recombinant DNA technology.

(A) I only

(B) III only

(C) I and II only

(D) II and III only

(E) I, II, and III

9c. Which of the following is true of the measurement of the 24 U Lantus dose?

(A) The patient must withdraw 0.24 mL from the Lantus vial.

(B) The patient must withdraw 2.4 mL from the Lantus vial.

(C) The amount the patient must withdraw from the vial depends on the volume of the syringe.

(D) 24 U is an excessive dose and should not be used.

(E) Precise measurement of 24 U cannot be made with an insulin syringe.

9d. In examining the patient, the physician notes that the patient complains of polydipsia. This refers to

(A) overgrowth of subcutaneous fat in the area of insulin injection

(B) excessive appetite

(C) excessive weight gain

(D) excessive urination

(E) excessive thirst

9e. Which of the following would be considered a normal fasting blood glucose level for this patient?

(A) 90 mg/L

(B) 100 μg/L

(C) 80 μg/dL

(D) 1 μg/mL

(E) 85 mg/dL

9f. Which of the following insulins is (are) suitable for administration by IV infusion?

I. aspart

II. lispro

III. regular

(A) I only

(B) III only

(C) I and II only

(D) II and III only

(E) I, II, and III

9g. Which of the following is MOST similar to Lantus Insulin?

(A) Levemir

(B) Humulin R

(C) Humulin N

(D) Novalog

(E) Apidra

9h. The patient asks the pharmacist about a product she has read about called Symlin. Which of the following is TRUE of Symlin?

I. incretin mimetic agent

II. should be stored at room temperature

III. indicated for treatment of type 1 and type 2 diabetics

(A) I only

(B) III only

(C) I and II only

(D) II and III only

(E) I, II, and III

9i. Which of the following insulins does NOT have a pH of 7.4?

(A) Lantus

(B) Lispro

(C) Aspart

(D) Regular

(E) NPH

9j. To use the Ascensia Elite device properly, patients must also use

I. lancets

II. a tuberculin syringe

III. an alpha-glucosidase inhibitor

(A) I only

(B) III only

(C) I and II only

(D) II and III only

(E) I, II, and III

9k. The patient's use of Sudafed PE tablets may

(A) precipitate ketoacidosis

(B) increase the patient's insulin requirement

(C) increase the chance of lipohypertrophy

(D) increase the chance of lipoatrophy

(E) decrease the patient's insulin requirement

9l. B-D Micro-Dose+ syringes have a capacity of

I.   0.3 mL

II. 0.5 mL

III. 0.7 mL

(A) I only

(B) III only

(C) I and II only

(D) II and III only

(E) I, II, and III

9m. Which of the following antidiabetic products can be classified as a non-sulfonylurea insulin secretagogue?

I.   DiaBeta

II. Prandin

III. Starlix

(A) I only

(B) III only

(C) I and II only

(D) II and III only

(E) I, II, and III

9n. A serious potential complication in the use of metformin HCl (Glucophage) in the treatment of diabetes mellitus is

(A) lactic acidosis

(B) pancreatitis

(C) nephropathy

(D) lipodystrophy

(E) thrombocytopenia

9o. Which of the following best describes the mechanism of action of pioglitazone?

(A) increases insulin production

(B) interferes with glucose absorption in the GI tract

(C) promotes glycogenolysis

(D) increases insulin receptor sensitivity

(E) antagonizes glucagon receptors

▪PROFILE NO. 10

Community Pharmacy Medication Record

Patient Name: Betty Tuviac
Address: 404 Eastern Avenue
Age: 39   Height: 5′9″
Sex: F   Weight: 168 lb
Allergies:

DIAGNOSIS

Primary	Secondary
1. Venous thrombosis	1.
2. Hypothyroidism	2.
3.	3.

MEDICATION RECORD

Date	Rx No.	Physician	Drug and Strength	Quantity	Sig	Refills
1. 5/3	89322	Schwartz	Warfarin 5 mg	10	1 daily	
2. 5/12	90109	Schwartz	Warfarin 7.5 mg	30	1 daily	
3. 5/21	91202	Schwartz	Warfarin 7.5 mg	30	1 daily	3
4. 6/18	91202	Schwartz	Refill			2
5. 7/15	91202	Schwartz	Refill			1
6. 8/1	94388	Wilson	Thyrolar—½	60	1 daily	5
7. 8/29	99733	Waxman	Synalgos-DC 30 mg	30	1 b.i.d.	

DIRECTIONS (Questions 10a through 10j): Each of the numbered items or incomplete statements in this section is followed by answers or completions of the statement. Select the ONE lettered answer or completion that is BEST in each case.

10a. Which of the following parameters should be monitored in a patient receiving warfarin?

   I. TTP

  II. PT

 III. INR

(A) I only

(B) III only

(C) I and II only

(D) II and III only

(E) I, II, and III

10b. Administration of which of the following drugs is likely to DECREASE warfarin activity in this patient?

   I. cimetidine

  II. carbamazepine

 III. rifampin

(A) I only

(B) III only

(C) I and II only

(D) II and III only

(E) I, II, and III

10c. An appropriate antidote for the treatment of warfarin overdose is

(A) EDTA

(B) streptokinase

(C) phytonadione

(D) potassium thiosulfate

(E) protamine sulfate

10d. This patient asks the pharmacist for a recommendation for an OTC analgesic for her tennis elbow. Which of the following agents would be appropriate to recommend?

    I. Advil

    II. Datril

    III. Tylenol

    (A) I only

    (B) III only

    (C) I and II only

    (D) II and III only

    (E) I, II, and III

10e. Which of the following is (are) associated with hypothyroidism?

    I. goiter

    II. weight gain

    III. cardiac palpitations

    (A) I only

    (B) III only

    (C) I and II only

    (D) II and III only

    (E) I, II, and III

10f. If a radiation dose of 200 mCi of radioactive iodine ($k = 0.23$ h^{-1}) is administered to a patient at 8 AM how long would it take for the amount of radiation emitted by the dose to fall below 25 mCi?

    (A) 9 hours

    (B) 4.6 hours

    (C) 6 hours

    (D) 0.23 hours

    (E) 3 hours

10g. The use of Thyrolar by this patient is likely to

    (A) increase the dosage requirement for warfarin

    (B) prevent the oral absorption of warfarin

    (C) increase the likelihood of renal damage

    (D) decrease the dosage requirement for warfarin

    (E) increase the likelihood of hepatic damage

10h. In a radiation emergency, which of the following would be appropriate to administer?

    (A) sodium nitrite

    (B) liothyronine

    (C) cholestyramine

    (D) potassium iodide

    (E) propylthiouracil

10i. Thyroid hormone synthesis is controlled by

    (A) thyroglobulin releasing cells in the pancreas

    (B) oxytocin from the posterior pituitary

    (C) FSH from the anterior pituitary

    (D) TSH from the anterior pituitary

    (E) LH from the anterior pituitary

10j. The use of Synalgos-DC by this patient is likely to

    (A) increase the action of the Thyrolar

    (B) decrease the action of Thyrolar

    (C) decrease the action of warfarin

    (D) cause thyroid storm

    (E) increase the action of warfarin

■ PROFILE NO. 11

Hospital Pharmacy Medication Record

Patient Name: Laura Smiler
Room Number: 874B
Age: 59   Height: 5′3″
Sex: F   Weight: 148 lb
Allergies: Aspirin, codeine

DIAGNOSIS

Primary   Secondary
1. Chronic UTI   1. Migraines
2. Conjunctivitis   2. PMS
3.

LAB TESTS

Date   Test and Results
1. 7/14   Urinalysis, pyuria, C & S = 1×10^6 *Escherichia coli*
2.
3.

MEDICATION RECORD

Date   Drug and Strength   Sig
1. 7/15   Cipro 200 mg IV   q12h × 7 days
2. 7/15   Uristat (OTC)   1 t.i.d.
3. 7/23   TMP-SMX   1q 12 h
            80/400 mg

PHARMACIST'S NOTES AND OTHER PATIENT INFORMATION

Date   Comment
1. 7/25   Patient discharged with Rx Septra DS #20 1q 12 h

DIRECTIONS (Questions 11a through 11t): Each of the numbered items or incomplete statements in this section is followed by answers or completions of the statement. Select the ONE lettered answer or completion that is BEST in each case.

11a. The term pyuria indicates the presence of what substance in the urine?

(A) pyruvate
(B) pyridoxine
(C) pus
(D) RBCs
(E) pyrogens

11b. *Escherichia coli* may be described as

(A) pneumococci
(B) a systemic fungal organism
(C) gram-positive bacilli
(D) gram-negative bacilli
(E) a virus

11c. Which of the following is (are) drugs of choice for the treatment of a urinary tract infection (UTI) caused by *E. coli*?

I. trimethoprim-sulfamethoxazole
II. ofloxacin
III. spectinomycin

(A) I only

(B) III only

(C) I and II only

(D) II and III only

(E) I, II, and III

11d. The physician's order for TMP-SMX may be filled using

I. Trimox

II. Bactrim

III. Septra

(A) I only

(B) III only

(C) I and II only

(D) II and III only

(E) I, II, and III

11e. Which of the following products are classified as fluoroquinolones?

I. Avelox

II. Levaquin

III. Kantrex

(A) I only

(B) III only

(C) I and II only

(D) II and III only

(E) I, II, and III

11f. Patients consuming Septra should be advised to

I. drink large amounts of fluids

II. maintain a very acidic urine

III. avoid the use of folic acid containing products

(A) I only

(B) III only

(C) I and II only

(D) II and III only

(E) I, II, and III

11g. The patient wishes to test her urine to determine the presence of bacteriuria. An appropriate test will detect which one of the following chemicals?

(A) ketones

(B) glucose

(C) nitrates

(D) nitrites

(E) HCG

11h. Uristat and similar products can most accurately be classified as a (an)

(A) urinary antiseptic

(B) antimicrobial agent

(C) buffer

(D) antispasmodic

(E) analgesic

11i. This patient should be advised that Phenazopyridines may cause

(A) discoloration of the urine

(B) migraines

(C) temporary weight gain

(D) dizziness

(E) temporary infertility

11j. Pyridium should not be administered for longer than

(A) 2 days

(B) 5 days

(C) 10 days

(D) 14 days

(E) 30 days

11k. Symptoms of premenstrual syndrome (PMS) may include all of the following EXCEPT

(A) backache

(B) cramping

(C) edema

(D) irritability

(E) weight loss

11l. Which of the following ingredients is (are) included in OTC PMS products?

    I. caffeine

    II. pamabrom

    III. subtilisin

    (A) I only

    (B) III only

    (C) I and II only

    (D) II and III only

    (E) I, II, and III

11m. On 7/28, the physician's office calls concerning the patient's conjunctivitis, which is getting worse. The prescriber wants a fluoroquinolone ophthalmic solution. Which of the following products could be suggested?

    I. Tobrex

    II. Levaquin

    III. Ciloxan

    (A) I only

    (B) III only

    (C) I and II only

    (D) II and III only

    (E) I, II, and III

11n. Ms. Goodsmith asks if it is possible to split tablets such as the statin drugs being used by her mother to reduce their expense. Which of the following characteristics may support this practice?

    I. elongated scored tablets

    II. splitting one tablet at the time when needed

    III. presence of drugs with short half-lives

    (A) I only

    (B) III only

    (C) I and II only

    (D) II and III only

    (E) I, II, and III

11o. Which one of the following is NOT a risk factor for macular degeneration?

    (A) aging

    (B) hypertension

    (C) male species

    (D) prolonged exposure to sunlight

    (E) smoking

11p. All of the following dietary supplements have shown some effectiveness in reducing the risk of age-related macular degeneration (AMD) EXCEPT:

    (A) lutein

    (B) calcium

    (C) vitamin C

    (D) vitamin E

    (E) zinc + copper

11q. Other methods of reducing the incidence of AMD include all of the following EXCEPT

    (A) smoking cessation

    (B) reduction of hypertension

    (C) sunglasses

    (D) daily dosing of antioxidants

    (E) use of high-fiber diet

11r. Which of the following factors contribute to why females are more prone to incontinence than males?

    I. have a longer urethra

    II. have a less well-defined internal sphincter

    III. greater dependence on body estrogens

    (A) I only

    (B) III only

    (C) I and II only

    (D) II and III only

    (E) I, II, and III

11s. Which of the following urinary catheters is (are) suitable for Ms. Goodsmith?

   I. Foley

   II. intermittent

   III. Texas

(A) I only

(B) III only

(C) I and II only

(D) II and III only

(E) I, II, and III

11t. What percentage concentration of acetic acid in normal saline is usually ordered by the nursing staff for bladder irrigation?

(A) 0.01–0.09

(B) 0.1–1

(C) 2–5

(D) 10

(E) 36

▪PROFILE NO. 12

Hospital Pharmacy Medication Record

Patient Name: Michael Wishengrad
Room Number: 422–4

Age: 68   Height: 5'11"
Sex: M   Weight: 180 lb Estimated surface area = 1.6 m^2
Allergies: NK

DIAGNOSIS

Primary   Secondary
1. Chronic lymphocytic leukemia   1. Oral candida
2.
3.

LAB TESTS

Date	Test and Results
1. 6/4	Lymphocytosis 12,000/μL; K = 4.5; Na = 138
2. 6/10	Lymphocytosis 8,000/μL; K = 2.6; Na = 128

MEDICATION RECORD

Date	Drug and Strength	Sig
1. 6/4	Allopurinol (Zyloprim) 100 mg	1 t.i.d.
2. 6/4	Zolpidem 5 mg	1 hs p.r.n.
3. 6/4	Leukeran 14 mg	PO b.i.d.
4. 6/4	D/C Leukeran	
5. 6/4	Fludarabine 25 mg/m^2 in D$_5$W	Daily for 5 days
6. 6/4	Nystatin Susp.	q 4 h for 2 days
7. 6/7	Mitrolan tabs chew	1 q 4 h p.r.n.

PHARMACIST'S NOTES AND OTHER PATIENT INFORMATION

6/4 Admissions history—patient has been on a regimen of Leukeran tablets for CLL.

DIRECTIONS (Questions 12a through 12 k): Each of the numbered items or incomplete statements in this section is followed by answers or completions of the statement. Select the ONE lettered answer or completion that is BEST in each case.

12a. Leukeran can BEST be classified as a (an)

(A) antimetabolite

(B) antibiotic

(C) cell cycle specific agent

(D) alkylating agent

(E) hormone

12b. How many milligrams of fludarabine phosphate (Fludara) is needed for the 5 days of therapy?

(A) 25

(B) 40

(C) 80

(D) 125

(E) 200

12c. The patient's body surface area (BSA) in square meters can best be determined with the use of a

(A) nomogram

(B) tape measure

(C) picogram

(D) caliper

(E) micrometer

12d. Which one of the following drug products would be the most appropriate substitute for zolpidem?

(A) ProSom

(B) Dalmane

(C) Lunesta

(D) Halcion

(E) Restoril

12e. In which age range is acute lymphocytic leukemia (ALL) most prevalent?

(A) <15 years

(B) 20–30 years

(C) 30–50 years

(D) 50–70 years

(E) >70 years

12f. Chemotherapeutic drugs classified as anti-metabolites include

   I. methotrexate

  II. carmustine

 III. cyclophosphamide

(A) I only

(B) III only

(C) I and II only

(D) II and III only

(E) I, II, and III

12g. Allopurinol is pharmacologically classified as a (an)

(A) xanthine oxidase inhibitor

(B) MAO inhibitor

(C) beta-adrenergic agonist

(D) antimetabolite

(E) alkylating agent

12h. Patients using allopurinol should be advised to

(A) drink adequate fluids

(B) avoid dairy products

(C) expect urine discoloration

(D) avoid bruising

(E) take at least 1 g of vitamin C daily

12i. In order to monitor the use of allopurinol, determinations should be made of

(A) serum potassium

(B) serum folate

(C) urinary glucose

(D) serum uric acid

(E) urinary 5-HT

12j. An appropriate instruction for the use of nystatin suspension would be to

(A) take with a large glass of water

(B) swish and swallow

(C) take on an empty stomach

(D) mix it with fruit juice before administration

(E) allow product to stand until it thickens

12k. Mr. Wishengrad had been purchasing products from his local health food store. Which of the following ingredients are claimed to be sleep aids?

   I. ginseng

  II. L-tryptophan

 III. melatonin

(A) I only

(B) III only

(C) I and II only

(D) II and III only

(E) I, II, and III

■ PROFILE NO. 13

Hospital Pharmacy Medication Record

Patient Name: Sondra Johnson
Room Number: 406–3
Age: 25   Height: 5′3″
Sex: F (NG)   Weight: 150 lb
Allergies: Pollen, opiates

DIAGNOSIS

Primary   Secondary
1. Suspected appendicitis   1. Frequent headaches
   (abdominal pain)   2. Anemia? (pallor)

LABORATORY TESTS

Date	Test	Results with (normal ranges)
6/4	Hemo profile	WBC 12,000/μL (4000–10,000), Hb 8 g/dL (12–16), Hct 24% (36–47), MCH 20 pg (27–32), MCV 20 (82–98), Glucose 135 mg/dL

MEDICATION RECORD

Date	Physician	Drug and Strength	Sig
6/4	Gavin	APAP 325 mg	1 or 2 PO q 4 h
		Colace	100 mg q AM p.r.n.
		Alternagel	15 mL q 4 h p.r.n.
		Ambien	5 mg hs

PHARMACIST'S NOTES AND OTHER PATIENT INFORMATION

Date	Comment
6/4	Patient's pain appears to have subsided; still very pale in appearance; complains of increasing frequency of headaches which are relieved by daily use of aspirin (3–10 tabs total); has morbid fear of needles, very anxious to leave hospital; BP 105/70 (AM) 110/72 (PM)

DIRECTIONS (Questions 13a through 13r): Each of the numbered items or incomplete statements in this section is followed by answers or completions of the statement. Select the ONE lettered answer or completion that is BEST in each case.

13a. All of the following signs are consistent with a diagnosis of acute appendicitis EXCEPT

(A) nausea and vomiting

(B) elevated WBC counts

(C) high fever

(D) abdominal pain in the lower right quadrant

(E) shift in WBCs to the right

13b. When questioned, Ms. Johnson states that she has been very pale and tired for several months. The paleness is likely to be due to which one of the following?

(A) anemia

(B) high WBC count

(C) low WBC count

(D) polycythemia

(E) drug allergies

13c. Ms. Johnson's medical history suggests which of the following?

  I. type 2 diabetes
  II. pernicious anemia
  III. hypertension

(A) I only
(B) III only
(C) I and II only
(D) II and III only
(E) I, II, and III

13d. A patient with an abnormally elevated number of erythrocytes is described as having

(A) aplastic anemia
(B) polycythemia
(C) macrocytic anemia
(D) microcytic anemia
(E) sickle cell anemia

13e. Before discharging this patient, what drug will the intern likely prescribe for treating the anemia?

(A) ferrous sulfate
(B) ferric sulfate
(C) folic acid and iron salt
(D) iron dextran
(E) vitamin B_{12}

13f. How many milligrams of iron is present in every 300 mg ferrous sulfate tablet? (Ferrous sulfate: $FeSO_4$ 7 H_2O = 278; Fe = 56; S = 32; O = 16; H = 1)

(A) 18
(B) 35
(C) 60
(D) 100
(E) 300

13g. The resident changes the above order of 300 mg ferrous sulfate to ferrous gluconate, which may be less irritating. What strength tablet should be ordered? (Ferrous sulfate: $FeSO_4$ 7 H20 = 278; Ferrous gluconate: $C_{12}H_{22}FeO_{14}$ 2 H_2O = 482; Fe = 56)

(A) 100
(B) 150
(C) 250
(D) 300
(E) 500

13h. Which one of the following tests could have been ordered to determine if pernicious anemia was present?

(A) Direct Coomb's
(B) Indirect Coomb's
(C) Total bilirubin
(D) Benedict's
(E) Schilling

13i. If the intern suspects malnutrition in Ms. Johnson, which one of the following blood assays will most quickly confirm such a diagnosis?

(A) ALT
(B) AST
(C) albumin levels
(D) prealbumin levels
(E) troponins

13j. Which one of the following drugs may contribute to the iron deficiency anemia?

(A) aspirin
(B) ampicillin
(C) multivitamins
(D) tetracycline
(E) vitamin B complex

13k. The designation of "NG" in Ms. Johnson's medical history indicates her status with respect to

(A) gastric condition
(B) health insurance
(C) pregnancy
(D) presence of HIV
(E) possible presence of a sexual transmitted disease such as gonorrhea

13l. Based on Ms. Johnson's blood glucose values, which of the following actions should be taken?

(A) place the patient on a low carbohydrate diet

(B) prescribe insulin

(C) prescribe metformin

(D) prescribe a combination of metformin and insulin

(E) prescribe a low dose of glyburide

13m. What is the targeted hemoglobin A_{1c} value for a diabetic patient?

(A) less than 7%

(B) 7–10%

(C) greater than 10%

(D) less than 120 mg/dL

(E) less than 200 mg/dL

13n. Ms. Johnson's fear of insulin injections might be relieved if the pharmacist explains that the needle size is likely to be which of the following?

(A) 21G 1/8 in

(B) 21G 1/2 in

(C) 21G 5/8 in

(D) 25G 1 in.

(E) 28G 5/8 in

13o. Ms. Johnson admits that she will have trouble monitoring her glucose levels if she has to undergo painful finger sticks for blood samples. What is a possible alternative that the pharmacist may suggest to maintain accurate monitoring?

(A) Use the One Touch Fast Take instrument.

(B) Use the Glucometer Elite instrument.

(C) Use any digital glucose monitor but cut the strip in half so that less blood is needed.

(D) Use urine samples in the glucose monitor.

(E) Have someone else perform the finger stick.

13p. During her hospital discharge, the patient mentions that both of her parents suffered from macular degeneration. What part of the body does this condition affect?

(A) brain

(B) eyes

(C) heart

(D) kidneys

(E) muscles

13q. Which one of the following dietary supplements appears to help slow or prevent the development of macular degeneration?

(A) glucosamine

(B) homocysteine

(C) lutein

(D) selenium

(E) zinc

13r. A week after discharge from the hospital, Sondra returns to the emergency department with complaints of severe abdominal pains. High blood levels of which of the following may indicate bile duct blockage?

I. unconjugated bilirubin

II. conjugated bilirubin

III. total bilirubin

(A) I only

(B) III only

(C) I and II only

(D) II and III only

(E) I, II, and III

■ PROFILE NO. 14

Community Pharmacy Medication Record

Patient Name: Patrick Shannon
Address: 456 Park Ave

Age: 68   Height: 5'10"
Sex: M   Weight: 180 lb
Allergies: Pollen

DIAGNOSIS

Primary	Secondary
1. Obsessive-compulsive disorder	1. Early stages Alzheimer's disease
2. Type 2 diabetes (under control)	2. Complaints of heartburn (potential of peptic ulcer?)

MEDICATION RECORD

Date	Rx No.	Physician	Drug and Strength	Quantity	Sig	Refills
1/3	453078	T. Lewis	Tofranil 150 mg	30	1 daily	ref #2
3/2	454100	T. Lewis	Digoxin 0.25 mg	60	1 AM	6×
4/4	455500	"	Zoloft 100 mg	30	1 daily	3×
	455501	"	Pepcid 20 mg	90	1 t.i.d.	1×
4/12	456670	T. Lewis	Nasonex Nasal	1 bt	1–2 sprays p.r.n.	3×
5/6	454100		Digoxin	30	1 AM	ref #1
5/8	455258		Zoloft 25 mg	30	1–2 daily for panic	ref #1

PHARMACIST'S NOTES AND OTHER PATIENT INFORMATION

Date	Comment
1/15	Patient complains of dryness of mouth and other side effects due to Tofranil. Suggest he consult with Dr. Lewis

DIRECTIONS (Questions 14a through 14t): Each of the numbered items or incomplete statement in this section is followed by answers or completions of the statement. Select the ONE lettered answer or completion that is BEST in each case.

14a. Under which one of the following categories would Zoloft be classified?

  (A) antihyperlipidemic
  (B) MAOI
  (C) selective serotonin reuptake inhibitor (SSRI)
  (D) tetracyclic antidepressant
  (E) tricyclic antidepressant

14b. Four days after starting therapy with Zoloft, Mr. Shannon complains that he is displeased with the high cost of Zoloft and claims that it is not helping him. The pharmacist should advise him that

  (A) the drug is less expensive than many others
  (B) the drug often takes 2–4 weeks before noticeable improvement occurs
  (C) it is his imagination that the drug is not working
  (D) he should be switched to another SSRI
  (E) he should be switched back to the tricyclic antidepressant previously used

14c. The patient shows the pharmacist the results of a cholesterol test performed in a shopping mall health fair. The stated level is 240 mg/dL. What is this value in terms of millimoles per liter (mol. wt. cholesterol = 387)?

(A) 0.62
(B) 6.2
(C) 62
(D) .062
(E) 0.0062

14d. The following week Mr. Shannon brings a copy of his cholesterol screening performed at a medical clinic. The listed levels are

Cholesterol	260 mg/dL
Triglycerides	98 mg/dL
HDL	73 mg/dL
VLDL	19.6
Direct LDL	114
Chol/HDL ratio	3.6

He is worried that all of the values sound high to him. Which one value is MOST encouraging?

(A) cholesterol
(B) high-density lipoprotein (HDL)
(C) low-density lipoprotein (LDL)
(D) triglycerides
(E) VLDL

14e. Last year, Mr. Shannon had a prescription filled for one of the statins, but claims that he stopped taking this medication because of the cost. Which one of the following OTC drugs may be suggested to him for lowering his cholesterol?

(A) aspirin
(B) glucosamine
(C) niacin
(D) thiamine
(E) saw palmetto

14f. Mr. Shannon has noticed some increases in his blood pressure measurements but cannot afford expensive heart medicines. The phar-macist should explain that the physician is most likely to initiate therapy for borderline hypertension with which of the following?

(A) ACE inhibitors
(B) calcium channel blockers
(C) diuretics
(D) potassium supplements
(E) direct vasodilators

14g. Which of the following statements concerning support (compression) stockings is (are) true?

  I. Stockings should be put on first thing in the morning.
 II. Stockings designated as antiembolism stockings exert only 20 mm of pressure.
III. Stockings with gradient pressures exert the greatest pressure on the lower extremities.

(A) I only
(B) III only
(C) I and II only
(D) II and III only
(E) I, II, and III

14h. Which of the following advice should the pharmacist give to Mr. Shannon when dispensing each bottle of Nasonex Nasal Spray?

  I. prime each new bottle by pumping about 10 times
 II. use in each nostril for most effective activity
III. administer every day to maximize the product's prophylactic activity

(A) I only
(B) III only
(C) I and II only
(D) II and III only
(E) I, II, and III

14i. Today, the patient presents a new prescription for clarithromycin 500 mg #42 Sig: 1 t.i.d. and omeprazole 20 mg #14 Sig: one tablet q AM. This combination is most likely being used to treat which one of the following conditions?

(A) *Helicobacter pylori*

(B) *Staphylococcus aureus*

(C) otitis media

(D) community-acquired pneumonia

(E) SARS

14j. Which one of the following drug interactions may occur with Mr. Shannon's therapy?

(A) decreased levels of digoxin due to the clarithromycin

(B) increased levels of digoxin due to the clarithromycin

(C) decreased levels of digoxin due to the omeprazole

(D) increased levels of digoxin due to the omeprazole

(E) no reaction with either drug is expected

14k. Mr. Shannon is very concerned because his 48-year-old wife is experiencing a constant redness on her cheeks that has lasted for over 1 month. Which of the following is the MOST likely explanation for this phenomenon?

(A) chronic alcoholism

(B) hypertension

(C) shingles

(D) rosacea

(E) menopause

Answer questions 14l through 14o using the following prescription.

Burow's solution	10 mL
salicyclic acid	4%
phenol	1%
white petrolatum qs	60 g
Sig: Apply to affected area t.i.d.	

14l. What is the active ingredient in Burow's solution?

(A) aluminum acetate

(B) acetic acid

(C) aluminum chloride

(D) calcium hydroxide

(E) hydrogen peroxide

14m. When preparing the above prescription, the pharmacist may wish to include which of the following in the formula?

 I. alcohol

 II. polysorbate 80

III. Aquaphor

(A) I only

(B) III only

(C) I and II only

(D) II and III only

(E) I, II, and III

14n. The function of salicylic acid in this product is as a (an)

(A) analgesic

(B) local anesthetic

(C) abrasive

(D) keratolytic

(E) preservative

14o. Patrick refuses to listen to his wife who advocates receiving the "Shingles vaccine." He states that he never had chickenpox and is not susceptible since he is older than 50 years. The pharmacist may inform him of which of the following?

 I. Often, childhood chickenpox is mild and not noticeable.

 II. People in the 40–70 age bracket are more susceptible than those older than 70.

III. People that never had chickenpox are most susceptible to shingles.

(A) I only

(B) III only

(C) I and II only

(D) II and III only

(E) I, II, and III

Answer questions 14p through 14t based on the following scenario. Mrs. Shannon has been experiencing a productive cough and high fever for several days. Now she has chest pain, chills, dyspnea, and increased high fever. The local clinic takes an X-ray and suggests that she enter the local hospital for further tests since the tentative diagnosis is community-acquired pneumonia (CAP).

14p. Which one of the following lab tests should be ordered for her?

- (A) ALT
- (B) C & S
- (C) creatine clearance
- (D) PTT
- (E) I & O

14q. Which one of the following antibiotics is least appropriate for its effectiveness against CAP?

- (A) azithromycin
- (B) clarithromycin
- (C) doxycycline
- (D) levofloxicin
- (E) penicillin K

14r. If the above patient is resistant to the antibiotic therapy being provided, one may suspect MRSA (methicillin-resistant *S. aureus*). Which one of the following drugs may then be suggested?

- (A) amoxicillin
- (B) cefprozil
- (C) clindamycin
- (D) diclofenac
- (E) vancomycin IV

14s. Assuming that vancomycin is being infused into the patient, what minimum serum concentration (mg/L) must be maintained?

- (A) 10
- (B) 15
- (C) 20
- (D) 40
- (E) 50

14t. A dose of 500 mg vancomycin every 6 hours has been ordered by the intern. Which of the following routes of administration is (are) appropriate?

- I. 500 mg in 100 mL D_5W, infuse over 1 hour
- II. 250 mg IV bolus followed by second dose 3 hours later
- III. 500 mg deep IM injection

- (A) I only
- (B) III only
- (C) I and II only
- (D) II and III only
- (E) I, II, and III

■PROFILE NO. 15

Community Pharmacy Medication Record

Patient Name: Leslie Schwartzman
Address: 43 West Main Street
Age: 11   Height: 4'11"
Sex: F   Weight: 88 lb
Allergies: Peanuts, sulfa

DIAGNOSIS

Primary	Secondary
1. Cystic fibrosis	1.
2. ADHD	2.

MEDICATION RECORD

Date	Rx No.	Physician	Drug and Strength	Quantity	Sig	Refills
1. 7/4	19287	Rodriguez	Mucomyst	3 × 30 mL	p.r.n. with nebulizer	3
2. 8/22	23388	Rodriguez	Cotazym	60	1 t.i.d.	5
3. 9/1	27003	Dixon	Concerta 18 mg	60	2 q AM	0

PHARMACIST'S NOTES AND OTHER PATIENT INFORMATION

Date	Comment
1.	
2.	

DIRECTIONS (Questions 15a through 15i): Each of the numbered items or incomplete statements in this section is followed by answers or completions of the statement. Select the ONE lettered answer or completion that is BEST in each case.

15a. The cause of cystic fibrosis can best be described as

   (A) viral

   (B) autoimmune

   (C) fungal

   (D) bacterial

   (E) genetic

15b. Which of the following tests are done to diagnose the presence of cystic fibrosis?

   (A) sweat test

   (B) chemical stress test

   (C) pulmonary function test

   (D) mucopolysaccharide test

   (E) Schilling's Test

15c. Mucomyst is generally administered orally for the treatment of

   (A) cystic fibrosis

   (B) aspirin overdose

   (C) drug-resistant tuberculosis

   (D) acetaminophen overdose

   (E) GERD

15d. Children with cystic fibrosis often have difficulty in absorbing

   (A) protein

   (B) fat

   (C) carbohydrate

   (D) electrolytes

   (E) water-soluble vitamins

15e. This patient should be advised to take the Cotazym

(A) an hour before or 2–3 hours after meals
(B) at bedtime
(C) while standing
(D) with each meal
(E) with an antacid

15f. Concerta contains the same active ingredient as

  I. Adderall
 II. Daytrana
III. Methylin

(A) I only
(B) III only
(C) I and II only
(D) II and III only
(E) I, II, and III

15g. The major advantage of Concerta over Ritalin is that Concerta

(A) is available as a transdermal patch.
(B) does not cause as much CNS stimulation.
(C) does not cause as much CNS depression.
(D) is a sustained-release product.
(E) is available in a liquid and solid dosage form.

15h. Which of the following adverse effects is MOST likely to occur when using Concerta?

(A) aplastic anemia
(B) hemolytic anemia
(C) hypertrichosis
(D) bradycardia
(E) tachycardia

15i. Which of the following drug products are NOT indicated for the treatment of attention deficit hyperactivity disorder (ADHD)?

  I. Orap
 II. Namenda
III. Strattera

(A) I only
(B) III only
(C) I and II only
(D) II and III only
(E) I, II, and III

■ PROFILE NO. 16

Community Pharmacy Medication Record

Patient Name: Joan Lewis
Address: 27 Green St. Apt 4
Age: 32   Height: 5'4"
Sex: F   Weight: 120 lb
Allergies: Bee stings, sulfas?

DIAGNOSIS

Primary   Secondary
1. Psychotic disorders   1. Borderline diabetic
2. Mild hypertension   2. Frequent UTIs

PHARMACIST'S NOTES AND OTHER PATIENT INFORMATION

1. Ms. Lewis has had drinking binges resulting in some depression. She now claims that she does not drink any alcohol.

DIRECTIONS (Questions 16a through 16r): Each of the numbered items or incomplete statements in this section is followed by answers or completions of the statement. Select the ONE lettered answer or completion that is BEST in each case.

16a. Ms. Lewis confides to the pharmacist that she thinks that she is going crazy because of some of her behavior. She constantly worries about not locking the front door, leaving the stove on, and has a strong desire to rearrange her furniture and kitchen cabinets. What condition should the pharmacist suspect?

(A) Alzheimer's disease
(B) senile dementia
(C) bipolar disorder
(D) obsessive-compulsive disorder (OCD)
(E) schizophrenia

16b. Which one of the following is commonly employed when initiating treatment for a patient with OCD?

(A) long-acting barbiturate
(B) serotonin reuptake inhibitor
(C) lithium carbonate
(D) tricyclic drug
(E) clomipramine

16c. Which one of the following is a brand name product of citalopram?

(A) Celexa
(B) Coreg
(C) Clozaril
(D) Paxil
(E) Serzone

16d. Which of the following drugs is MOST likely to be prescribed for a patient who has a history of panic attacks but with no comorbid major depression?

(A) phenytoin
(B) phenobarbital
(C) lithium carbonate
(D) prazepam
(E) venlafaxine

16e. Ms. Lewis is concerned that one of her tablets lists magnesium stearate as an ingredient. What is the purpose of this chemical?

(A) antioxidant
(B) coating agent
(C) disintegration agent
(D) lubricant
(E) nutritional source of magnesium

16f. Ms. Lewis presents a new prescription for a diaphragm. How will the prescriber likely indicate the desired size?

(A) small, medium, or large
(B) 2, 3, or 4 in
(C) 60, 70, or 75 mm
(D) 20, 25, or 30 French
(E) 16, 20, or 25 gauge

16g. When dispensing the diaphragm, the pharmacist should suggest concurrent use of a product containing which of the following?

(A) benzalkonium chloride
(B) boric acid
(C) lanolin
(D) mineral oil
(E) nonoxynol-9

16h. Ms. Lewis's 4-year-old child, Larry, appears to have behavior abnormalities including hyperactivity, short attention span, and abdominal colic. He also appears to be learning-impaired. Which of the following causes may explain these symptoms?

I.   Alzheimer's disease
II. ADHD
III. lead poisoning

(A) I only
(B) III only
(C) I and II only
(D) II and III only
(E) I, II, and III

16i. The Centers for Disease Control and Prevention define childhood lead poisoning as when the lead levels in the blood are at 10 μg/dL or higher. What is this concentration in parts per million?

(A) 0.1 ppm
(B) 1 ppm
(C) 10 ppm
(D) 100 ppm
(E) 1,000 ppm

16j. Which of the following products may be used for the treatment of lead poisoning?

I.   BAL
II. succimer
III. Mucomyst

(A) I only
(B) III only
(C) I and II only
(D) II and III only
(E) I, II, and III

16k. Ms. Lewis has been experiencing some redness in both eyes. Which one of the following ingredients present in her contact lens products is most likely responsible?

(A) homosalate
(B) polyvinyl alcohol
(C) subtilisin
(D) sodium carboxymethylcellulose
(E) thimerosol

16l. Further discussion with Ms. Lewis reveals that she has been preparing pint quantities of her own contact lens soaking solution using salt tablets as the main ingredient. Which one of the following microorganisms presents a specific danger for an eye infection?

(A) *Acanthamoeba*
(B) *E. coli*
(C) *S. aureus*
(D) *Streptococcus*
(E) *Aspergillus niger*

16m. Ms. Lewis asks the pharmacist about the sedative Lunesta which is being advertised on TV. Which of the following descriptions is not correct?

(A) generic name is Eszopiclone
(B) intended for short-term use (<30 days)
(C) not classified as a benzodiazepine
(D) half-life is approximately 6 hours
(E) metabolized in the liver

16n. Ms Lewis's 62 year-old mother Ethel accompanies her into the pharmacy. All of the following observations concerning Ethel would lead the pharmacist to believe she is suffering from Parkinson disease EXCEPT

(A) drooping eyelids
(B) hand tremors
(C) forward tilting of the head
(D) dementia
(E) slow, shuffling gait

16o. When attempting to detect drug-induced Parkinsonism, the pharmacist may question Ethel concerning her medication history. Which one of the following classes of drugs is known to cause secondary Parkinsonism?

(A) ACE antihypertensives
(B) antidepressants
(C) antihyperlipidemics
(D) antipsychotics
(E) sedatives

16p. Ms. Lewis agrees to participate in a clinical trial for a new drug. The clinical pharmacist prepares an IM injection using the water-soluble disodium salt and evaluates the following information: [mol. wt. disodium salt = 460; Na = 23; disassociation constant = 2.4; desired concentration = 40 mg/mL]. What will be the approximate osmolarity (mOm/L) of this injection if no other ingredients are present?

(A) 100
(B) 200
(C) 250
(D) 300
(E) 400

16q. Although the pharmacist adjusted the above solution to isotonicity with sodium chloride, the patient complains of stinging at the injection site when 2 mL IM injection is given. Which one of the following is the most likely explanation for the irritation?

(A) poor nursing technique
(B) presence of sodium chloride
(C) volume of 2 mL is too large for IM injection
(D) high pH
(E) absence of an antimicrobial preservative

16r. Studies on the above antibiotic in several patients indicate a clearance rate of 0.064/h. What is the approximate plasma half-life of this drug?

(A) <5 hours
(B) 6 hours
(C) 11 hours
(D) 15 hours
(E) >15 hours

■ PROFILE NO. 17

Hospital Pharmacy Medication Record

Patient Name: Lee Albright
Room Number: 604–2

Age: 16   Height: 5'6"
Sex: M   Weight: 100 lb
Allergies: None known

DIAGNOSIS

Primary	Secondary
Sickle cell anemia	General malaise and weakness

LABORATORY TESTS

Date	Test	Results
8/15	Electrolytes	Sodium 145 mEq/L; potassium 3.5 mEq/L; chloride 100 mmol/L; calcium 7 mg/dL; bicarbonate 24 mmol/L; albumin 4 g/dL; BUN 28 mg/dL; glucose 105 mg/dL
8/16	Serum Cr	0.8 mg/dL

MEDICATION RECORD

Date	Physician	Drug and Strength	Sig
8/15	Dandree	Morphine sulf 0.2 mg/kg SC. STAT then 0.15 mg/kg SC.	q 4 h p.r.n. for 4 days
		Start $D_5W/1/2$ NS	1 L q 8 h
		Colace 100 mg	1 q AM as needed
		Zolpidem 5 mg	1 h.s. p.r.n.
		Multivitamin	1 daily
8/16	Dandree	D/C electrolytes	
		Start standard TPN, 2 L per day at 08:00 and 14:00 with flow rate 125 mL/h if tolerated.	
		Amino acid sol 5% + $D_{50}W$ aa 500 mL NaCl 50 mEq; KCl 40 mEq;	
		MVI Ped 5 mL CaGluconate 8.6 mEq + Trace Metals-5 2 mL	
8/18	Dandree	Anticipate discharge; convert IV morphine to morphine in PCA unit; arrange visiting nurse coverage	
		PM—Discharge with PCA unit containing 100 mL morphine sulfate with flow set at 0.02 mg/kg MS q h for 3 days.	

PHARMACIST'S NOTES AND OTHER PATIENT INFORMATION

Date	Comment
8/16	Reviewed patient's previous medical history plus present history and complaints; needs further evaluation to determine need for TPN

DIRECTIONS (Questions 17a through 17n): Each of the numbered items or incomplete statements in this section is followed by answers or completions of the statement. Select the ONE lettered answer or completion that is BEST in each case.

17a. All of the following are methods used to assess the patient's nutritional state EXCEPT

(A) albumin levels

(B) AST levels

(C) anthropometric

(D) proalbumin levels

(E) transferrin levels

17b. Which of the following diseases is (are) associated with malnutrition?

I. Graves

II. Kwashiorkor

III. Marasmus

(A) I only

(B) III only

(C) I and II only

(D) II and III only

(E) I, II, and III

17c. Which one of the following drugs is most likely to be ordered for the treatment of sickle cell anemia?

(A) fluorouracil

(B) hydroxyurea

(C) iron dextran

(D) levothyroxine

(E) propylthiouracil

17d. Which of the following is true about the prescriber's order for zolpidem?

(A) Because it is a benzodiazepine, zolpidem is contraindicated for patients taking morphine.

(B) The route of administration, oral, or parenteral, must be specified.

(C) The drug will duplicate the action of morphine.

(D) Administration of the drug should be 2 hours before bedtime.

(E) None of the above are correct.

17e. After the original STAT dose, how many milliliters of morphine sulfate (10 mg/mL) should be administered per dose?

(A) 0.15

(B) 0.7

(C) 1

(D) 1.5

(E) 2.8

17f. How many nonprotein kilocalories is the patient receiving per hour if the TPN solution is infused over an 8-hour period?

(A) 100

(B) 120

(C) 240

(D) 800

(E) 850

17g. How many grams of nitrogen is being infused into the patient daily?

(A) 4

(B) 8

(C) 16

(D) 25

(E) 50

17h. Which of the following methods are appropriate for administering the TPN solutions to Lee Albright?

I. through a central catheter

II. through a PICC line in the arm

III. directly through a peripheral vein

(A) I only

(B) III only

(C) I and II only

(D) II and III only

(E) I, II, and III

17i. Which one of the following equations would enable the pharmacist to estimate the renal creatinine clearance in Mr. Albright?

(A) Cockroft Gault

(B) Harris Benedict

(C) Henderson Hasselbalch

(D) Loo Riegelman

(E) Method of least residuals

17j. What will be the estimated creatinine clearance rate in this patient?

(A) 60

(B) 80

(C) 100

(D) 120

(E) 160

17k. Which one of the following types of amino acid formulas is specifically designed for patients under high stress or with liver impairment?

(A) inclusion of homocysteine

(B) increased levels of all nonessential amino acids

(C) increased levels of all of the essential amino acids

(D) higher levels of branched chained amino acids (BCAA)

(E) addition of taurine

17l. Which one of the following ions as a trace metal is not included in TPN formulas?

(A) aluminum

(B) copper

(C) manganese

(D) chromium

(E) zinc

17m. How many milliliters of morphine sulfate (10 mg/mL) should be used to fill the PCA device?

(A) 0.14

(B) 2.2

(C) 6.6

(D) 66

(E) 14.4

17n. Reasons why the physician may have chosen the employment of a PCA for infusion rather than an elastomeric infusion device include all of the following reasons EXCEPT

(A) can change the dosing while the unit is attached to the patient

(B) patient may remain ambulatory

(C) can program bolus dosing if desired

(D) unit is less expensive to use and maintain

(E) unit can deliver subcutaneous dosing while the elastomeric cannot

▪PROFILE NO. 18

Hospital Pharmacy Medication Record

Patient Name: Anthony Costello
Room Number: 621
Age: 42   Height: 5'4"
Sex: M   Weight: 132 lb
Allergies: Aspirin, hay fever

DIAGNOSIS

Primary	Secondary
1. Hodgkin's disease	1. Graves' disease
2.	2. Essential hypertension (under control with diet)
3.	3. Allergies

LAB TESTS

Date	Test and Results
1. 6/12	SMA-12

MEDICATION RECORD

Date	Drug and Strength	Sig
1. 6/12	Propylthiouracil 50 mg	2 b.i.d.
2.	Mechlorethamine 6 mg/m^2 on day 1	
3.	Procarbazine 100 mg/m^2	
4.	Prednisone 40 mg	1 daily
5.	Vincristine 2 mg on day 1	
6.	Lorazepam 2 mg	1 h.s. p.r.n.
7.	Colace 100 mg	1 q d
8.	APAP 325 mg	2 tabs p.r.n. fever

PHARMACIST'S NOTES AND OTHER PATIENT INFORMATION

Date	Comment
1. 6/12	Start MOPP therapy on 6/14 if blood work results are normal.

DIRECTIONS (Questions 18a through 18o): Each of the numbered items or incomplete statements in this section is followed by answers or completions of the statement. Select the ONE lettered answer or completion that is BEST in each case.

18a. Which of the drugs used by this patient is indicated for the treatment of Graves disease?

(A) mechlorethamine

(B) prednisone

(C) procarbazine

(D) propylthiouracil

(E) vincristine

18b. Which of the following drugs is (are) administered orally during MOPP treatment?

I. mechlorethamine (Mustargen)

II. procarbazine (Matulane)

III. prednisone

(A) I only

(B) III only

(C) I and II only

(D) II and III only

(E) I, II, and III

18c. Which one of the following forms of cancer is LEAST responsive to chemotherapy?

(A) hepatocellular
(B) Hodgkin's
(C) ovarian
(D) prostate
(E) testicular

18d. The nursing staff invites the pharmacist to a meeting for reviewing the SOAP for Mr. Costello. This acronym refers to which one of the following?

(A) evaluation of his treatment program
(B) general cleanliness of the patient
(C) special bathing needs
(D) special operational procedure for administering chemotherapy
(E) specific procedures for discharging the patient

18e. The intern reports that Mr. Costello is experiencing extravasation of the mechlorethamine (Mustargen). Which one of the following courses of treatment should be initiated?

(A) Apply warm compresses immediately.
(B) Infiltrate 1/6 mol. sodium thiosulfate into area and apply ice compresses.
(C) Infiltrate epinephrine 1/1,000 into area.
(D) Infuse heparin sodium 20,000 units into area.
(E) Withdraw infusion needle and apply compresses of sodium thiosulfate 10% w/v

18f. How many grams of sodium thiosulfate USP is needed to prepare 100 mL of 1/6 mol. solution? (mol. Wt. of $Na_2S_2O_3$ 5 H20 = 248; mol. wt. of water = 18)

(A) 2.1
(B) 4.1
(C) 7.5
(D) 14.9
(E) 24.8

18g. The pharmacy has only the anhydrous form of sodium thiosulfate. How many grams of this form is needed to obtain a 10% w/v sodium thiosulfate USP solution? (mol. wt. of $Na_2S_2O_3$ 5 H_2O = 248; mol. wt. of water = 18)

(A) 3
(B) 6.4
(C) 13.5
(D) 4
(E) 0 (because anhydrous form cannot be used)

18h. Which one of the following is a serious delayed toxic effect of many chemotherapeutic drugs?

(A) bone marrow depression
(B) cardiotoxicity
(C) nausea and vomiting
(D) peripheral neuropathy
(E) respiratory depression

18i. By which of the following routes of administration may the 2 mg of vincristine be administered?

I. into a running IV line
II. intramuscular injection
III. intrathecally by syringe

(A) I only
(B) III only
(C) I and II only
(D) II and III only
(E) I, II, and III

18j. Which of the following agents would be appropriate to administer to a patient on chemotherapy with mechlorethamine?

I. Epogen (epoetin alfa)
II. Neupogen (filgrastim)
III. Plavix (clopidogrel)

(A) I only
(B) III only
(C) I and II only
(D) II and III only
(E) I, II, and III

18k. The physician orders weekly injections of cyanocobalamin (vitamin B_{12}). Which of the following routes of administration are appropriate for this agent?

I. subcutaneous

II. intramuscular

III. intravenous

(A) I only

(B) III only

(C) I and II only

(D) II and III only

(E) I, II, and III

18l. Mr. Costello requires an antihistamine for the treatment of his allergies. Which of the following is an antihistamine suitable for Mr. Costello's needs?

I. Zyrtec (cetirizine)

II. Clarinex (desloratadine)

III. Allegra (fexofenadine)

(A) I only

(B) III only

(C) I and II only

(D) II and III only

(E) I, II, and III

18m. Mr. Costello's wife is presently taking lisinopril (Prinivil) and complains of a involuntary coughing. Which one of the following drugs is probably more suitable for her?

(A) Acupril

(B) Altace

(C) Benicar

(D) Lotensin

(E) Zestril

18n. Which one of the following is most similar to Prinivil?

(A) Accupril

(B) Benazepril

(C) Captopril

(D) Vasotec

(E) Zestril

18o. When performing a prospective review of a new prescription for an ACE inhibitor, the pharmacist should recognize potential problems in women during which of the following stages of pregnancy?

I. first trimester

II. second trimester

III. third trimester

(A) I only

(B) III only

(C) I and II only

(D) II and III only

(E) I, II, and III

▪ PROFILE NO. 19

Hospital Pharmacy Medication Record

Patient Name: Laura Hockford
Room Number: 202B

Age: 52   Height: 5'10"
Sex: F   Weight: 140 lb
Allergies: Peanuts

DIAGNOSIS

Primary	Secondary
1. CA ovaries	1. Essential HTN
2. Diabetes	2.
3.	3.

MEDICATION RECORD

Date	Drug and Strength	Sig
1. 5/2	HCTZ 50 mg	1 PO q d
2.	Colace 100 mg	1 every AM
3.	Restoril 15 mg	1 h.s. p.r.n.
4.	Hytrin 2 mg	1 h.s.
5. 5/4	Paclitaxel 150 mg/m², infuse over 24 h followed by Cisplatin 30 mg/m²	

PHARMACIST'S NOTES AND OTHER PATIENT INFORMATION

Date	Comment
1. 5/4	Patient declines radiotherapy; drug therapy to be scheduled
2. 5/6	Anticipate discharge tomorrow, schedule follow-up therapy every 3 weeks for a total of three more sessions with usual blood work.

DIRECTIONS (Questions 19a through 19n): Each of the numbered items or incomplete statements in this section is followed by answers or by completions of the statement. Select the ONE lettered answer or completion that is BEST in each case.

19a. Paclitaxel is available under which of the following trade names?

   I. Tazidime

   II. Taxotere

   III. Taxol

   (A) I only

   (B) III only

   (C) I and II only

   (D) II and III only

   (E) I, II, and III

19b. Which one of the following procedures is NOT appropriate when dispensing injectable paclitaxel?

   (A) storing the solution in polyvinyl chloride (PVC) bags

   (B) storing unopened vials in the refrigerator

   (C) dispensing the solution in a glass bottle

   (D) administering the solution by infusion through an in-line filter

   (E) dispensing a slightly hazy, diluted solution

19c. The pharmacist may wish to suggest the addition of dolasetron mesylate to Ms. Hockford's therapy. This drug is used as a (an)

(A) antiemetic

(B) antihistamine

(C) local anesthetic

(D) antidepressant

(E) antivesicant

19d. Which of the following statements concerning cisplatin is (are) true?

   I. available under the tradename of Paraplatin

   II. classified as an alkylating agent

   III. often causes nausea and vomiting

(A) I only

(B) III only

(C) I and II only

(D) II and III only

(E) I, II, and III

19e. Assuming that the patient's BSA was determined to be 1.85 m^2, how many milliliters of paclitaxel injection will be needed if 50 mL multidose vials (6 mg/mL) are available?

(A) 5

(B) 23

(C) 43

(D) 46

(E) 50

19f. The literature reports that major side effects for paclitaxel (Taxol) include bone marrow depression, cardiac toxicity, and peripheral neuropathy. Which one of the following chemotherapeutic agents does not cause bone marrow depression?

(A) cytarabine (Cytosar-U)

(B) lomustine (CeeNU)

(C) mitomycin (Mutamycin)

(D) tamoxifen (Nolvadex)

(E) vinblastine (Velban)

19g. Which one of the following is the best description of peripheral neuropathy?

(A) degenerative state of peripheral nerves

(B) severe, localized headache

(C) inflammation of peripheral veins

(D) numbness of the feet

(E) vasodilation of peripheral blood vessels

19h. Adverse effects of chemotherapeutic agents, such as bone marrow depression, pass through three stages: onset, maximum depression, and recovery to normal. Which one of the following terms is used to indicate the time for maximum depression?

(A) climb

(B) lag time

(C) retention time

(D) nadir

(E) suppression time

19i. Which of the following suggestions should the pharmacist make to the physician before the start of cisplatin therapy?

   I. DC the Hytrin

   II. DC the HCTZ

   III. Start infusions of 2 L D$_{2.5}$W/1/2NS 12 hours before the cisplatin infusion

(A) I only

(B) III only

(C) I and II only

(D) II and III only

(E) I, II, and III

19j. On 5/10, Ms. Hockford is readmitted to the hospital. The admitting physician observes weight loss, rales, FUO, N & V, and coughing with a greenish mucus. She orders chest X-rays, SMA 16, and blood tests for culture and sensitivity. Which one of the following drugs may be ordered for the diagnosis of FUO?

(A) APAP

(B) biscodyl

(C) diazepam

(D) insulin

(E) IV nitroprusside

19k. The pharmacy receives an order for Augmentin 1 g IVMB stat, then q 6 h. For which of the following reasons must the pharmacist consult with the prescriber?

   I. Augmentin is not available as a parenteral dosage form.

   II. The strength ordered is an excessive amount.

   III. The drug is not a broad-spectrum antibiotic.

(A) I only
(B) III only
(C) I and II only
(D) II and III only
(E) I, II, and III

19l. Culture and sensitivity lab report indicates the following MICs: Antibiotic A > 4 μg/mL; B $= 4$ μg/mL; C < 4 μg/mL; D $= 8$ μg/mL; E < 8 μg/mL Assuming similar toxicities, which antibiotic is probably the best choice for Ms. Hockford's infection?

(A) antibiotic A
(B) antibiotic B
(C) antibiotic C
(D) antibiotic D
(E) antibiotic E

19m. The prescriber is considering using parenteral vancomycin on the patient. Which of the following reactions is (are) likely to occur if a nurse infuses vancomycin too rapidly?

   I. red man syndrome

   II. hypotension

   III. pseudomembranous colitis

(A) I only
(B) III only
(C) I and II only
(D) II and III only
(E) I, II, and III

19n. The order for an antibiotic indicates an infusion "100 mg q 8 h + SASH." This acronym relates to which of the following?

(A) covering the injection site with a cold compress
(B) covering the injection site with a warm compress
(C) infusing 100 mL normal saline after the antibiotic
(D) subjective observation of the patient 30 minutes after the infusion
(E) use of a heparin well

∎PROFILE NO. 20

Community Pharmacy Medication Record

Patient Name: Catherine Chaudry
Address: 12 Congress St. Fairhaven VT

Age: 35   Height: 5'6"
Sex: F   Weight: 124 lb
Allergies: Pollen

DIAGNOSIS

Primary	Secondary
1. Hypertension	1. High total cholesterol
2. Diabetes	2.
3.	

MEDICATION RECORD

	Date	Rx No.	Physician	Drug and Strength	Quantity	Sig	Refills
1.	1/5	59535	Lewis	Hytrin 2 mg	60	1 daily	3×
2.		59536	Collins	*Ortho*-Tri-Cyclen	3 pack	1 q AM	6 mos
3.		59537	Lewis	Glyburide 2.5 mg	60	1 q d	3×
4.	2/12	64012	Collins	TMP-SMZ, Regular		1 q 12 h for 10 d	1×
5.	3/5	66156	Lewis	Lipitor 20 mg	30	1 h.s.	1×
6.		59535	Lewis	Hytrin 2 mg	60	1 daily	Refill 1/3
7.		59537		Glyburide 2.5 mg	60	1 q d	Refill 1/3

PHARMACIST'S NOTES AND OTHER PATIENT INFORMATION

	Date	Comment
1.	4/1	Patient purchased niacin 250 mg
2.		

DIRECTIONS (Questions 20a through 20q): Each of the numbered items or incomplete statements in this section is followed by answers or completions of the statement. Select the ONE lettered answer or completion that is BEST in each case.

20a. To what class of drugs does Hytrin belong?

   (A) alphal-adrenergic blockers
   (B) ACE inhibitors
   (C) calcium channel blockers
   (D) diuretics
   (E) angiotensin II-receptor antagonists

20b. When the pharmacist originally filled the prescription for Hytrin, he should have warned the patient about the "first-dose" effect. This refers to which of the following?

   (A) loss of appetite for 1–3 days
   (B) hypertension that may occur after the first dose
   (C) postural hypotension
   (D) drowsiness that diminishes after two doses
   (E) a flushing of the face

20c. Ms. Chaudry is unhappy with the side effects that she attributes to the Ortho-Tri-Cyclen. She asks about a drug her mother is taking, Evista, which she read was a different type of hormone. Which of the following comments should the pharmacist offer concerning this drug?

    I. It may be used in premenopausal women to regulate their menstrual cycle.

    II. It is classified as a selective estrogen receptor modulator.

    III. Its main intent is for the prevention of osteoporosis in postmenopausal women.

    (A) I only

    (B) III only

    (C) I and II only

    (D) II and III only

    (E) I, II, and III

20d. The pharmacist could suggest that Ms. Chaudry approach her OB/GYN doctor suggesting a switch from Ortho-Tri-Cyclen to which of the following?

    (A) Microgestin Fe

    (B) Ortho-Evra

    (C) Ortho-Novum

    (D) Ortho-Cyclen

    (E) Estraderm

20e. Ms. Chaudry's husband just returned from a business trip to Canada where he received a prescription written by trade name to treat a peptic ulcer. In which of the following references may the pharmacist locate the generic name of the drug product?

    (A) Facts and Comparisons

    (B) Martindale (The Extra Pharmacopeia)

    (C) Merck Index

    (D) PDR

    (E) USP DI

20f. When picking up her prescriptions, the patient mentions that the family is going to the beach and will need a sunscreen lotion with an SPF of 8. All of the following sunscreen agents are suitable EXCEPT

    (A) benzones

    (B) homosalate

    (C) mineral oil + iodine

    (D) PABA

    (E) padimates

20g. During the past 2 years, Mr. Chaudry has been treated for schizophrenia. His last stay at a clinic included treatment with fluphenazine decanoate injection 25 mg, which he claims was an injection at 2-week intervals for 2 months. Upon discharge, which one of the following drugs would most likely be prescribed as an oral medication?

    (A) divalproex (Depakote)

    (B) haloperidol (Haldol)

    (C) metaxalone (Skelaxin)

    (D) risperidone (Risperdal)

    (E) quetiapine (Seroquel)

20h. What is the best explanation for the administration of the fluphenazine decanoate only once every 2 weeks?

    (A) The toxicity of the drug precludes more frequent administration.

    (B) The injection is a sustained-release dosage form.

    (C) Schizophrenia is an occasional occurrence and does not need more frequent administration.

    (D) Probably the patient was mistaken and does not remember the daily injections.

    (E) The drug itself has a very long half-life.

20i. Ms. Chaudry's diabetes is under control and she determines her blood glucose levels every other day. At what minimum time interval should a test for glycated hemoglobin be performed?

(A) every other day

(B) weekly

(C) every month

(D) every 3–6 months

(E) every year

20j. When picking up her refills, Catherine expresses concern since her mother was just admitted to the hospital with the diagnosis of ascites. Which one of the following best describes this condition?

(A) a parasite infection

(B) an accumulation of serous fluid in the peritoneal cavity

(C) collection of fluid in the lungs

(D) a fever of unknown origin

(E) a skin condition caused by mites

20k. Catherine's mother also suffers from ankylosing spondylitis. This condition affects which of the following body areas?

(A) ankles

(B) knee joints only

(C) fingers and wrists

(D) spine and large body joints

(E) neck

20l. Which of the following statements concerning alcohol are true?

I. Marked mental impairment occurs when blood levels are >100 mg/dL.

II. Alcohol is oxidized to acetaldehyde in the body.

III. The metabolism of alcohol follows first-order kinetics exclusively.

(A) I only

(B) III only

(C) I and II only

(D) II and III only

(E) I, II, and III

20m. A friend suggests the use of Lotrimin Ultra for recurrent athlete's foot. Which one of the following drugs is the active ingredient in this nonprescription product?

(A) butenafine

(B) clotrimazole

(C) miconazole

(D) tolnaftate

(E) zinc undecylenate

20n. The order for "TMP-SMZ, Regular" may be filled with which of the following?

I. Bactrim

II. cotrimoxazole

III. trimethobenzamide

(A) I only

(B) III only

(C) I and II only

(D) II and III only

(E) I, II, and III

20o. Ms. Chaudry's 70-year-old mother who lives alone has trouble placing drops into her eyes and is not sure if she is actually getting the drop into the eye. The prescription reads: "2 drops in each eye every day." Which of the following is useful advice that the pharmacist might offer?

I. Quickly place two drops in the eye, then keep the eye open.

II. Store in refrigerator before using.

III. Separate the drops by approximately 2 minutes and close eye between drops.

(A) I only

(B) III only

(C) I and II only

(D) II and III only

(E) I, II, and III

20p. Ms. Chaudry comments that she is starting a new diet, which includes several glasses of grapefruit juice daily. Which of the following communications with the patient may be helpful when she asks if it is true that drinking grapefruit juice may affect certain of her drugs?

   I. Any problem may be avoided by drinking orange juice.

  II. Since the blood levels of the drugs may decrease, increase your dose by one-half

 III. Delay taking the drug for 2 hours after drinking the grapefruit juice.

20q. Which one of the following herbs has also been shown to affect CYP3A4 enzyme?

(A) echinacea

(B) ginger

(C) ginseng

(D) St. John's wort

(E) valerian

■ PROFILE NO. 21

Community Pharmacy Medication Record

Patient Name: Laura Jackson
Address: 12 Comfort Lane
Age: 70   Height: 5'4"
Sex: F   Weight: 112 lb
Allergies: Sensitive to aspirin, sulfas; limit chocolates

DIAGNOSIS

Primary	Secondary
1. Parkinsonism	1. Mild anemia
2. Glaucoma	2. Stroke (1 year ago)
3. CHF	3.

MEDICATION RECORD

Date	Rx No.	Physician	Drug and Strength	Quantity	Sig	Refills
1. 8/4	82542	Puleo	Fe Sulfate 250 mg	60	1 q AM	2×
2.	82543	Puleo	Levoxyl 100 μg	30	1 q AM	2×
3.	82544	Puleo	Digoxin 0.25 mg	60	1 q d	1×
4.	82545	Puleo	Furosemide 40 mg	30	1 qod	1×
5. 9/28	82543 ref	Puleo	Levoxyl 100 μg	60	1 q AM	1/2
6.	87555 ref	Puleo	Fe Sulfate 250 mg	100	2 q AM	2×
7.	82545 ref	Puleo	Furosemide	30		1/2
8. 10/4	82544 ref	Puleo	Digoxin	60		1/1
9. 10/28	82545 ref	Puleo	Furosemide	30		2/2

PHARMACIST'S NOTES AND OTHER PATIENT INFORMATION

Date	Comment
1.	Do not use child-resistant closures.
2.	Laura is sometimes confused; explain all medicines to her. Whenever possible, suggest she take medications first thing in the AM with breakfast.
3.	OTCs—Mylanta 15 mL q AM and PM; Tums 1 or 2 every night; vitamin C 500 mg q AM

DIRECTIONS (Questions 21a through 21o): Each of the numbered items or incomplete statements in this section is followed by answers or completions of the statement. Select the ONE lettered answer or completion that is BEST in each case.

21a. Levoxyl was prescribed to control

(A) hypothyroidism

(B) hyperthyroidism

(C) Graves' disease

(D) hyperparathyroidis

(E) hypoparathyroidism

21b. If Mrs. Jackson misses a dose of Levoxyl, she should be instructed to

(A) double the following morning's dose

(B) take 1 ½ tablets the following morning

(C) increase her intake of iodized salt

(D) call her physician for advice

(E) continue with normal dosing the following morning

21c. Which of the following drug products contain the same active ingredient as Levoxyl?

    I. Cytomel

    II. Thyrolar

    III. Synthroid

    (A) I only

    (B) III only

    (C) I and II only

    (D) II and III only

    (E) I, II, and III

21d. The pharmacist should question Mrs. Jackson concerning her compliance with which of the following drugs?

    I. Levoxyl

    II. furosemide

    III. digoxin

    (A) I only

    (B) III only

    (C) I and II only

    (D) II and III only

    (E) I, II, and III

21e. For which one of the following reasons may a patient be interested in purchasing a bottle of glucosamine chondroitin tablets?

    (A) relief of arthritis

    (B) control of blood sugar

    (C) provide proteins (amino acids) for muscles

    (D) a dietary supplement to help gain weight

    (E) an adaptogen and general energizer

21f. Mrs. Jackson's daughter is worried that her mother is showing symptoms of Alzheimer's disease. Which one of the following is the earliest symptom of this disease?

    (A) incontinence

    (B) inability to learn new skills

    (C) loss of recent memory

    (D) loss of remote memory

    (E) wandering

21g. All of the following drugs are currently used for treating Alzheimer's disease EXCEPT:

    (A) selegiline (Eldepryl)

    (B) memantine (Namenda)

    (C) donepezil (Aricept)

    (D) galantamine (Razadyne)

    (E) rivastigmine (Exelon)

21h. When questioned about her recent weight loss, Mrs. Jackson admitted that her breakfast and lunch consisted of two pieces of toast and herbal tea sweetened with Equal. The active ingredient in Equal is

    (A) lactulose

    (B) aspartame

    (C) fructose

    (D) saccharin

    (E) sucrose

21i. Factors contributing to Mrs. Jackson's poor blood iron levels may be

    I. consumption of herbal tea

    II. antacid consumption

    III. daily consumption of vitamin C

    (A) I only

    (B) III only

    (C) I and II only

    (D) II and III only

    (E) I, II, and III

21j. For this patient, the evening dose of Tums is probably intended to

    (A) decrease gastric secretions

    (B) decrease gastroesophageal reflux

    (C) prevent osteoporosis

    (D) provide magnesium ions

    (E) improve the absorption of digoxin

21k. Pharmacokinetic changes in the elderly often include increases in

    I. proportional amount of body fat

    II. plasma albumin levels

    III. renal clearance

(A) I only

(B) III only

(C) I and II only

(D) II and III only

(E) I, II, and III

21l. Based on the following data, determine how many milliliters of digoxin elixir is needed to replace a daily 0.25-mg dose of digoxin tablets.

	Strength	"F value"
Digoxin tablet	0.25 mg	0.6
Digoxin elixir	0.05 mg/mL	0.75

(A) 3

(B) 3.8

(C) 4

(D) 5

(E) 6.4

21m. An early sign of digoxin toxicity in Mrs. Jackson is likely to be

(A) hazy vision

(B) hearing impairment

(C) tinnitus

(D) yellowish skin

(E) increased appetite

21n. The pharmacist may need to suggest an adjustment in the dosing of digoxin if the patient is placed on

    I. amiodarone

    II. quinidine

    III. verapamil

(A) I only

(B) III only

(C) I and II only

(D) II and III only

(E) I, II, and III

▪PROFILE NO. 22

Hospital Pharmacy Medication Record

Patient Name: Paula Riley
Room Number: ER
Age: 28   Height: 5'6"
Sex: F   Weight: 145 lb
Allergies: Penicillin, sulfas

DIAGNOSIS

Primary	Secondary
1. Gravid	1. Colitis
2. Severe cramps	2. COPD (since childhood)
3.	3.

LAB TESTS

Date	Test & Results
1. 7/12	SMA-12
2.	Blood profile
3.	Blood typing

MEDICATION RECORD

Date	Drug and Strength	Sig
1. 7/13	D_5W 1 L daily	KVO
2.	Terbutaline 25 µg/min then 0.5 mg sc q4h	
3.	Zolpidem 5 mg	1 h.s. p.r.n.
4.	Colace 100 mg	1 qd
5.	Advil 200 mg	1–2 tabs p.r.n.
6. 7/15	KCl 40 mEq in 1 L D_5NS	Infuse t.i.d.
7.	Barium sulfate	Admin per usual/Dr. Cooper orders
8. 7/16	Atropine 4 mg + chlorpromazine 12.5 mg	Preop order

PHARMACIST'S NOTES AND OTHER PATIENT INFORMATION

Date	Comments
1. 7/13	Patient being transfered to room 434b. Continue tocolytic therapy.

DIRECTIONS (Questions 22a through 22p): Each of the numbered items or incomplete statements in this section is followed by answers or completions of the statement. Select the ONE lettered answer or completion that is BEST in each case.

22a. Terbutaline is being used as a tocolytic agent. The term tocolytic refers to a drug that

(A) increases GI tract tone
(B) reduces GI tract motility
(C) reduces uterine contractility
(D) prevents emesis
(E) dilates bronchioles

22b. Under which one of the following trade names is terbutaline available?

(A) Alupent
(B) Brethine
(C) Hytrin
(D) Proventil
(E) Ventolin

22c. The pharmacist places 2 mL of terbutaline injection (1 mg/mL) into 250 mL of D_5W. How many drops per minute will be needed to deliver the terbutaline if the administration set delivers 15 drops to the milliliter?

(A) 6
(B) 11
(C) 23
(D) 46
(E) 120

22d. Over what period of time will the terbutaline admixture last?

(A) 40 minutes
(B) 80 minutes
(C) 100 minutes
(D) 160 minutes
(E) 480 minutes

22e. Which one of the following is the active ingredient in Advil?

(A) aspirin
(B) acetaminophen
(C) ibuprofen
(D) ketoprofen
(E) naproxen

22f. Paula complains to the family physician that her husband often kicks her while he is asleep. The following morning he does not recall the events and resents the accusation that he is developing anger and hostility toward her. What is the most likely diagnosis for these occurrences?

(A) narcolepsy
(B) night terrors
(C) non-REM sleep disorder
(D) REM sleep disorder
(E) too much late TV

22g. Which of the following concerning barium sulfate is (are) true?

  I. practically insoluble in water
  II. administered by the oral route
  III. administered by the rectal route

(A) I only
(B) III only
(C) I and II only
(D) II and III only
(E) I, II, and III

22h. The purpose of the pre-op atropine is to

(A) relieve the patient's anxiety
(B) reduce secretions
(C) cause vasoconstriction of small blood vessels
(D) constrict the bronchioles
(E) produce a state of "twilight sleep"

22i. The pharmacist should question the atropine/chlorpromazine order because of

  I. an acid–base reaction between the two ingredients
  II. the combination is irrational
  III. the high dose of atropine requested

(A) I only
(B) III only
(C) I and II only
(D) II and III only
(E) I, II, and III

Questions 22j through 22n: Mrs. Riley is discharged from the hospital on 7/21 with prescriptions for a Foley catheter, ostomy pouches, translucent drain dressings, Valium 2 mg 1 t.i.d. p.r.n., Prinivil 5 mg b.i.d. ProSom 1 mg in AM, Sonata 5 mg 2 hours before bedtime, psyllium 1 dose in AM, and a multivitamin for pregnancy.

22j. For which of the following items is a prescription actually needed?

    I.   Foley catheter

    II. ostomy pouches

    III. translucent drain dressings

    (A) I only
    (B) III only
    (C) I and II only
    (D) II and III only
    (E) I, II, and III

22k. An ileostomy differs from a colostomy in which of the following characteristics?

    I.   The discharge from an ileostomy is more viscous.

    II. The stoma is significantly larger.

    III. The discharge is more irritating to the skin.

    (A) I only
    (B) III only
    (C) I and II only
    (D) II and III only
    (E) I, II, and III

22l. Which of the following is (are) suitable products for the psyllium order?

    I.   Metamucil

    II. Fibercon

    III. Mitrolan

    (A) I only
    (B) III only
    (C) I and II only
    (D) II and III only
    (E) I, II, and III

22m. Mrs. Riley should be counseled to administer the Metamucil by

    (A) mixing the granules with 8 oz of water, stirring, and drinking immediately

    (B) mixing the granules with 1 pt of water, stirring, and drinking immediately

    (C) mixing the granules with 8 oz water, stirring, letting mixture sit for 20 minutes before drinking

    (D) swallowing the granules, then drinking 8 oz of water

    (E) allowing the granules to effervesce in 8 oz of water before drinking

22n. Which of the following drugs in Mrs. Riley's discharge orders should be questioned by the pharmacist?

    I.   Prinivil

    II. ProSom

    III. Sonata

    (A) I only
    (B) III only
    (C) I and II only
    (D) II and III only
    (E) I, II, and III

22o. If Mrs. Riley's physician decides to initiate antihypertensive therapy, which one of the following antihypertensive agents is probably the best choice for use during pregnancy?

    (A) captopril
    (B) enalapril
    (C) hydrochlorothiazide
    (D) methyldopa
    (E) nifedipine

22p. After 2 months, Ms. Riley appears to have adjusted well to her ileostomy. However, on the following Monday morning she presents the following signs: loss of appetite with nausea and vomiting, blurred vision, muscle cramps, and some confusion. Which one of the following conditions is most likely to be occurring?

    (A) bactermia
    (B) hyponatremia
    (C) hypernatremia
    (D) hyperkalemia
    (E) sepsis

PROFILE NO. 23

Community Pharmacy Medication Record

Patient Name: Lola Woolbright
Address: 7 Evan Road
Age: 31   Height: 5'4"
Sex: F   Weight: 210 lb
Allergies: Penicillin

DIAGNOSIS

Primary	Secondary
1. Vaginal infection	1. Anemia
2. Endometriosis	2. PMS (painful)
3.	3. Anxiety
	4. Obesity

MEDICATION RECORD

	Date	Rx No.	Physician	Drug and Strength	Quantity	Sig	Refills
1.	4/4	34765	Coughlin	Mycelex G	1	1 qn	1×
2.	4/4	34766	"	Ativan 1 mg	30	1 b.i.d. p.r.n.	0
3.	4/4	34767	"	Triphasil 28	1 pack	ut dict	1×
4.	4/27	37102	"	Ativan 1 mg	30	1 b.i.d. p.r.n.	1×
5.	4/27	37103	"	Xenical 120 mg	90	1 t.i.d. p.r.n.	1×
5.	4/27	37104	"	Feldene 20 mg	90	1 t.i.d.	1×

PHARMACIST'S NOTES AND OTHER PATIENT INFORMATION

	Date	Comment
1.	4/7	Atkins Diet
2.		

DIRECTIONS (Questions 23a through 23s): Each of the numbered items or incomplete statements in this section is followed by answers or completions of the statement. Select the ONE lettered answer or completion that is BEST in each case.

23a. The Mycelex G prescription is probably being used to treat

(A) candidiasis
(B) aspergillosis
(C) gonorrhea
(D) genital herpes
(E) syphilis

23b. The most common causative microorganism of nongonococcal urethritis is

(A) *Candida cryptococcus*
(B) *Chlamydia trachomatis*
(C) *Klebsiella aerogenes*
(D) *Proteus mirabilis*
(E) *Treponema pallidum*

23c. The drug usually considered the first choice to treat all stages of syphilis in a penicillin-allergic individual is

(A) doxycycline
(B) ceftriaxone
(C) fluconazole
(D) erythromycin
(E) ciprofloxacin

23d. The drug(s) usually considered as first choice(s) in the treatment of Chlamydia infections include

    I. azithromycin

    II. gentamicin

    III. fluconazole

(A) I only

(B) III only

(C) I and II only

(D) II and III only

(E) I, II, and III

23e. Ms. Woolbright calls her physician to find out what can be done to avoid unwanted pregnancy since she had unprotected sexual intercourse last night. Which of the following should her physician recommend?

(A) a spermicidal cream

(B) Progestasert

(C) Evra

(D) Plan B

(E) Clomid

23f. Which of the following are acceptable lubricants for use with a condom or diaphragm?

    I. White Vaseline

    II. Koromex Clear Gel

    III. K-Y jelly

(A) I only

(B) III only

(C) I and II only

(D) II and III only

(E) I, II, and III

23g. Ms. Woolbright's endometriosis is best treated by the use of

(A) Advil

(B) Deltasone

(C) Danocrine

(D) Kytril

(E) Mifeprex

23h. Ms. Woolbright's father-in-law suddenly dies at home. He had no symptoms of illness and his only medical problem was a 20-year history scenario of type 2 diabetes. Which one of the following is the most likely cause of death?

(A) diabetic ketoacidosis

(B) septicemia bacterial infection

(C) kidney failure

(D) myocardial infarction

(E) pneumonia

23i. The action of Xenical can best be described as a (an)

(A) anxiolytic agent

(B) COMT inhibitor

(C) lipase inhibitor

(D) amylase inhibitor

(E) CNS stimulant

23j. Ms. Woolbright's husband has suffered from type 2 diabetes for 15 years. To which one of the following conditions is he most susceptible?

(A) fatty liver

(B) HTN

(C) motor neuropathy

(D) neuralgia

(E) retinopathy

23k. Benzodiazepines are often used to treat generalized anxiety disorders. Which one of the following is NOT a benzodiazepine?

(A) methylphenidate (Ritalin)

(B) chlordiazepoxide (Librium)

(C) alprazolam (Xanax)

(D) clorazepate (Tranxene)

(E) lorazepam (Ativan)

23l. The mechanism of action of the benzodiazepines is believed to be

(A) alpha$_1$ blockade

(B) potentiation of the inhibitory neuro-transmitter GABA

(C) blockade of dopamine receptor sites

(D) blockade of the reuptake of dopamine

(E) beta-adrenergic blockade

23m. The Atkins diet is based on the consumption of a diet that contains

(A) low fat

(B) low carbohydrate

(C) mostly citrus fruits

(D) low protein

(E) high carbohydrate

23n. If Ms. Woolbright acutely overdosed on her Ativan, which of the following would be appropriate to administer?

(A) EDTA

(B) disulfiram

(C) naloxone

(D) flumazenil

(E) naltrexone

23o. Ms. Woolbright is trying to count calories. She reads the labeling of a food product that indicates that each serving of the product contains 3 g of fat, 8 g of carbohydrate, and 1 g of protein. How many calories are in each serving of this product?

(A) 48

(B) 63

(C) 86

(D) 24

(E) 240

23p. Lola's 1-year-old child has been constipated for the past 3 days. Which one of the following laxatives is most appropriate?

(A) Dulcolax suppositories

(B) Fleet's Phospho-Soda

(C) glycerin suppositories

(D) milk of magnesia

(E) mineral oil

23q. Lola's husband has been advised by his physician to consider the use of a TENS device. What is the main function of the device?

(A) to allow continuous infusion of a solution

(B) to increase a patient's mobility

(C) to regulate infusion rates

(D) relieve pain

(E) to counteract depression

23r. Mrs Woolbright brings in a new prescription for Vytorin for her husband. Which of the following active ingredients are present in this product?

(A) atorvastatin + simvastatin

(B) ezetimibe + simvastatin

(C) ezetimibe + fluvastin (Lescol)

(D) lovastatin mevacor + atorvastatin

(E) lovastatin + fluvastin

23s. Because of her husband's many allergies, she is concerned when she notices that the Vytorin capsule label indicates the presence of butylated hydroxyanisole. The pharmacist should assure her that this chemical is present as a (an)

(A) antioxidant

(B) antimicrobial preservative

(C) coloring agent

(D) filler

(E) hygroscopic agent

■ PROFILE NO. 24

Community Pharmacy Medication Record

Patient Name: Harold White
Address: 869 Elm St.

Age: 3   Height: 36″

Sex: M   Weight: 40 lb

Allergies: Chocolate, salicylates

DIAGNOSIS

Primary	Secondary
1. Recurrent earaches; colds	1. Frequent
2. Strep. throat	2. Allergies?
3. Colitis	3.

MEDICATION RECORD

Date	Rx No.	Physician	Drug and Strength	Quantity	Sig
1. 9/2	83043	McLaughlin	Bactrim Susp	6 oz	2 tsp b.i.d.
2. 10/6	84665	McLaughlin	Pen Vee K Susp 250	200 mL	1 tsp q.i.d.
3. 11/5	86956	Steen	Cromolyn eye drops	30 mL	2 gtts OD t.i.d.

PHARMACIST'S NOTES AND OTHER PATIENT INFORMATION

Date	Comment
1.	

DIRECTIONS (Questions 24a through 24p): Each of the numbered items or incomplete statements in this section is followed by answers or completions of the statement. Select the ONE lettered answer or completion that is BEST in each case.

24a. Causative organisms of otitis media include

  I. *H. pylori*

  II. *Hemophilus influenzae*

  III. *Streptococcus pneumoniae*

  (A) I only

  (B) III only

  (C) I and II only

  (D) II and III only

  (E) I, II, and III

24b. Drugs often used for the treatment of otitis media include

  I. amoxicillin

  II. trimethoprim-sulfamethoxazole

  III. doxycycline

  (A) I only

  (B) III only

  (C) I and II only

  (D) II and III only

  (E) I, II, and III

24c. When asked to suggest a nonprescription product to reduce Harold's fever and headache, the pharmacist could select products containing

  I. aspirin

  II. ibuprofen

  III. acetaminophen

(A) I only

(B) III only

(C) I and II only

(D) II and III only

(E) I, II, and III

24d. Chemically, ibuprofen is a derivative of

(A) fibric acid

(B) phenylacetic acid

(C) propionic acid

(D) salicylic acid

(E) xanthines

24e. When used to reduce fever, ibuprofen should not be used

(A) for more than 3 days

(B) for more than 10 days

(C) for less than 3 days

(D) for less than 10 days

(E) if the fever is greater than 104°F

Questions 24f through 24h: The eye drop prescription filled on 11/5 reads as follows:

Rx	
Cromolyn sodium 2.5%	30 mL
Dispense a sterile isotonic solution	
Sig: gtt ii OD t.i.d.	

24f. The pharmacist dilutes the commercially available 4% cromolyn solution with purified water. How many milligrams of sodium chloride is needed to render the solution isotonic, assuming that the 4% solution was isotonic?

(A) 100

(B) 170

(C) 330

(D) 540

(E) 900

24g. What pore size filter (in microns) should the pharmacist use to obtain a sterile solution?

(A) 0.22

(B) 0.45

(C) 1.0

(D) 5.0

(E) 10

24h. What direction should the pharmacist place on the prescription label for the Sig of "OD"?

(A) every day

(B) affected eye

(C) left eye

(D) both eyes

(E) right eye

24i. Cromolyn solutions are used in the eyes to

I. treat *Pseudomonas* infections

II. relieve glaucoma

III. treat conjunctivitis

(A) I only

(B) III only

(C) I and II only

(D) II and III only

(E) I, II, and III

24j. For approximately how many days will the ophthalmic solution last assuming that the product is being used continuously? The dropper delivers 15 drops per 1 mL.

(A) 30

(B) 38

(C) 45

(D) 75

(E) 100

24k. Which one of the following values is most accurate when determining an appropriate dose for a child?

(A) age in rounded years

(B) age in months

(C) height compared to an adult

(D) surface area

(E) weight compared to an adult

24l. When Ms. White asks how to administer the ophthalmic solution to Harold, the pharmacist may suggest

   I. quickly place the two drops directly onto the cornea

   II. after instillation, gently squeeze inner corner of eye nearest the nose for a minute

   III. place one drop into the lower inside lid of the eye, then follow with the second drop after a few minutes

(A) I only

(B) III only

(C) I and II only

(D) II and III only

(E) I, II, and III

24m. Which one of the following tricyclic antidepressants has been used successfully in treating nocturnal enuresis in children?

(A) amitriptyline (Elavil)

(B) doxepin (Sinequan)

(C) imipramine (Tofranil)

(D) nortriptyline (Pamelor)

(E) trimipramine (Surmontil)

24n. Buildup of cerumen in the ear may be removed with the aid of which of the following OTC products?

   I. Debrox

   II. S.T. 37

   III. Anbesol

(A) I only

(B) III only

(C) I and II only

(D) II and III only

(E) I, II, and III

24o. The allergist believes that Harold may be sensitive to tartrazine. Tartrazine is present in some pharmaceuticals as a (an)

(A) antioxidant

(B) antimicrobial preservative

(C) antiseptic

(D) buffer

(E) coloring agent

24p. Claritin Reditabs purchased by Mr. White may be described as being ORD (orally dissolving) tablets. Advantages of this dosage form include all of the following EXCEPT

(A) no need for water

(B) suitable for elderly

(C) suitable for children

(D) do not have to swallow the tablet

(E) can readily be stored in a Kleenex tissue before using

■ PROFILE NO. 25

Nursing Home Pharmacy Medication Record

Patient Name: Jacob Mezpit
Room Number: 334-B

Age: 74   Height: 5'11"
Sex: M   Weight: 191 lb
Allergies:

DIAGNOSIS

Primary   Secondary
1. Borderline hypertension   1. Recovering alcoholic
2. Gout   2. Smoker
3.
4.

MEDICATION RECORD

Date	Physician	Drug and Strength	Sig	DC'd
1. 2/6	Waters	Allopurinol 300 mg	1 daily	6 mos
2.	Waters	Nadolol 80 mg	b.i.d.	2 mos
5. 2/8	Waters/per phone	Mylanta Liq.	15 mL p.r.n.	

PHARMACIST'S NOTES AND OTHER PATIENT INFORMATION

Date	Comment
1. 2/9	Evaluated Mr. Jacobs—refuses to stop smoking.

DIRECTIONS (Questions 25a through 25n): Each of the numbered items or incomplete statements in this section is followed by answers or completions of the statement. Select the ONE lettered answer or completion that is BEST in each case.

25a. The immediate primary goal(s) for the treatment of acute gout will be to

  I. reduce uric acid levels
  II. administer high doses of an uricosuric agent
  III. relieve the pain of the attack

(A) I only
(B) III only
(C) I and II only
(D) II and III only
(E) I, II, and III

25b. Drugs of choice for treating acute attacks of gout include

  I. indomethacin
  II. ibuprofen
  III. colchicine

(A) I only
(B) III only
(C) I and II only
(D) II and III only
(E) I, II, and III

25c. Drugs of choice for controlling hyperuricemia include

    I. colchicine
    II. febuxostat
    III. allopurinol

(A) I only
(B) III only
(C) I and II only
(D) II and III only
(E) I, II, and III

25d. The nursing staff should be advised that the allopurinol

    I. should be consumed with a large amount of fluid
    II. may initially precipitate an attack of gout
    III. must be taken on an empty stomach to assure absorption

(A) I only
(B) III only
(C) I and II only
(D) II and III only
(E) I, II, and III

25e. Some Mylanta products contain simethicone. This agent acts to

(A) dispel gas in the GI tract
(B) inhibit the production of acid in the stomach
(C) inhibit the production of gastrin in the stomach
(D) neutralize excess stomach acid
(E) prevent constipation

25f. Simethicone can be found as the major active ingredient in

    I. Tums
    II. Phazyme
    III. Mylicon

(A) I only
(B) III only

(C) I and II only
(D) II and III only
(E) I, II, and III

25g. A pharmacist wishes to identify a tablet brought into the institution by the patient. Which of the following reference sources does NOT contain a color guide for commercial tablets?

(A) *USP DI Volume I*
(B) *USP DI Volume III*
(C) *Facts and Comparisons*
(D) *PDR*
(E) *Red Book*

25h. The patient asks the pharmacist if there are any drugs that can treat his alopecia. Which of the following may be used in this patient to correct alopecia?

    I. minoxidil
    II. finasteride
    III. fluticasone

(A) I only
(B) III only
(C) I and II only
(D) II and III only
(E) I, II, and III

25i. Nadolol is most similar in action to

(A) Avapro
(B) Mavik
(C) Benicar
(D) Cozaar
(E) Levatol

25j. Which one of the following agents has the MOST lipophilic activity?

(A) acebutolol
(B) propranolol
(C) nadolol
(D) carvedilol
(E) bisoprolol

25k. Mr. Mezpit shows signs of peripheral neuropathy. This may be caused by a deficiency of

(A) tocopherol

(B) riboflavin

(C) inositol

(D) thiamine

(E) phytonadione

25l. Which of the following nutrients is (are) considered to be an antioxidant?

I. phytonadione

II. riboflavin

III. alpha-tocopherol

(A) I only

(B) III only

(C) I and II only

(D) II and III only

(E) I, II, and III

25m. A drug that has the tendency to impart an orange color to urine, sweat, and tears is

(A) carbamazepine

(B) rifampin

(C) verapamil

(D) clindamycin

(E) isoniazid

25n. Which of the following drugs is (are) suitable for long-term prevention of gout?

I. allopurinol

II. aspirin

III. NSAIDs

(A) I only

(B) III only

(C) I and II only

(D) II and III only

(E) I, II, and III

■ PROFILE NO. 26

Community Pharmacy Medication Record

Patient Name: Bernard Milkoff
Address: 644 Benson Road
Age: 54   Height: 5′10″
Sex: M   Weight: 195 lb
Allergies:

DIAGNOSIS

Primary	Secondary
1. Manic-depressive illness	1.
2.	2.
3.	3.

MEDICATION RECORD

Date	Rx No.	Physician	Drug and Strength	Quantity	Sig	Refills
1. 8/9	78977	Kramer	Zoloft 50 mg	30	1 daily	3
2. 9/4	78977	Kramer	Refill			2
3. 10/1	78977	Kramer	Refill			1
4. 10/24	80434	Kramer	Lithium carbonate 300 mg	60	1 t.i.d.	4
5. 11/12	81773	Davis	hydrochlorothiazide 25 mg	60	1 b.i.d.	
6. 11/24	82140	Davis	Azulfidine 500 mg	100 2 q.i.d.	100	3
7. 11/24	82141	Kramer	Wellbutrin 100 mg	60 b.i.d.	60	3

PHARMACIST'S NOTES AND OTHER PATIENT INFORMATION

Date	Comment
1. 11/12	Low-sodium diet, uses Ex-Lax and Mitrolan

DIRECTIONS (Questions 26a through 26r): Each of the numbered items or incomplete statements in this section is followed by answers or completions of the statement. Select the ONE lettered answer or completion that is BEST in each case.

26a. Which of the following drugs is most similar in action to Zoloft?

(A) Loxitane

(B) Zofran

(C) Nardil

(D) Celexa

(E) Clozaril

26b. The active ingredient in Wellbutrin is indicated for which of the following:

   I. antidepressant

  II. seasonal affective disorder.

 III. nocturnal enuresis

(A) I only

(B) III only

(C) I and II only

(D) II and III only

(E) I, II, and III

26c. Wellbutrin contains the same active ingredient as

(A) Cerebyx

(B) Zyban

(C) Lamictal

(D) Habitrol

(E) Sublimaze

26d. Patients receiving lithium carbonate should be advised to

(A) avoid taking the drug at bedtime

(B) avoid taking the drug with milk

(C) consume a low-potassium diet

(D) consume a low-sodium diet

(E) drink 8–12 glasses of water per day while on the drug

26e. In using lithium products, toxicity commonly occurs when serum lithium levels exceed

(A) 1.5 mg/dL

(B) 1.5 mEq/L

(C) 1.5 mg/L

(D) 15 mg/L

(E) 300 μg/mL

26f. The addition of hydrochlorothiazide to the patient's regimen is likely to

(A) have no effect on lithium action

(B) decrease serum lithium levels

(C) decrease the absorption of lithium

(D) increase the absorption of lithium

(E) increase serum lithium levels

26g. In monitoring serum lithium levels, blood samples are usually drawn

(A) in the morning

(B) at bedtime

(C) just prior to taking a dose

(D) 1–3 hours after taking a dose

(E) at the midpoint between two doses

26h. Lithotab 300 mg tablets each contain how many milliequivalents (mEq) of lithium? ($Li_2CO_3 = 74$; $Li = 7$)

(A) 4

(B) 8

(C) 16

(D) 21

(E) 43

26i. Hydrochlorothiazide can best be described as a (an)

(A) thiazide diuretic

(B) osmotic diuretic

(C) thiazide-like diuretic

(D) carbonic anhydrase inhibitor

(E) loop diuretic

26j. Which one of the following drugs has the greatest potential for causing new memory impairment (anterograde amnesia)?

(A) flurazepam

(B) temazepam

(C) triazolam

(D) estazolam

(E) quazepam

26k. Mr. Milkoff is having difficulty in falling asleep but does not wake up during the night. Which one of the following is probably the best choice of hypnotic?

(A) estazolam

(B) temazepam

(C) eszopiclone

(D) flurazepam

(E) zolpidem

26l. The Azulfidine received by Mr. Milkoff is used in the treatment of

(A) respiratory infection

(B) irritable bowel syndrome

(C) systemic infection

(D) inflammatory bowel disease

(E) impotence

26m. A therapeutic substitute for sulfasalazine is

(A) Bentyl

(B) Buspar

(C) Lialda

(D) Imodium

(E) Lomotil

26n. Mr. Milkoff's physician indicates that he wishes to start him on some Nardil. What recommendation would you make to the prescriber about Mr. Milkoff's drug regimen?

(A) Have Mr. Milkoff discontinue the Zoloft at least 2 weeks before starting Nardil.

(B) Immediately discontinue the hydrochlorothiazide.

(C) The dose of Zoloft and Nardil should be at least 4–6 hours apart.

(D) Lithium will counteract the effect of the Nardil.

(E) Nardil is not indicated for this patient.

26o. Diphenhydramine should not be recommended to an elderly patient who is suffering from

I. incontinence

II. diarrhea

III. prostatitis

(A) I only

(B) III only

(C) I and II only

(D) II and III only

(E) I, II, and III

26p. A lab test that aids in the diagnosis of cancer of the prostate is

(A) PSA

(B) GGT

(C) ESR

(D) SGOT

(E) PTT

26q. Mitrolan is prescribed for the treatment of which of the following disorders?

I. GERD

II. diarrhea

III. constipation

(A) I only

(B) III only

(C) I and II only

(D) II and III only

(E) I, II, and III

26r. The active ingredient in Ex-Lax is

(A) calcium polycarbophil

(B) phenolphthalein

(C) methylcellulose

(D) senna

(E) bisacodyl

■ PROFILE NO. 27

Community Pharmacy Medication Record

Patient Name: Lauren Schroeder
Address: 501 Easterly Drive
Age: 62
Sex: F
Allergies:

Height: 5'3"
Weight: 178 lb

DIAGNOSIS

Primary	Secondary
1. Osteoarthritis	1.
2. Hyperlipidemia	2.
3. Menopause	3.

MEDICATION RECORD

Date	Rx No.	Physician	Drug and Strength	Quantity	Sig	Refills
1. 2/27	34987	Garth	Oxaprozin 600 mg	60	2 t.i.d.	5
2. 3/15	35875	Garth	Ultram	40	1 q.i.d.	5
4. 5/29	39887	Garth	Miacalcin	1	As directed	
5. 7/4	45799	Garth	Pravastatin 40 mg	90	1 daily	3

PHARMACIST'S NOTES AND OTHER PATIENT INFORMATION

Date	Comment
1. 3/6	Aleve Tablets (OTC)
2. 3/17	Tums Chewable 500 mg

DIRECTIONS (Questions 27a through 27k): Each of the numbered items or incomplete statements in this section is followed by answers or completions of the statement. Select the ONE lettered answer or completion that is BEST in each case.

27a. In dispensing the prescription for oxaprozin, the pharmacist should have dispensed which of the following products?

(A) Daypro
(B) Motrin
(C) Ansaid
(D) Clinoril
(E) Mobic

27b. Oxaprozin is believed to act by

(A) antagonizing dopamine receptors
(B) stimulating dopamine receptors
(C) inhibiting xanthine oxidase
(D) decreasing the production of prostaglandins
(E) increasing the production of prostaglandins

27c. Which of the following statements is (are) true?

I. The active ingredient of Aleve is naproxen sodium.
II. Aleve should be administered two to three times daily.
III. Antacids should not be used within 2 hours of taking Aleve.

(A) I only
(B) III only
(C) I and II only
(D) II and III only
(E) I, II, and III

27d. Tums chewable contains

(A) magnesium oxide
(B) silicon dioxide
(C) aluminum hydroxide
(D) simethicone
(E) calcium carbonate

27e. The pharmacist should advise this patient that Miacalcin should be administered

(A) intranasally
(B) by inhalation
(C) sublingually
(D) orally
(E) rectally

27f. When the oxaprozin prescription was filled, the pharmacist should have advised the physician that

(A) it is not available in a 600 mg strength
(B) it is only used on a p.r.n. basis for acute pain
(C) it should not be used for more than 10 days
(D) it is not to be used in patients with osteoarthritis
(E) it should not be administered three times daily

27g. Which of the following is true of pravastatin?

I. It is the safest statin for use in pregnant women
II. It should be taken in the evening
III. It can cause rhabdomyolysis

(A) I only
(B) III only
(C) I and II only
(D) II and III only
(E) I, II, and III

27h. Misoprostol (Cytotec) can best be described as a (an)

I. synthetic prostaglandin analog
II. inhibitor of gastric acid secretion
III. H_2-receptor antagonist

(A) I only
(B) III only
(C) I and II only
(D) II and III only
(E) I, II, and III

27i. Misoprostol (Cytotec) is contraindicated for use in

(A) the elderly
(B) patients using aspirin
(C) patients with osteoarthritis
(D) pregnant women
(E) patients with hypertension

27j. Which of the following is true of Ultram?

I. It is an NSAID.
II. It is only administered parenterally.
III. It works in the CNS.

(A) I only
(B) III only
(C) I and II only
(D) II and III only
(E) I, II, and III

27k. Which of the following would NOT be appropriate to use in treating this patient's osteoarthritis?

I. Feldene
II. Humira
III. Enbrel

(A) I only
(B) III only
(C) I and II only
(D) II and III only
(E) I, II, and III

■PROFILE NO. 28

Community Pharmacy Medication Record

Patient Name: James Donnelly
Address: 4 Obsidian Way
Age: 82   Height: 5'7"
Sex: M   Weight: 193 lb
Allergies:

DIAGNOSIS

Primary	Secondary
1. Hypertension	1.
2. CHF	2.
3.	3.

MEDICATION RECORD

Date	Rx No.	Physician	Drug and Strength	Quantity	Sig	Refills
1. 6/23	90988	Quagmeyer	Digoxin 0.25 mg	30	1 daily	3
2. 6/23	90989	Quagmeyer	Lasix 40 mg	60	1 b.i.d.	3
3. 6/23	90990	Quagmeyer	Klor-Con 10 mEq	60	1 daily	3
4. 8/10	90988	Quagmeyer	Refill			
5. 8/10	90989	Quagmeyer	Refill			
6. 8/10	93889	Thomas	Amiloride 5 mg tab	30	1 daily in AM	3

PHARMACIST'S NOTES AND OTHER PATIENT INFORMATION

Date	Comment
1. 7/15	Baking soda to settle stomach

DIRECTIONS (Questions 28a through 28i): Each of the numbered items or incomplete statements in this section is followed by answers or completions of the statement. Select the ONE lettered answer or completion that is BEST in each case.

28a. Digoxin can be described as an agent that produces a

   I. negative chronotropic effect

   II. positive inotropic effect

   III. vagomimetic effect

(A) I only

(B) III only

(C) I and II only

(D) II and III only

(E) I, II, and III

28b. Patients with congestive heart disease who begin using digoxin are likely to experience

(A) classic angina pain

(B) edema

(C) decreased force of cardiac contraction

(D) slowed heart rate

(E) orthostatic hypotension

28c. Which of the following drugs is most closely related to digoxin?

(A) hydralazine

(B) mexiletine

(C) flecainide

(D) terazosin

(E) milrinone

28d. If this patient's medication were changed from digoxin tablets to Lanoxicaps, what would be an appropriate equivalent dose?

(A) 2.5 mg

(B) 25 μg

(C) 0.125 mg

(D) 0.25 mg

(E) 200 μg

28e. Which of the following are effects associated with digoxin toxicity?

I.   diarrhea

II. CNS stimulation

III. thrombocytopenia

(A) I only

(B) III only

(C) I and II only

(D) II and III only

(E) I, II, and III

28f. In dispensing amiloride, the pharmacist should recommend to the prescriber that

(A) the dose of digoxin be increased by 50%

(B) the Klor-Con be discontinued

(C) the dose of Klor-Con be raised by 50%

(D) the dose of digoxin be decreased by 50%

(E) the dose of Klor-Con be reduced by 50%

28g. Which of the following would be considered to be a normal serum potassium concentration?

(A) 3.9 mEq/L

(B) 9.4 mEq/L

(C) 7.2 mg/dL

(D) 4.4 mg/dL

(E) 120 mEq/L

28h. Lasix is most similar to

(A) acetazolamide

(B) hydrochlorothiazide

(C) Buprenex

(D) Dyrenium

(E) Demadex

28i. The profile for Mr. Donnelly reveals the possibility of

I.   substance abuse

II. chemical complexation

III. noncompliance

(A) I only

(B) III only

(C) I and II only

(D) II and III only

(E) I, II, and III

▪ PROFILE NO. 29

Community Pharmacy Medication Record

Patient Name: Sandor Melendez
Address: 4 Charleston Court
Age: 22
Sex: M
Allergies: Ragweed pollen

Height: 6'1"
Weight: 178 lb

DIAGNOSIS

Primary	Secondary
1. Bronchial asthma	1.
2. Head lice	2.
3. Psoriasis	3.

MEDICATION RECORD

Date	Rx No.	Physician	Drug and Strength	Quantity	Sig	Refills
1. 7/9	38383	Toolie	Benadryl 25 mg	30	b.i.d.	1
2. 7/9	38384	Toolie	RID Shampoo	2 oz	Apply ut dict	1
3. 7/15	39439	Toolie	betamethasone dipropionate Cream 0.05%	15 g	Apply as needed	

PHARMACIST'S NOTES AND OTHER PATIENT INFORMATION

Date	Comment
1. 7/9	Hydrocortisone cream 0.5% (OTC)

DIRECTIONS (Questions 29a through 29k): Each of the numbered items or incomplete statements in this section is followed by answers or completions of the statement. Select the ONE lettered answer or completion that is BEST in each case.

29a. Benadryl may have been prescribed for this patient as a (an)

   I. antipruritic

   II. sedative

   III. antihistamine

(A) I only

(B) III only

(C) I and II only

(D) II and III only

(E) I, II, and III

29b. An active ingredient of RID Shampoo is

(A) lindane

(B) pyrethrins

(C) piperonyl butoxide

(D) crotamiton

(E) eucalyptol

29c. In counseling the parent of the patient receiving RID Shampoo, the pharmacist should stress the importance of avoiding

   I. contact with the skin longer than 5 minutes

   II. the use of metallic combs

   III. contact with the eyes

(A) I only

(B) III only

(C) I and II only

(D) II and III only

(E) I, II, and III

29d. Another name for head lice is

(A) *Sarcoptes scabiei*
(B) *Tinea versicolor*
(C) *Pediculus capitis*
(D) *Tinea capitis*
(E) *Pediculus pubis*

29e. RID Shampoo is usually administered

(A) once in 7 days
(B) once daily for 5 days
(C) once daily for 3 days
(D) twice daily for 2 days
(E) twice daily for 3 days

29f. Diprosone cream contains

(A) fluoxymesterone
(B) betamethasone dipropionate
(C) dexamethasone
(D) triamcinolone acetonide
(E) fluocinonide

29g. Betamethasone dipropionate cream should NOT be used in patients with

I. psoriasis
II. herpes simplex infection
III. *Candida* infection

(A) I only
(B) III only
(C) I and II only
(D) II and III only
(E) I, II, and III

29h. Which of the following products for the treatment of head lice may be purchased OTC?

I. A-200 Pyrinate
II. Nix
III. Eurax

(A) I only
(B) III only
(C) I and II only
(D) II and III only
(E) I, II, and III

29i. Patients with ragweed allergy should avoid lice remedies that contain

(A) pyrethrins
(B) organic solvents
(C) lindane
(D) parabens
(E) pyrogens

29j. Scabies is a condition caused by a

(A) protozoan
(B) tick
(C) flea
(D) mite
(E) fungus

29k. Which of the following products are indicated for the treatment of psoriasis?

I. Synalar cream
II. Soriatane
III. Stelara

(A) I only
(B) III only
(C) I and II only
(D) II and III only
(E) I, II, and III

▪PROFILE NO. 30

Community Pharmacy Medication Record

Patient Name: Kathleen Irelander
Address: 72 Mountain Ash Road
Age: 34   Height: 5'7"
Sex: F   Weight: 122 lb
Allergies:

DIAGNOSIS

Primary	Secondary
1. Heroin abuse	1. PCP
2. AIDS-HIV	2.
3.	3.

MEDICATION RECORD

Date	Rx No.	Physician	Drug and Strength	Quantity	Sig	Refills
1. 5/16	39998	Goldman	Norvir 100 mg	120	6 b.i.d.	2
2. 5/16	39999	Goldman	Retrovir 300 mg	60	1 b.i.d.	2
3. 5/16	40000	Goldman	Epivir 150 mg	60	1 b.i.d.	2
2. 7/9	48749	Goldman	Pentam 300	10	Bring to office	2

PHARMACIST'S NOTES AND OTHER PATIENT INFORMATION

Date	Comment
1. 6/1	Robitussin DM (OTC)

DIRECTIONS (Questions 30a through 30l): Each of the numbered items or incomplete statements in this section is followed by answers or completions of the statement. Select the ONE lettered answer or completion that is BEST in each case.

30a. Which of the following agents would be appropriate to use in treating a patient with acute heroin overdose?

(A) flumazenil
(B) naloxone
(C) cuprimine
(D) tolazamide
(E) physostigmine

30b. Another name for heroin is

(A) diacetylmorphine
(B) oxycodone
(C) ethylmorphine
(D) oxymorphone
(E) methylmorphine

30c. "PCP" in the profile refers to

(A) phencyclidine
(B) pronounced cardiac pronation
(C) *Pneumocystis carinii* pneumonia
(D) postcoronary patient
(E) precancerous psoriasis

30d. Another name for Retrovir is

    I. zidovudine

    II. AZT

    III. ribavirin

(A) I only

(B) III only

(C) I and II only

(D) II and III only

(E) I, II, and III

30e. Patients receiving Retrovir must be monitored carefully for the development of

(A) blood dyscrasias

(B) malignant hypertension

(C) edema

(D) pneumothorax

(E) pulmonary fibrosis

30f. Which of the drug products used by this patient is/are a protease inhibitor?

    I. Norvir

    II. Retrovir

    III. Epivir

(A) I only

(B) III only

(C) I and II only

(D) II and III only

(E) I, II, and III

30g. Patients on Retrovir should avoid the use of

(A) acetaminophen

(B) benzodiazepines

(C) penicillins

(D) iron products

(E) vitamin A

30h. Pentamidine (Pentam) is available in which of the following dosage forms?

    I. capsules

    II. aerosol

    III. injection

(A) I only

(B) III only

(C) I and II only

(D) II and III only

(E) I, II, and III

30i. Patients using Pentam must be monitored for the development of

(A) GI ulceration

(B) *Pseudomonas* infection

(C) kidney failure

(D) liver failure

(E) severe hypotension

30j. Which of the following are active ingredients in Robitussin DM?

    I. codeine

    II. dextromethorphan HBr

    III. guaifenesin

(A) I only

(B) III only

(C) I and II only

(D) II and III only

(E) I, II, and III

30k. Which of the following are adverse effects associated with the use of Epivir?

    I. lactic acidosis

    II. hypertensive crisis

    III. Stevens–Johnson syndrome

(A) I only

(B) III only

(C) I and II only

(D) II and III only

(E) I, II, and III

30l. Patents using Norvir should be monitored for clinically significant drug interactions with

    I. amiodarone

    II. triazolam

    III. pimozide

(A) I only

(B) III only

(C) I and II only

(D) II and III only

(E) I, II, and III

Answers and Explanations

Numbers within parentheses at the end of the answers refer to the numbered references that are listed in the front matter.

PROFILE NO. 1

1a. **(E)** Metolazone (Zaroxolyn) is a thiazide-like drug that inhibits reabsorption of sodium and chloride in the ascending limb of the loop of Henle and the early distal tubules. Choices (A) and (C) are loop diuretics, choice (B) is a carbonic anhydrase inhibitor, and choice (D) is not a diuretic. *(10)*

1b. **(D)** The prostate-specific antigen (PSA) is a protein produced by the cells of the prostate gland. PSA test measures the level of PSA in the blood. When the prostate gland enlarges, PSA levels in the blood tend to rise. Such an elevation can be caused by cancer or benign conditions such as BPH. Generally, a PSA level of 0 to 4 ng/mL is considered to be normal. Values higher than this level suggest the need for further evaluation to determine the cause of the elevation. *(16)*

1c. **(C)** Candesartan (Atacand) is an angiotensin II-receptor blocker. This class of drugs has somewhat fewer adverse effects associated with it than the ACE inhibitors (eg, nonproductive cough, angioedema). However, like the ACE inhibitors, angiotensin II antagonists are not safe to use during the second and third trimester of pregnancy. *(6)*

1d. **(A)** Thiazide diuretics are best taken in the morning to avoid being awakened during the night because of an urge to void. Patients should also be advised to maintain adequate hydration and to take the drug with food or milk. *(3)*

1e. **(E)** Dutasteride (Avodart) is an agent that interferes with the enzyme that converts testosterone to dihydrotestosterone in the body. Since prostate development and size is dependent upon dihydrotestosterone, the use of dutasteride will cause a reduction of prostate size. Drugs that reduce DHT production, such as Avodart and Proscar, may take as long as 6 months to achieve maximal shrinkage of prostate size. *(3)*

1f. **(D)** Dutasteride as well as finasteride (Proscar) are classified in pregnancy category X. They should, therefore, not be used in women or even come in contact with the skin of pregnant women. Dutasteride and finasteride also have the ability to stimulate hair growth in some patients and possibly cause hirsutism. Finasteride is also available for the treatment of alopecia by the name Propecia. *(3)*

1g. **(E)** The use of thiazide diuretics such as hydrochlorothiazide is associated with the potential for causing hypokalemia, hypomagnesemia, and hypercalcemia. *(6)*

1h. **(E)** Thiazide drugs such as hydrochlorothiazide may exhibit a cross-sensitivity with sulfa drugs. *(3)*

1i. **(D)** Mr. Wallace should be advised to avoid the use of Claritin-D because this product contains pseudoephedrine, a sympathomimetic drug that could cause his blood pressure to rise. Many companies that have included pseudoephedrine in their formulations may have reformulated these products to contain other decongestants because of the realization that pseudoephedrine can be used as a precursor in the synthesis of methamphetamine. *(11)*

1j. **(C)** Doxazosin (Cardura) and alfuzosin (Uroxatral) are alpha₁-adrenergic blocking agents. They are useful in treating BPH because they relax the smooth muscle of the prostate and of the bladder sphincter, thereby allowing better urine flow. Eplerenone (Inspra) is an aldosterone blocker used in the treatment of hypertension. *(3)*

1k. **(B)** Nitroprusside (Nitropress) is used in the treatment of hypertensive emergency. It is generally administered by IV infusion. Nitroprusside decreases both preload and afterload and is particularly useful in patients with impaired left ventricular function. Nitroprusside solutions are very easily degraded by light and must be protected from light by using an opaque covering on infusion containers. Treprostinil (Remodulin) is only indicated for the treatment of pulmonary arterial hypertension. Tebuxostat (Uloric) is used to treat gout *(3)*

1l. **(D)** Methyldopa is considered to be the safest antihypertensive agent for pregnant women, of those listed. The others may have a higher propensity for causing fetal damage. *(5)*

PROFILE NO. 2

2a. **(C)** Celecoxib (Celebrex) is a nonsteroidal anti-inflammatory drug (NSAID) that is believed to act by inhibiting prostaglandin synthesis by inhibiting cyclooxygenase-2 (COX-2). COX-2 inhibitors are believed to cause less GI upset than COX-1 NSAIDs. Their effects on renal dysfunction and platelet inhibition, however, are comparable with COX-1 agents. *(3)*

2b. **(C)** A creatinine clearance (CL_{Cr}) level of <25 mL/min would indicate the presence of

severe renal impairment. None of the NSAIDs should be used in such patients because NSAIDs may decrease renal blood flow and may exacerbate renal impairment. *(14)*

2c. **(B)** Nitroglycerin sublingual tablets are required by the FDA to be packaged in a glass container with a tight metal cap in order to reduce the loss of drug. The tablets should also be kept in a cool, dry place, not refrigerated. *(3)*

2d. **(B)** Prinzmetal's angina or vasospastic angina is characterized by spasm of the smooth muscle of the proximal coronary arteries, often leading to an angina attack of long duration. Such attacks often occur at night and without a stress component. *(14)*

2e. **(A)** Cosamin DS contains glucosamine and chondroitin. Glucosamine is believed to promote the formation and repair of cartilage. Chondroitin is a substance that is believed to promote water retention and elasticity in cartilage and inhibit enzymes that breakdown cartilage. These agents are available OTC in many different combinations. *(11)*

2f. **(D)** Misoprostol (Cytotec) is a drug that can produce an antisecretory effect in the stomach and can elicit a mucoprotective effect by increasing mucus and bicarbonate production. It is indicated for the prevention of NSAID-induced peptic ulcers and should be used for the duration of NSAID therapy. Misoprostol is categorized as a pregnancy category X drug. *(3)*

2g. **(C)** The use of nitroglycerin sublingual tablets may cause a number of effects. Because of its vasodilating effect, nitroglycerin may cause hypotension and headache. Many patients also state that the use of nitroglycerin sublingual tablets produces a slight burning sensation when placed under the tongue. *(3)*

2h. **(A)** Nitroglycerin is available in a number of different dosage forms, including a sublingual, translingual, transdermal, ointment, IV, and an oral sustained-release form. It is not available as a suspension dosage form. *(3)*

2i. **(C)** Tramadol (Ultram) is a centrally acting analgesic agent that may be useful for this patient. Because of its central action, however, tramadol may cause dizziness, somnolescence, and sweating. *(14)*

2j. **(C)** Senokot products contain senna, an anthraquinone, which produces a mild stimulant effect on the GI tract. The advantage of senna is that it is not significantly systemically absorbed from the GI, thereby reducing the likelihood of systemic adverse effects. *(11)*

2k. **(A)** Nitrolingual spray is a metered-dose aerosol-containing nitroglycerin. It is sprayed onto or under the tongue upon onset of an angina attack. An advantage that this product has over nitroglycerin sublingual tablets is that the pressurized packaging of the nitroglycerin in the Nitrolingual spray reduces the likelihood of drug loss by volatility. *(3)*

2l. **(C)** When any nitroglycerin products are used, patients should be advised to avoid the use of alcoholic beverages, sildenafil (Viagra), vardenafil (Levitra), tadalafil (Cialis), or any other drugs than can cause vasodilation. The combined use of these drugs and nitroglycerin may result in the development of hypotension, dizziness, and/or syncope. *(10)*

PROFILE NO. 3

3a. **(E)** Micronor is a progestin-only oral contraceptive product that contains norethindrone. Such products are somewhat less effective than combination products that contain both an estrogen and progestin. Progestin-only products are taken daily rather than cyclically. *(3)*

3b. **(D)** Ortho Gynol II Extra Strength Jelly is a contraceptive product. It also has some vaginal lubricant properties as well. It may be used either alone or in conjunction with a condom or diaphragm product. *(3)*

3c. **(C)** Generalized tonic–clonic seizures have also been referred to as grand mal seizures.

Such seizures are characterized by alternating tonic and clonic muscle activity. *(16)*

3d. **(C)** Carbamazepine (Tegretol) and valproic acid (Depakene) are anticonvulsants used for the treatment of many convulsive disorders including generalized tonic–clonic seizures. Lamotrigine is indicated for the treatment of partial seizures. *(3)*

3e. **(C)** Dilantin Kapseals contain extended phenytoin sodium. This product is suitable for single daily dosing or divided daily dosing because the peak concentration of the drug is reached approximately 12 hours after administration. Products that contain phenytoin sodium, prompt, are suitable only for divided daily dosing because the peak concentration is reached after only 1 to 3 hours. *(3)*

3f. **(B)** Gingival hyperplasia is a condition characterized by an overgrowth of gum tissue. Unless quickly treated, this condition can result in tooth loss and further gum disease. *(16)*

3g. **(A)** Michaelis–Menten or saturation kinetics is exhibited by some drugs including phenytoin. Such kinetics is characterized by slower metabolism of a drug at high doses than at low doses because of the saturation of metabolic enzymes. *(5)*

3h. **(D)** The therapeutic plasma concentration of phenytoin is 10 to 20 μg/mL. A phenytoin plasma concentration of 5 μg/mL several weeks after initiating therapy may indicate inadequate dosing or patient noncompliance. *(14)*

3i. **(D)** Phenytoin use may decrease the pharmacological effect of the Micronor by increasing the hepatic metabolism of the progestin in Micronor. Because progestin-only products such as Micronor tend to be somewhat less effective in preventing pregnancy, this may result in an unwanted pregnancy. *(3)*

3j. **(D)** Fosphenytoin (Cerebyx) is a phenytoin ester that is a prodrug of phenytoin. Fosphenytoin causes less irritation at the IV injection site than phenytoin. It can be administered at three times the rate of phenytoin and, unlike phenytoin, is effective when given intramuscularly. Doses of fosphenytoin are stated in phenytoin equivalents (PE). *(31)*

3k. **(D)** The IM route for phenytoin sodium is generally avoided because the precipitation of phenytoin at the injection site may be painful and result in erratic absorption. Phenytoin is easily precipitated in the presence of an acidic substance (such as multivitamins) in the IV admixture. The addition of phenytoin sodium to an IV infusion is therefore generally not recommended. *(3)*

3l. **(A)** A morbilliform rash is one that resembles that of measles. *(16)*

3m. **(E)** The usual drug of choice for the treatment of status epilepticus is lorazepam (Ativan). Other benzodiazepines such as midazolam (Versed) or diazepam (Valium) may also be used. Propofol (Diprivan) is a nonbenzodiazepine anesthetic agent that is also useful in treating refractory status epilepticus. *(3)*

3n. **(B)** Patients receiving chronic phenytoin therapy may develop folate deficiency because phenytoin reduces folic acid absorption. Folate supplementation may, therefore, be required in such patients. *(3)*

3o. **(E)** Nonoxynol-9 is a surfactant spermicide that is the active ingredient of Ortho Gynol II Extra Strength Jelly. *(3)*

3p. **(C)** Docusate sodium, the active ingredient of the stool softener Colace, is an anionic surfactant that promotes the penetration of water into the intestinal contents. This softens the contents and facilitates their evacuation. *(11)*

3q. **(E)** Lycopene is a pigment that gives tomatoes their characteristic red color. It has potent antioxidant properties and its use has been shown to reduce the incidence of prostate cancer. This agent has also been shown to reduce the levels of LDLs in the body. *(3)*

PROFILE NO. 4

4a. **(E)** Carbidopa serves as a dopa-decarboxylase inhibitor that prevents the peripheral decarboxylation of levodopa and permits a greater proportion of the levodopa dose to enter the brain in its intact form. The use of carbidopa in combination with levodopa permits the use of lower levodopa doses than would be used without carbidopa. *(32)*

4b. **(C)** Pyridoxine promotes the peripheral conversion of levodopa to dopamine by dopa-decarboxylase, thereby decreasing the activity of the administered levodopa. *(3)*

4c. **(A)** Darkening of the urine with the use of levodopa or Sinemet is normal and is a product of levodopa metabolism. The patient may disregard it. *(3)*

4d. **(C)** Akineton (Biperiden) is an anticholinergic agent used in the treatment of Parkinson's disease. Such agents reduce the incidence and severity of akinesia, rigidity, and tremor in patients with Parkinson's disease. Anticholinergic drugs are used as adjuncts to levodopa in the treatment of Parkinson's disease. *(3)*

4e. **(B)** Tiagabine (Gabitril) is an anticonvulsant. Selegiline (Eldepryl), rasagiline (Azilect), ropinirole (Requip), and bromocriptine (Parlodel) are dopaminergic agents used in treating Parkinson's disease. *(3)*

4f. **(D)** The on–off effect is a deterioration of levodopa activity, which is most prevalent just before the next dose is due. It may be caused by pharmacokinetic issues, altered sensitivity of dopaminergic receptors, or by other alterations in the CNS. The on–off effect can be reduced by reducing the dosing interval used (ie, give the levodopa more frequently) or by adding an MAO inhibitor such as selegiline (Eldepryl), which will reduce the metabolic breakdown of levodopa. *(3)*

4g. **(A)** Diplopia, or double vision, is sometimes experienced by patients receiving levodopa therapy. *(14)*

4h. **(C)** When a patient on levodopa is to be switched to Sinemet, at least 8 hours must be allowed to elapse from the last dose of levodopa to the first dose of Sinemet in order to decrease the likelihood of toxicity. Because the carbidopa in the Sinemet increases the proportion of intact levodopa that enters the brain, the dose of levodopa administered via Sinemet should be 75% to 80% less than that administered prior to the initiation of Sinemet therapy. *(3)*

4i. **(B)** The prolonged use of dibenzoxazepine antipsychotic drugs such as loxapine and phenothiazine drugs such as chlorpromazine may cause extrapyramidal effects such as Parkinson-like symptoms because these drugs act as dopamine antagonists. *(3)*

4j. **(A)** Carbidopa is available by itself as Lodosyn. This product should be employed in combination with levodopa to create a dosage combination for patients with Parkinson's disease. *(3)*

4k. **(B)** Biperiden (Akineton) is an anticholinergic drug that is used in the treatment of Parkinson's disease. It is believed to work by competitively antagonizing the effects of acetylcholine in the CNS, thereby correcting an imbalance between cholinergic and dopaminergic activity seen in Parkinson patients. Anticholinergic drugs such as biperiden may produce typical anticholinergic adverse effects such as constipation, dry mouth, and urinary retention. *(3)*

4l. **(E)** Selegiline (Eldepryl) is a selective irreversible inhibitor of MAO type B. MAO-B is located primarily in the CNS, and MAO-A is located primarily in the GI tract and in the liver. Therefore, MAO-B inhibitors are less likely to affect the metabolism of tyramine found in cheese and wine, or sympathomimetic agents such as those found in nasal decongestants. While use of moderate doses of selegiline are unlikely to cause such interactions, when higher doses are used the selectivity of selegiline may diminish, thereby causing inhibition of MAO-A. Since the threshold between MAO-A and MAO-B inhibition is not clear, it would be prudent to avoid tyramine containing foods as well as sympathomimetic drugs when using this drug. *(6)*

4m. **(D)** Emsam is a transdermal product that contains selegiline as its active ingredient and is indicated for the treatment of depression. Selegiline is a MAO-B inhibitor. *(32)*

PROFILE NO. 5

5a. **(E)** Timolol (Timoptic, Timoptic-XE) acts as a beta-adrenergic blocking agent that reduces the production of aqueous humor in the eye. *(3)*

5b. **(E)** Timoptic and metipranolol (Optipranolol) are both beta-adrenergic blocking agents. *(3)*

5c. **(A)** Intraocular pressure may vary considerably in the same individual, depending on the time of day that the measurement is taken as well as many other factors. A measurement of 14 mm Hg is well within the normal range of 10 to 20 mm Hg. *(14)*

5d. **(B)** Timoptic-XE is a sterile ophthalmic solution of timolol maleate. The solution also contains a substance known as Gelrite, which is a purified polysaccharide derived from gellan gum. When the Gelrite solution comes in contact with cations, such as the sodium found in tears, the solution forms a gel, which sustains the contact of the timolol with the eye. Eventually tears wash the gel away. *(10)*

5e. **(D)** Urticaria is a name for hives. These are usually caused by a hypersensitivity reaction and can be manifested as discolored, swollen areas of the body. *(16)*

5f. **(C)** Acetazolamide (Diamox) is a carbonic anhydrase inhibitor. Since carbonic anhydrase is an enzyme that promotes aqueous humor production, the use of an inhibitor of carbonic anhydrase will reduce the formation of aqueous humor and, thereby, reduce intraocular pressure. *(5)*

5g. **(B)** Bimatoprost (Lumigan) is a synthetic prostaglandin analog that reduces intraocular pressure by increasing outflow of aqueous humor from the eye. The most common adverse effects associated with this product are conjunctival hyperemia, growth of eyelashes, and ocular pruritis. *(31)*

5h. **(C)** Edetate disodium is a metal scavenger that binds free metal ions. This is used to reduce the chance of trace metal-catalyzed decomposition reactions. *(1)*

5i. **(B)** The active ingredient in Motrin IB and Advil is ibuprofen. Datril contains acetaminophen. Excedrin contains acetaminophen, aspirin and caffeine. Aleve contains naproxen. Anacin contains aspirin and caffeine. *(11)*

5j. **(D)** Visine-A Allergy Relief contains naphazoline as its active ingredient. This agent is decongestant that tends to exhibit $alpha_1$ agonist activity. Its use in the eye causes vasoconstriction, relief of "red eyes," and ophthalmic congestion. *(11)*

5k. **(B)** The use of a beta-adrenergic blocking agent such as Timoptic-XE or levobunolol (Betagan) by a patient with a history of respiratory illness and breathing difficulty may be hazardous because beta-adrenergic blockers may cause bronchoconstriction. Even the relatively small amount of drug that enters the systemic circulation via an ophthalmic administration has been reported to cause breathing difficulty in susceptible patients. *(3)*

5l. **(E)** Anticholinergic drugs may cause mydriasis (pupillary dilation). This is likely to result in elevated intraocular pressure and exacerbation of the patient's glaucoma symptoms. *(3)*

PROFILE NO. 6

6a. **(B)** The active ingredient in Benzac is benzoyl peroxide, an agent that appears to act by providing antibacterial activity, especially against *Propionibacterium acnes*, the predominant organism in acne lesions. *(11)*

6b. **(C)** Patients using tretinoin (Retin-A) products should be advised to avoid the use of the product near the eyes, mouth, angles of the nose, and mucous membranes because tretinoin may irritate these tissues. Patients using this product should also be advised to avoid excessive exposure to sunlight and sunlamps because the drug may increase the patient's susceptibility to burning. *(3)*

6c. **(E)** Butylated hydroxytoluene, or BHT, is an oil-soluble antioxidant that is commonly employed in food and topical products in order to reduce the likelihood of spoilage. *(1)*

6d. **(D)** Retin-A Micro is a gel that contains microspheres containing tretinoin. *(10)*

6e. **(A)** The systemic use of clindamycin, the active ingredient of Cleocin, has been associated with the development of diarrhea in some patients. If the diarrhea is severe and/or persistent, the patient's physician should be contacted because such a response may indicate the development of pseudomembranous enterocolitis, a serious and potentially life-threatening condition. *(3)*

6f. **(A)** A product that contains 10 mg of drug per milliliter will contain 1,000 mg, or 1.0 g/100 mL. This is equivalent to a 1% (wt./vol.) solution of the drug. *(1)*

6g. **(D)** Isotretinoin (Claravis) is an isomer of retinoic acid, a metabolite of retinol (vitamin A). Beta-carotene is provitamin A. *(3)*

6h. **(E)** Many adverse effects are associated with the use of isotretinoin (Claravis). Cheilitis, an inflammation around the margins of the lips, is very common. Conjunctivitis (inflammation of the conjunctival lining of the eye) is also a common adverse effect associated with the use of this drug. Hyperlipidemia, sometimes severe, can also occur in patients using isotretinoin. Isotretinoin is also in pregnancy category X. A pregnant woman should therefore never use it. *(10)*

6i. **(C)** Because of the many adverse effects associated with the use of isotretinoin (Claravis), and as part of the iPLEDGE program associated with the prescribing, dispensing, and use of this product, the pharmacist must dispense a patient package insert to any patient receiving this drug product. Patients are also required to sign an informed consent form before receiving the product. *(10)*

6j. **(E)** When puberty occurs, the level of sebaceous gland activity increases. This results in an increase in sebum production. When the fats in sebum are converted to free fatty acids by microorganisms such as *Corynbacterium acnes* in the pilosebaceous unit, they cause a localized inflammatory response, which, in turn, causes the development of the primary lesion of acne, the comedone. *(14)*

6k. **(B)** Aluminum oxide is a water-insoluble material that is employed in the Brasivol formulation as an abrasive. When rubbed onto the affected area, the abrasive property is meant to help remove the comedone plugs and allow better drainage of the comedone. *(11)*

6l. **(D)** Salicylic acid is a keratolytic agent, that is, it helps to remove keratin from the skin surface. This facilitates the opening of plugged comedones and decreases the likelihood of new comedone formation. *(11)*

6m. **(D)** Sebum is a lipid secretion of the sebaceous glands, which are associated with the hair follicle. Sebum acts as a protectant on the skin surface. When the esterified fatty acids of sebum are broken down to free fatty acids by microorganisms, the inflammatory lesion of acne may be formed. *(11)*

PROFILE NO. 7

7a. **(C)** Montelukast sodium (Singulair) and zafirlukast (Accolate) are both leukotriene antagonists. Salmeterol (Serevent) and albuterol (Ventolin HFA) are selective beta$_2$ agonists, cromolyn (Intal) is a mast cell stabilizer, and budesonide (Pulmicort) is a corticosteroid. *(3)*

7b. **(C)** Montelukast sodium (Singulair) is a leukotriene antagonist and is not effective in halting an acute asthma attack. Proventil-HFA contains a rapidly acting bronchodilator that will be more effective in treating an acute attack. *(3)*

7c. **(D)** Singulair and Flovent Diskus should not be administered on a p.r.n. basis. They are only useful for prophylaxis of an asthma attack. Lubiprostone (Amitiza) is a chloride channel activator used to increase fluid secretions in the intestine, thereby improving intestinal motility and reducing constipation. *(3)*

7d. **(E)** The Proventil-HFA Aerosol product contains albuterol, a selective beta$_2$ agonist. *(3)*

7e. **(E)** Older and younger patients who have difficulty in coordinating their inhalation of an aerosol may benefit from the use of a spacer device. *(3)*

7f. **(A)** The HFA in Proventil-HFA refers to a propellant in the hydrofluroalkane group. HFAs are a newer type of propellant used in *metered dose inhalers* for asthma. They replace the fluorochlorocarbon (CFC) group of propellants, which were phased out of use in 2008 because they were known to adversely affect the ozone layer of the earth. *(3)*

7g. **(A)** Rotacaps are a dosage form marketed by GlaxoSmithKline that contain a powder intended for inhalation. It is used with a device called a Rotahaler. *(3)*

7h. **(C)** The active ingredient in Flovent Discus is fluticasone, a corticosteroid. When administered by inhalation to asthmatic patients, Flovent Diskus reduces the likelihood of future acute asthmatic attacks. Flovent Diskus and other corticosteroids inhalations are not suitable for use during an acute asthma attack. *(3)*

7i. **(C)** When a bronchodilator such as Proventil-HFA is to be used with a corticosteroid inhalation such as Flovent Diskus, the patient should be advised to use the bronchodilator at least several minutes before the corticosteroid to promote better passage of the corticosteroid into the lower lung. *(3)*

7j. **(C)** Habitrol patches contain nicotine as their active ingredient. They are applied for a 24-hour period. A new site should be used for each application. *(32)*

7k. **(B)** Both Flovent Diskus and Advair HFA are inhalation products containing fluticasone propionate. *(3)*

PROFILE NO. 8

8a. **(C)** Nitrostat is a nitroglycerin sublingual tablet that has been stabilized in order to decrease the likelihood that loss of potency of the tablets will take place. As a result, Nitrostat appears to have a considerably longer shelf life than do nonstabilized nitroglycerin tablets. *(3)*

8b. **(A)** The pharmacist should dispense Nitrostat, as well as other oral nitroglycerin products, in its original container because such containers are designed to minimize the loss of nitroglycerin during storage. *(3)*

8c. **(B)** Transdermal nitroglycerin patches should be applied onto a hairless site. Site rotation is important with each administration in order to decrease the likelihood of skin irritation. Transdermal patches should not be applied to distal portions of the extremities because these areas do not permit as reliable absorption of the nitroglycerin as do other areas of the body. *(3)*

8d. **(C)** When discontinuing therapy with nitroglycerin transdermal systems, gradual reduction of both the dosage and frequency of application over a 4- to 6-week period is advisable in order to minimize the likelihood of sudden withdrawal reactions. *(16)*

8e. **(B)** Dipyridamole (Persantine), in addition to being used in the treatment of angina, is also employed as an antiplatelet agent. It appears to act in this regard by inhibiting cyclic nucleotide phosphodiesterase activity. *(3)*

8f. **(D)** Nitroglycerin administered orally undergoes extensive first-pass hepatic deactivation, thereby limiting the usefulness of this route of administration. *(31)*

8g. **(D)** The use of alcohol or tadalafil (Cialis) (and similar ED drugs) in combination with nitroglycerin may produce a hypotensive response because of the vasodilating action of all of these drugs. The hypotensive response may be manifested as dizziness, fainting, and/or weakness. *(3)*

8h. **(A)** Nitroglycerin may be adsorbed onto the PVC tubing used in most IV administration sets. This may result in loss of drug and inadequate dosing. Manufacturers of nitroglycerin for IV use supply non-PVC infusion tubing, which minimizes the adsorption of nitroglycerin. Such special tubing is generally recommended for use with nitroglycerin products. *(3)*

8i. **(B)** The dose of nitroglycerin topical ointment is measured in inches. It is applied to the skin with minimal rubbing, and the area to which it has been applied is covered with plastic wrap to facilitate drug absorption, and to prevent staining of clothing. *(3)*

8j. **(C)** Phenylephrine is an alpha$_1$ agonist. It causes constriction of blood vessels throughout the body, thereby causing a decongestant effect. Vascular constriction may also increase blood pressure and increase the likelihood of future angina attacks in this patient. *(6)*

PROFILE NO. 9

9a. **(B)** Patients with type 1 diabetes mellitus are generally insulin dependent. Their disease generally begins early in life and is characterized by little or no insulin production capability by the pancreas. *(14)*

9b. **(D)** Humalog contains insulin lispro, a human insulin analog that is prepared by recombinant DNA technology. Humalog is a rapid-acting insulin. It should be administered within 15 minutes of mealtime. Humalog is a clear product. *(3)*

9c. **(A)** The Lantus insulin contains 100 units of activity per milliliter. Twenty-four units of Lantus activity will therefore be contained in 0.24 mL of the product. *(3)*

9d. **(E)** Polydipsia refers to excessive thirst. This is frequently seen in type 1 diabetics because of the excessive urination (polyuria) that is associated with the body's attempt to eliminate excessive glucose in the blood. *(14)*

9e. **(E)** A fasting blood sugar of 85 mg/dL is well within the normal range of 70 to 110 mg/dL. *(3)*

9f. **(B)** Regular insulin is the only form of insulin suitable for IV infusion. All other insulins are unsuitable for IV administration either because they contain particulates (eg, NPH insulin) or have characteristics such as low pH, which make it unsuitable for IV use. *(3)*

9g. **(A)** Levemir (insulin detemir) is a long-acting basal insulin similar in action to Lantus. It appears to be less likely than Lantus to cause weight gain and can be stored at room temperature for 6 weeks. Novalog and Apidra are rapid-acting insulins. Humulin R is regular insulin and Humulin N is an intermediate-acting NPH insulin. *(3)*

9h. **(B)** Pramlintide (Symlin) is a synthetic analog of human amylin, a naturally occurring neuroendocrine hormone synthesized from pancreatic beta cells that contributes to glucose control during the postprandial period. Amylin is often deficient in diabetic patients. Symlin should be injected subcutaneously immediately prior to major meals. It is used in conjunction with insulin to control the patient's glucose levels in type 1 and type 2

diabetes. It should, however, never be mixed with insulins. Before a Symlin container is opened, it should be kept refrigerated. Once it is opened, it may be refrigerated or kept at room temperature for up to 28 days. *(31)*

9i. **(A)** Insulin glargine (Lantus) is manufactured with a pH of 4. It is, therefore, not compatible with other insulins. Lantus insulin is designed to precipitate when administered subcutaneously and will produce approximately 24 hours of action with a single dose. *(3)*

9j. **(A)** The Ascensia Elite device requires that a small amount of blood be used to measure the blood glucose level. To obtain this blood, the patient or caregiver must use a lancet device to puncture the skin. *(3)*

9k. **(B)** Sudafed PE tablets contain phenylephrine, a sympathomimetic decongestant that is capable of inducing the conversion of glycogen to glucose in the body. This may increase glucose levels in the blood and increase the patient's insulin requirement. *(3)*

9l. **(C)** B-D Micro-Fine+ Insulin syringes are available with a capacity of 0.3, 0.5, and 1.0 mL. The smaller sizes are useful in situations where a low dose (<50 units) of insulin must be administered because they permit more precise measurement of small amounts of insulin than do conventional insulin syringes, which contain a volume of 1.0 mL. *(1)*

9m. **(D)** Nateglinide (Starlix) and repaglinide (Prandin) are non-sulfonylurea insulin secretagogues. They are generally shorter acting than the first- or second-generation sulfonylureas. Glyburide (Diabeta, Glynase) is a second-generation sulfonylurea. *(32)*

9n. **(A)** Excessive lactate in the blood results from abnormal conversion of pyruvate into lactate. Lactic acidosis is the result of an increase in blood lactate levels when body buffer systems are overcome. Lactic acidosis may be caused by cardiopulmonary failure, side effects of drugs and toxins, and by various acquired and congenital diseases. Lactic acidosis is a rare but serious complication in the use of metformin HCl that may be fatal in 50% of patients who develop it. *(6)*

9o. **(D)** Pioglitazone (Actos), unlike many other oral hypoglycemic agents, acts by increasing insulin receptor sensitivity. Most of the other agents work by increasing insulin production by the beta cells of the pancreas. *(31)*

PROFILE NO. 10

10a. **(D)** Prothrombin Time (PT) and International Normalized Ratio (INR) are typically monitored in a patient on warfarin. PT evaluates the ability of blood to clot properly. It is often used in conjunction with the partial thromboplastin time (PTT) to evaluate the function of all coagulation factors. The INR is used to monitor the effectiveness of blood thinning drugs such as warfarin (Coumadin). *(3)*

10b. **(D)** The administration of rifampin (Rifadin) or carbamazepine (Tegretol) to a patient stabilized on warfarin is likely to result in decreased warfarin activity because of the ability of these drugs to increase the metabolism of warfarin. Cimetidine is an enzyme inhibitor and would, therefore, likely increase warfarin activity. *(3)*

10c. **(C)** Phytonadione (vitamin K_1) is a specific antidote for warfarin toxicity. Treatment of hemorrhage caused by oral anticoagulant therapy generally consists of the administration of 10 to 20 mg of phytonadione. *(6)*

10d. **(D)** Datril and Tylenol contain acetaminophen, an analgesic/antipyretic that does not appear to displace warfarin from plasma protein-binding sites. Advil contains ibuprofen, an agent that is capable of displacing warfarin from protein-binding sites, thus increasing warfarin activity. *(11)*

10e. **(C)** Patients who are hypothyroid will generally have elevated TSH levels, which can increase the size of the thyroid gland and produce a goiter. Since reduced thyroid hor-

mone levels will be likely to decrease metabolic rate, weight gain may occur in such patients. Cardiac palpitations are usually associated with hyperthyroidism. *(14)*

10f. **(A)** 9 hours; $t50 = 0.693/k = 0.693/0.23 = 3$ hours. Therefore, after 3 hours 100 mCi would remain, after 6 hours 50 mCi would remain, and after 9 hours 25 mCi would remain. *(1)*

10g. **(D)** Thyrolar and other thyroid hormone products appear to increase the catabolism of vitamin K-dependent clotting factors. This potentiates the action of warfarin and may decrease the warfarin dosage requirement. *(3)*

10h. **(D)** In a radiation emergency, the administration of potassium iodide would saturate the thyroid with nonradioactive iodide, thereby making it less likely that radioactive iodides created in the emergency would accumulate in thyroid tissue. *(6)*

10i. **(D)** Thyroid hormone production in the body is controlled by the level of TSH produced by the anterior pituitary. *(14)*

10j. **(E)** Synalgos-DC contains aspirin. The aspirin may displace warfarin from protein-binding sites and may increase warfarin activity in the body. *(3)*

PROFILE NO. 11

11a. **(C)** The term pyuria refers to pus in the urine. Such a condition is often associated with a UTI. *(27)*

11b. **(D)** *E. coli* is a gram-negative bacillus generally associated with the GI tract. It is commonly a causative organism in UTIs as well as in institutionally borne infections. *(5)*

11c. **(C)** Trimethoprim-sulfamethoxazole and ofloxacin products are popular drugs for the treatment of UTIs. Drug-resistant strains may necessitate switching to another antimicrobial agent. *(5)*

11d. **(D)** Both Septra and Bactrim are combination products of trimethoprim and sulfamethoxazole that have synergistic action against many microorganisms. The advantage of using such a combination as opposed to single-drug therapy is the ability of this combination to block two consecutive steps used by bacteria to produce tetrahydrofolic acid. Blocking two steps greatly diminishes the likelihood that bacterial resistance will develop. Trimox is one of the brand names for amoxicillin. *(3)*

11e. **(C)** Levaquin (levofloxacin) and Avelox (moxifloxacin) are fluoroquinolone drugs. Kanamycin (Kantrex) is an aminoglycoside. *(3)*

11f. **(A)** Patients using either Septra or other sulfa drugs should be advised to maintain adequate fluid intake in order to facilitate the urinary antimicrobial action of the product as well as to prevent precipitation of poorly soluble drugs in the urinary tract. Urinary acidification may accelerate the precipitation of sulfa drugs. There is no need for patients to avoid the use of folic acid containing foods. *(3)*

11g. **(D)** One of the causative microbes for UTIs is *E. coli*. This microbe reduces nitrates present in the urine to nitrites. Thus, elevated nitrite levels are indicative of the presence of bacteria in the urine (ie, bacteriuria). There are several commercial products such as AZO Test Strips, Uri-Test, and Microstix-3. When a strip is dipped into the urine, a color change will detect nitrites. Fortunately, the test is not affected by the presence of antimicrobial agents, thus can be used to monitor as to when the UTI is cleared. *(3)*

11h. **(E)** Phenazopyridine (Pyridium) is an azo dye employed as a urinary analgesic. It has no antiseptic activity. Phenazopyridine is often used to reduce pain in patients with UTIs prior to the successful control of bacteria by antimicrobial agents. *(3)*

11i. **(A)** Phenazopyridine is excreted unchanged into the urine. In doing so, it may cause a red-orange discoloration of the urine. *(3)*

11j. **(A)** When used with antimicrobial agents for the treatment of UTIs, Pyridium should not be used for more than 2 days. This permits Pyridium's analgesic action to be employed during the early period of therapy when the infection is not yet under control. After 2 days, the infection should be under control and the continued use of Pyridium should not be required. In addition, the use of Pyridium beyond 2 days would mask pain that might be an indication of the failure of the antimicrobial therapy. *(3)*

11k. **(E)** Probably the most common psychological symptom of PMS is tension characterized by irritability and depression, which occur in 70% to 90% of all women. Weight gain of several pounds may be observed due to water retention. Several OTC products contain mild diuretics to combat this bloating. *(3)*

11l. **(C)** Caffeine in doses of 100 to 200 mg every 3 to 4 hours is a safe and effective diuretic but may cause sleeplessness. Pamabrom, a derivative of theophylline, is also effective in doses of 50 mg up to four times a day. Pamabrom is the active ingredient in Midol PMS and Pamprin. Subtilisin is an incorrect answer since this chemical is only present in some contact lens products as an enzymatic cleanser. *(2; 3)*

11m. **(B)** Two possible choices would be ciprofloxacin (Ciloxan), which is available in a droptainer at a 3.5 mg/mL concentration, and ofloxacin (Ocuflox) available as a 0.3% concentration. Both are effective against gram-positive and gram-negative microorganisms including *Pseudomonas aeruginosa*. The microbes usually responsible for conjunctivitis are *S. aureus*, *S. epidermis*, and *S. pneumonia*. While Levaquin (levofloxacin) is a fluoroquinolone, it is not available as an ophthalmic solution. Tobrex (tobramycin) is not a fluoroquinolone. *(3)*

11n. **(C)** Studies have shown that splitting tablets may result in weight deviations as great as 37%. However, when properly instructed, patients could greatly improve the process, especially by using a tablet-splitting device. Best results occurred when breaking elongated tablets, especially if the tablets were scored. Only one tablet should be split at one time for a 1- or 2-day dosing. Also, drugs with relatively longer duration of action are ideal since more fluctuation of dosing is acceptable. There is greater danger in splitting tablets with short half-lives since one would expect more dosing variation. [*30:51:62 (2009)*]

11o. **(C)** Macular degeneration is an age-related disease in which central vision is lost although peripheral vision is still present. Thus, the affected patient can walk unassisted but suffers from visual distortion and blank spots. Risk factors increase for persons older than 55 years. Some sources claim males and females are equally affected while other sources claim more females are affected. *(6; 14)*

11p. **(B)** Calcium supplementation does not appear to reduce the incidence of AMD. All of the other choices appear to have some beneficial effects. *(5; 14)*

11q. **(E)** While high-fiber diets are beneficial for most individuals, it has not been shown to help prevent AMD. Eye protection from bright sunlight by the use of sunglasses is advisable. *(5; 14)*

11r. **(D)** The female internal sphincter has poor muscle control and the shorter urethra increases the incidence of incontinence. There is a relationship in the incidence in incontinence in postmenopausal women attributed to lowering of their estrogen levels. *(14; 22)*

11s. **(C)** The Foley and intermittent catheters are inserted through the urethra into the bladder to ease urine flow. They may be attached with tubing to a urinary leg bag or a bedside bag. The Texas catheter is an external catheter for males only. It is attached around the penis to allow urine flow. It may also be attached to a leg bag. *(1; 22)*

11t. **(B)** Diluted acetic acid solutions are good irrigating solutions. A 0.25% acetic acid solution can be suggested for disinfecting the urinary tract and catheter. *(1; 22)*

PROFILE NO. 12

12a. **(D)** Chlorambucil (Leukeran) is an alkylating agent that is a cell cycle nonspecific agent. It appears to alkylate DNA by causing breakage of strands and cross-linkages. It is administered orally as 2 mg tablets. *(3)*

12b. **(E)** The dose ordered was 25 mg/m^2 of body BSA. Since the estimated surface area of this patient is 1.6 m^2,

$$1.6 \times 25 \text{ mg} = 40 \text{ mg/d}.$$

Since 5 days of therapy was ordered,

$$40 \text{ mg} \times 5 \text{ mg} = 200 \text{ mg total.} \qquad (1)$$

12c. **(A)** A nomogram is a chart that permits the determination of a patient's BSA in square meters from the patient's known height and weight data. Nomograms are frequently employed in calculating doses for potent agents such as the antineoplastic drugs. *(1)*

12d. **(C)** Considering the patient's age, a short-acting sedative would be most appropriate. Eszopiclone (Lunesta), like zolpidem, is a nonbenzodiazepine, which is less likely to result in side effects the following day. Zaleplon (Sonata) is similar to zolpidem as well. The other choices are all benzodiazepines—ProSom (estazolam), Dalmane (flurazepam), Halcion (triazolam), and Restoril (temazepam). These drugs or their metabolites have relatively long half-lives in the body. Triazolam appears to cause a higher incidence of anterograde amnesia than the other choices. *(6)*

12e. **(A)** ALL represents about 80% of the acute leukemias in children and about 20% of the acute leukemias in adults. Long-term survival rates of greater than 70% are now obtained with chemotherapy. *(14)*

12f. **(A)** Methotrexate is an antimetabolite drug that inhibits dihydrofolic acid reductase. One of methotrexate's main uses is in psoriasis therapy. It is available in both oral and parenteral dosage forms. Carmustine (BCNU) inhibits synthesis of DNA and RNA and is classified as an alkylating agent, as is cyclophosphamide (Cytoxan). (3)

12g. **(A)** Allopurinol is a xanthine oxidase inhibitor. Inhibition of xanthine oxidase enzyme results in a reduction in the formation of uric acid, a common metabolite formed in patients being treated with antineoplastic drugs. Allopurinol is, therefore, commonly employed in the prevention or management of hyperuricemia. (3)

12h. **(A)** When allopurinol therapy is initiated, large quantities of uric acid may be mobilized in the body and enter the urinary tract. Without adequate hydration, urates are likely to precipitate in the tract, causing pain and inflammation. (3)

12i. **(D)** Because allopurinol is employed in managing uric acid levels in the body, the monitoring of serum urate levels will provide a means of determining the success of therapy. (3)

12j. **(B)** When nystatin oral suspension is employed in the treatment of oral candidiasis infection, it is important that sufficient contact time be allowed between the drug and the mucosal surface of the oral cavity. This can be accomplished by having the patient swish the suspension in the mouth for several minutes prior to swallowing it. (3)

12k. **(D)** Melatonin is an endogenous hormone that may affect human sleep patterns. Tryptophan has been advocated as a sleep aid, but its effectiveness has not been clearly established. (3)

PROFILE NO. 13

13a. **(E)** WBC counts are valuable in determining the presence of infection in the body. Usually there is a moderate increase in WBCs especially leukocytes. Counts of 12,000 to 18,000 cells per microliter are signs of leukocytosis, which characterizes appendicitis. Some hospitals use the jargon "a shift to the left" to reflect a high neutrophil count since most reports list neutrophils first in the series of WBC types. A "shift to the right" indicates a high lymphocyte count. Often in cases of acute appendicitis, the WBC count is not elevated. However, if the appendix ruptures, there is a significant danger of septicemia. (14)

13b. **(A)** Patients suffering from anemia will often have a pale complexion accompanying their feeling of lethargy. While Ms. Johnson has an elevated WBC count, that is unlikely to result in paleness. (14)

13c. **(A)** A blood glucose value of 135 mg/dL is above the targeted maximum value of 120. The patient is also overweight. It is unlikely that she is suffering from pernicious anemia, which would have been reflected in a high mean corpuscular volume (MCV). Her low hemoglobin (Hb) values of 4 to 5 g/dL most likely reflect an iron deficiency. Hypertension is unlikely since her blood pressure values are normal and there is no history of taking antihypertensive drugs. (14; 16)

13d. **(B)** Polycythemia vera is a relatively rare disease characterized by an excess of RBCs which thickens the blood resulting in slower passage through small blood vessels. Bleeding from the gums and a red appearance of the face are common. (16)

13e. **(A)** Various iron salts in the reduced forms (ferrous) may be used for iron deficiencies. The sulfates, fumarates, and gluconates are three available forms. It is probably not necessary to subject Ms. Johnson to an intramuscular injection of iron dextran. Vitamin B_{12} is prescribed for pernicious anemia. Folic acid is especially useful in preventing megaloblastic anemia. (1; 14)

13f. **(C)**

$$\text{mg of Fe} = 300 \text{ mg} \times \frac{\text{Atomic wt. iron}}{\text{Formula wt. ferrous sulfate}}$$

$$= 300 \text{ mg} \times \frac{56}{278}$$

$$= 60.4 \text{ mg.} \qquad (1, 23)$$

13g. **(E)** From the previous question, it was determined that 60 mg elemental iron was present in every 300 mg tablet. To obtain 60 mg of iron from the ferrous gluconate, one would calculate

$$\frac{56 \text{ Fe}}{482 \text{ Fe gluconate}} = \frac{60 \text{ mg Fe}}{x \text{ mg Fe gluconate}}$$

$$\therefore x = 516 \text{ mg} \qquad (1, 23)$$

13h. **(E)** The Schilling test involves oral administration of a small amount of radioactive vitamin B_{12}, followed by urine assay. Intrinsic factor and vitamin B_{12} are then administered. A diagnosis of pernicious anemia may be made if there is an increase in serum vitamin B_{12} when the intrinsic factor is present. *(14)*

13i. **(D)** Prealbumin, also called transthyretin, is a transporter protein for thyroid hormone. Normal serum levels of prealbumin are 16 to 40 mg/dL with <16 associated with malnutrition. Values may be monitored by taking blood samples twice a week for patients with values between 11 and 15 mg/dL. Values below 11 mg/dL indicate high-risk patients. TPN patients should have increases in prealbumin of 2 mg/dL per day with normal values reached in 8 days. The half-life of prealbumin is 2 to 3 days, thus a better marker of malnutrition than albumin that has a half-life of 20 days. Now considered the standard for assessing and monitoring nutritional status, prealbumin is less affected by liver disease than other serum proteins. *(6; 29)*

13j. **(A)** Constant daily use of large doses of aspirin may increase GI tract irritation with a corresponding increase in bleeding. *(5; 14)*

13k. **(C)** The notation of "G" indicates "gravid," which means pregnant. Nonpregnant females may be designated as "NG" or "nongravid." *(1; 14)*

13l. **(A)** A blood glucose value of 135 suggests that the patient may have type 2 diabetes. Further questioning concerning symptoms such as thirst, frequent urination, and family history may be helpful. Since the patient is overweight, a reasonable strategy will be for self-monitoring of glucose values plus some adjustments in diet. A lower carbohydrate diet coupled with exercise may be sufficient without the use of insulin or oral hypoglycemic drugs. Before discharge, the glycosylated hemoglobin (hemoglobin A_{1C}) should be determined. This value reflects blood sugar levels for the previous 2 to 3 months. *(6; 14)*

13m. **(A)** The hemoglobin A_{1C} indicates whether the patient's blood sugar levels have been under control over the previous 2 to 3 months. Normal patients have values less than 7% which is the targeted level for diabetics that are under good control. Values above 9% show poor control and levels above 12% call for more aggressive therapy. Tests for glycosylated hemoglobin should be performed every 3 to 6 months. *(6; 14)*

13n. **(E)** Needle sizes are based on two measurements: the length in inches, and the diameter based on an arbitrary system in which the smaller the diameter, the larger the number. Since most insulin injections are administered subcutaneously, a short needle of 3/8 to 5/8 in and small gauge of 25 to 27 is used. *(13; 25)*

13o. **(A)** One Touch Fast Take (LifeScan) is a strip and meter that requires drawing of only 1.5 mcL of blood from the arm rather than finger; thus the blood sampling is less painful. *(10; 25)*

13p. **(B)** Macular degeneration is a condition in which there is deterioration of the macula, which is the central area of the retina. Painless loss of vision occurs. It is more common in the elderly but tends to run in families. *(14; 16)*

13q. **(C)** Lutein is a natural carotenoid found in the retina. There is evidence that supplements of lutein may help prevent the development of macular degeneration, which is characterized by painless loss of vision. Although the adult daily requirement has not been established, suggested levels of lutein are in the range of 1 to 6 mg. The lutein contents of Ocuvite formulas are 2 to 6 mg while many multi-vitamins contain doses of only 250 μg or none of lutein. Lutein is also available as a single-entity product. *(1; 14; 25)*

13r. **(D)** Bilirubin is a breakdown product formed from the breakdown of hemoglobin. It is also known as "indirect" bilirubin and is character-ized by its poor water solubility and difficulty in being accurately assayed. Fortunately, it is metabolized by the liver's glycuronic acid into conjugated bilirubin or "direct" bilirubin that is water soluble and excreted in the bile. High direct bilirubin indicates blockage of the bile ducts (cholestasis). High blood levels of indirect bilibubin indicate a hemolytic disor-der or liver damage that is preventing the needed metabolism. *(6; 17)*

PROFILE NO. 14

14a. **(C)** The generic name for Zoloft is sertraline. The drug is classified as an SSRI and is effec-tive for the treatment of OCD. This condition is characterized by recurrent and persistent ideas, thoughts, and impulses that are often time-consuming and interfere with normal social functioning. Zoloft is available as 25-, 50-, and 100-mg tablets plus an oral concen-trate. *(3; 25)*

14b. **(B)** Antidepressants often take 2 weeks or more before significant improvement may be observed. The pharmacist should suggest that the patient continue on therapy for a longer period of time. *(3; 14)*

14c. **(B)** 240 mg/dL equals 2,400 mg/L or 2.4 g/L.

$$\frac{2.4\ g}{387\ g/mol} = 0.0062\ mol\ or\ 6.2\ mM/L. \quad (23)$$

14d. **(B)** Mr. Shannon's HDL value is desirable when compared to his LDL, triglycerides, and total cholesterol values. Most cholesterol pro-files include a LDL/HDL ratio in which a low value is desirable. Another meaningful ratio is the cholesterol/HDL value. In this patient,

a ratio of 3.6 is fairly low since the usual range is 4 to 7. Again, a low ratio is desirable. Mr. Shannon's direct LDL is high with a normal range usually considered 0 to 100. *(14; 16)*

14e. **(C)** Patients with hyperlipidemia have been successfully treated with daily intake of niacin, especially if the statins do not appear to work well. While niacin is relatively safe, daily doses as high as 3,000 mg may be neces-sary. Side effects of flushing, peptic ulcera-tion, and jaundice may occur. *(2)*

14f. **(C)** The first approach for reduction of blood pressure should be the combination of diet and diuretics. If the condition does not improve within a couple of months, more aggressive and expensive treatment may be required. *(6; 14)*

14g. **(E)** Compression stockings are intended to be worn during the day and should be fitted first thing in the morning on arising. While available in several pressures, those stock-ings known as antiembolism stockings usually exert only 20 mm of pressure and are, theoret-ically, intended for the bedridden patient. However, many ambulatory clients use them. Better grade stockings have graduated pressure with the highest pressure on the lower leg and lesser pressure on the thighs. This gradient aids in the return of blood to the heart.

14h. **(C)** Nasonex Nasal (mometasone furoate) spray is a corticosteroid anti-inflammatory product intended for the treatment of sea-sonal or perennial allergic rhinitis with dos-ing of one or two sprays daily in each nostril. Daily use of this product is not required when pollen counts are low. A new unit must be primed by actuating the pump 10 times before using. If the unit is not used for a week or more, the priming must be repeated. *(10)*

14i. **(A)** The combination of clarithromycin (Biaxin) and omeprazole 20 mg (Prilosec) is one of the therapies used to eradicate *H. pylori*. The dura-tion of therapy is usually 28 days with Biaxin taken during the first 14 days, then Prilosec from days 15 through 28. *(14; 18a)*

14j. **(B)** In some patients, especially the elderly, digoxin levels may increase when clarithromycin is administered. This is believed to be due to the inhibition of P-glycoprotein by clarithromycin. P-glycoprotein is believed to promote renal clearance of digoxin. *(3; 10; 25)*

14k. **(D)** Rosacea is a condition characterized by redness in the cheeks and other areas of the face. Left untreated, the color increases with dilation of small blood vessels. The condition worsens when the patient is exposed to the sun or is under stress. Usually the tetracyclines or metronidazole is used as treatment since there is some evidence of bacterial involvement. *(28, April 2003)*

14l. **(A)** Burow's solution contains 5% aluminum acetate. It is used topically as an astringent dressing. Conditions such as athlete's foot, diaper rash, dry skin, and various types of dermatitis such as poison ivy may be treated with this product. *(1)*

14m. **(B)** Aquaphor is a good absorbent of liquids such as Burow's solution and will ease its incorporation into the oleaginous petrolatum ointment base. Alcohol should not be included in the formula since it will have a tendency to evaporate and cause migration of the salicylic acid to the surface of the ointment. Polysorbate 80 is a nonionic surfactant which would have no useful purpose in the formula. *(1; 4; 19)*

14n. **(D)** Salicylic acid is used in topical products as a keratolytic agent, which is an agent that aids in loosening and removing dead skin cells (keratin). *(1; 4)*

14o. **(A)** Shingles most often appears after the age of 50. The disease presents as large blisters covering large areas, especially face, trunk, shoulders, neck, and legs. Eruptions follow the path of the infected nerve on only one side of the body. The severity of chickenpox in childhood has no bearing on later shingles.

Some children never realize that they have chickenpox, but the virus lies dormant for many years. Treatment for shingles often involves APAP, acyclovir, and valacyclovir. Capsaicin cream may relieve the pain. All people older than 60 years should definitely receive the vaccine. *(9; 29)*

14p. **(B)** C & S refers to culture and sensitivity. This allows for evaluation of the microorganisms that may be present and the likely antimicrobial agents that will counteract the infection. *(5; 7)*

14q. **(E)** The major causative microbes for CAP (community acquired pneumonia) are *P. aeruginosa* and *S. aureus* both of which are very resistant to penicillin. The disease is often treated with azithromycin, the macrolides, and doxycyline. While the fluoroquinolones may be effective, bacterial resistance is now common. Other forms of pneumonia may be treated with regular penicillin or penicillinase-resistant penicillin. However, in all instances, cultures should be obtained to determine which antibiotics will be effective. *(6; 7; 17)*

14r. **(E)** While either vancomycin or linezolid ((Zyvox) are the next line of defense, the incidences of MRSA being resistant to vancomycin have increased. Both are administered as intravenous infusions.

14s. **(A)** Dosing of vancomycin should be based on the present serum level of the drug in the body. The trough concentration just before the next dose should be at least 10 mg/L with targeted levels of 15 to 20 mg/L to improve drug penetration and the clinical outcomes. Dosing every 8 to 12 hours is now recommended recognizing that toxicity begins near the 20 mg/L level.

14t. **(A)** Vancomycin is a very irritating drug and may cause necrosis. Thus, it is not injected intramuscularly. Extravasation must be avoided with infusions. Usually 500 mg to 1 g is added to 100 to 200 mL of D_5W or N/S and administered over at least 1 hour. *(1; 9; 21)*

PROFILE NO. 15

15a. **(E)** Cystic fibrosis is an inherited disease that affects the lungs, digestive system, sweat glands, and male fertility. Its name is derived from the fibrous scar tissue that develops in the pancreas, one of the principal organs affected by the disease. The disease is characterized by the production of thicker than normal mucus in various parts of the body. The organ systems most severely affected by cystic fibrosis are the digestive system and the respiratory system. *(14)*

15b. **(A)** While genetic testing can be performed to diagnose cystic fibrosis, the sweat test is one of the easiest and most accurate tests for this disease. People with cystic fibrosis have a higher than normal salt concentration in their sweat. In performing this test, a drug such as pilocarpine is applied to the skin. Then an electric current is applied to the area to enhance pilocarpine absorption. This causes sweating in the area of drug application. Measurement of the salt content of the sweat can identify the disease. *(14)*

15c. **(D)** While acetylcysteine (Mucomyst) is generally administered by inhalation as a mucolytic agent in treating cystic fibrosis, oral acetylcysteine is considered to be the antidote of choice in treating acetaminophen overdose. Acetylcysteine supplies the sulfhydryl groups that are necessary to provide normal and safe metabolism of acetaminophen. *(6)*

15d. **(B)** From early infancy, children with cystic fibrosis have difficulty in absorbing dietary fats. This is caused by the obstruction of pancreatic and biliary ducts that would otherwise deliver pancreatic lipase and other enzymes that are involved with fat absorption. Such patients, therefore, frequently suffer from steatorrhea, the presence of excessive fat in the stools. *(14)*

15e. **(D)** Cotazym is a product that contains pancreatic enzymes such as lipase, amylase, and protease from porcine (pig) origin. It should be taken orally with each meal in order to help digest the food that is being consumed. The product may be administered in a capsule form, or the contents of the capsule may be emptied into food or liquid. *(3)*

15f. **(D)** The active ingredient in Concerta, Methylin, and Daytrana is methylphenidate. Ritalin and Methylin are used orally. Daytrana is a transdermal patch that is applied once daily and worn for 9 hours. Adderall contains different amphetamine salts. *(3)*

15g. **(D)** Concerta is a product that is a sustained-release form of methylphenidate. The method used to provide sustained-release action is an osmotic pump (OROS) system that causes the drug to be released gradually as it passes through the GI tract. *(3)*

15h. **(E)** Concerta contains methylphenidate, an amphetamine-like compound that can cause CNS and cardiac stimulation, resulting in adverse effects such as insomnia, nervousness, loss of appetite, and tachycardia. *(3)*

15i. **(C)** Pimozide (Orap) is an antipsychotic agent and is not indicated for the treatment of ADHD. Memantine HCl (Namenda) is a drug used to treat Alzheimer's disease. Atomoxetine (Strattera) is a nonstimulant selective norephinephrine reuptake inhibitor used to treat ADHD. *(3)*

PROFILE NO. 16

16a. **(D)** OCD is a condition characterized by obsessive thoughts and compulsive behavior that hinder everyday functioning. Usually, the condition has a gradual onset in early adulthood. Bipolar disorders usually are characterized by unpredictable mood swings from excessive social extroversion to depression. The schizophrenic patient is usually socially withdrawn with periods of delusions or hallucinations. *(14)*

16b. **(B)** The SSRIs are usually considered the first-line treatment for OCD patients. Patient response may vary from one product to another. Usual starting doses are 50 mg/d for fluvoxamine and 20 mg for citalopram, paroxetine, or fluoxetine. After a few days of observation, it may be necessary to adjust the dose, usually upward. The tricyclic drug, clomipramine, is also effective but has more side effects and presents a greater danger if overdosed. The patient should also be informed that behavioral improvements may take several weeks while taking these drugs. *(14)*

16c. **(A)** Celexa is Forest's brand of citalopram. This SSRI is available as 10-, 20-, and 40-mg tablets with the usual daily dose of 20 to 60 mg. There is also an oral solution (10 mg/5 mL), which allows greater flexibility in dosing. *(10)*

16d. **(E)** Venlafaxine (Effexor) is probably the best choice. Dosing of 37.5 mg daily with upward dosing may be necessary. A second mode of therapy may be the use of SSRIs in low doses. Some patients may be given one of the benzodiazepines, but this is not considered first-line therapy, especially if the patient's history includes alcoholism or other substance abuse. *(3; 10)*

16e. **(D)** Magnesium stearate is a lubricant added to many commercial tablet formulations. It serves as a lubricant to permit better flow of tablet granulations into tablet machines and to reduce the likelihood that compressed tablets will stick in the tablet machine. *(3)*

16f. **(C)** Diaphragms are a prescription-only item that are originally fitted by a physician. Their sizes are in millimeter, which refer to the diameter of the diaphragm. *(1; 10; 11)*

16g. **(E)** Nonoxynol-9 is a nonionic surface active agent that is classified as a spermicide. Women using a diaphragm as a contraceptive method should coat the unit with a cream or jelly containing nonoxynol-9. The diaphragm should be left in place for 6 hours after intercourse. *(1; 10; 11)*

16h. **(D)** Larry may be exhibiting signs of ADHD. Further signs would be impulsive behavior. The young age of the boy precludes the likelihood

of Alzheimer's disease, but the symptoms described may also suggest lead poisoning. The pharmacist should query the mother further concerning the possibility that her child has consumed paint chips containing lead. The most serious symptom of lead poisoning is acute encephalopathy. The high toxicity of lead is primarily due to its strong attraction to sulfhydryl (SH) groups found in some proteins. The pharmacist should urge the mother to contact the boy's pediatrician for further evaluation. *(14; 16)*

16i. **(A)**

$$10 \ \mu g = 0.01 \ mg = 0.00001 \ g \text{ and } 1 \ dL = 100 \ mL$$

$$\frac{0.00001 \ g}{100 \ mL} = \frac{x \ g}{1{,}000{,}000} \ \therefore x = 0.1 \ ppm. \quad (23)$$

16j. **(C)** The standard for treating lead poisoning has been intravenous administration of BAL (dimercaprol) followed by disodium calcium edetate. A new therapy is the use of succimer, a drug that contains 2,3-dimercaptosuccinic acid (DMSA), which is administered by the oral route. *N*-Acetylcysteine (Mucomyst) is not effective for this poisoning.

16k. **(E)** Although its popularity has decreased, thimerosol has been used in pharmaceutical products such as parenteral and ophthalmic solutions as an antimicrobial preservative. Some people exhibit great sensitivity to this mercury-containing chemical. *(1; 2)*

16l. **(A)** Acanthamoeba is an opportunistic protozoan with a very resistant cyst. If an eye becomes infected, keratitis may develop. *(2)*

16m. **(B)** Unlike Zolpidem (Ambien) and zalepion (Sonata), eszopiclone (Lunesta) is not being restricted by the FDA to short-term use. It is a nonbenzodiazepine and classified in controlled drug schedule IV. Available strengths are 1, 2, and 3 mg tablets with the starting dose usually 2 mg, but only 1 mg in the elderly. *(25)*

16n. **(D)** While some patients with Parkinson's disease, especially the elderly, may exhibit signs of dementia, many have full mental faculties. The other listed choices are characteristics of individuals suffering from the disease. *(28, March 2006)*

16o. **(D)** Antipsychotics especially haloperidol and chlorpromazine will block dopamine receptors causing symptoms similar to parkinsonism. *(28, March 2006)*

16p. **(B)** 40 mg/mL = 40,000 mg/L

40,000 mg/460 = 87 millimoles

87 mmoles × 2.4 = 209 mOsm/L   *(1; 23)*

16q. **(D)** The disodium salt of a drug is likely to have a high pH that may cause irritation at the injection site. Perhaps the pH could be reduced closer to 7 to 8 with hydrochloric acid. *(19; 21)*

16r. **(C)** Half-life = 0.693/CL

$$= 0.693/0.064/h$$

$$= 10.8 \text{ hours} \qquad (17; 23)$$

PROFILE NO. 17

17a. **(B)** Elevated levels of aspartate aminotransferase enzyme (AST) are an indication that the patient is experiencing a myocardial infarction or a liver disease such as viral hepatitis. Anthropometic assessment consists of physically measuring the patient's muscle mass. Obviously, malnourished patients will have less lean muscle, which is also reflected in high blood or urine nitrogen levels. Recent unexplained weight loss should have been part of the original patient history. *(14; 16)*

17b. **(D)** Kwashiorkor presents as malnutrition with the presence of a fatty liver and edema. Marasmus is a more generalized starvation with a loss of body fat and protein. Graves disease is an incorrect answer since it is related to hyperthyroidism, a hypermetabolic state, psychiatric disturbances, and muscular tremors. This condition may be controlled with drugs such as propylthiouracil, propranolol, or oral iodides. *(14)*

17c. **(B)** Sickle cell disease is characterized by anemia with RBC hemolysis accompanied by severe pain due to microvascular inclusions. The erythrocytes have a crescent shape. Acute attacks are treated by keeping the patient well hydrated and using oral or parenteral morphine (0.1–0.15 mg/kg) every 3 to 4 hours for the pain. Recent studies have shown that hydroxyurea will increase levels of HbF (fetal hemoglobin), thus decreasing sickle cell polymerization and erythrocyte sickling. *(3; 14; 16)*

17d. **(E)** While the safety and efficacy of zolpidem has not been definitely established, the dose of 5 mg is reasonable as a mild hypnotic or sedative. The drug is marketed under the trade name of Ambien and is available as 5- and 10-mg tablets. Because of its relatively fast onset of action, it is taken at bedtime, not 2 hours before. Chemically, zolpidem is not a benzodiazepine. *(25)*

17e. **(B)** The original order was for subcutaneous administration of morphine sulfate 0.15 mg/kg of body weight every 4 hours when needed.

$$\frac{100 \text{ lb} \times 1 \text{ kg}}{2.2 \text{ lb}} = 46 \text{ kg.}$$

0.15 mg/kg × 46 kg = 6.9 mg.   *(1; 23)*

$$\frac{6.9 \text{ mg}}{x \text{ mL}} = \frac{10 \text{ mg}}{1 \text{ mL}}$$

$$\therefore x = 0.69 \text{ or } 0.7 \text{ mL.}$$

17f. **(A)** Each 1,000 mL of TPN contains 500 mL of 50% dextrose, or 250 g dextrose with a flow rate of 125 mL/h.

$$\frac{250 \text{ g}}{1,000 \text{ mL}} = \frac{x \text{ g}}{125 \text{ mL}}$$

$$\therefore x = 31.25 \text{ g of dextrose.}$$

Caloric density of dextrose is 3.4 kcal/g. Therefore, 31.25 g × 3.4 kcal/g = 106 kcal. *(4; 13)*

17g. **(B)** 1,000 mL of 5% amino acid solution will contain 50 g of amino acids. Since the average nitrogen content of amino acids is 16%, 50 g $\times$ 16% = 8 g. (4; 13)

17h. **(C)** The prescribed TPN solution is hypertonic. Any solution containing more than 10% glucose should not be administered peripherally because of potential damage to the veins in the arm. Originally, administration of these solutions were limited to central catheters, mainly into the subclavian vein, which has a high blood flow. The development of PICC lines (peripherally inserted central catheters) allows the use of veins in the arm since the line is threaded further into the vein to an area with high blood flow. A further advantage of the PICC line is that it may be inserted by health professionals without employing a surgical cut-down for insertion. (13; 22)

17i. **(A)** The Cockroft–Gault equation is very useful in estimating creatinine clearance. The equation reads

$$Cl_{Cr} = \frac{(140 - age) \times body\ weight}{72\,S_{Cr}},$$

where age is in years and weight is in kg.

A correction factor of 0.85 is placed before the (140−age) expression for females. (5; 17)

17j. **(C)** The serum creatinine value reported on 8/16 was 0.8 mg/dL. The male patient is 16 years old and weighs 100 lb (45.5 kg). Therefore,

$$Cl_{Cr} = \frac{(140 - age) \times body\ weight}{72\,S_{Cr}},$$

$$Cl_{Cr} = \frac{(140 - 16)(45.5\ kg)}{72\,(0.8)}$$

$$Cl_{Cr} = 98\ mL/min.$$

If the patient is female, a correction factor of 0.85 is placed before the (140−age) expression. (5; 17)

17k. **(D)** Studies indicate that the BCAAs are more readily assimilated into the body. Formulas with the BCAAs are used in stressed patients and those with liver impairment. Commercial products include HepatAmine, FreeAmine

HBC, Branch Amine, and Aminosyn-HBC. (3; 4)

17l. **(A)** No daily requirement for aluminum in the human body has been established. In fact, the USP/NF has established upper limits for aluminum in LVPs as a trace impurity.

17m. **(C)** The PCA order issued on August 18 reads "0.02 mg morphine sulfate per kilogram of body weight infused each hour for 3 days."

0.02 mg/kg/h $\times$ body weight of 100 lb (46 kg) = 0.92 mg/h

0.92 mg/h $\times$ 24 h $\times$ 3 days = 66.2 mg total.

$$\frac{10\ mg}{1\ mL} = \frac{66.2\ mg}{x\ mL} \qquad (23)$$

$$\therefore x = 6.6\ mL\ of\ morphine\ sulfate\ solution.$$

17n. **(D)** Elastomeric devices are used as infusion delivery systems for ambulatory patients in many situations. These disposable pumps such as Baxter's Intermates and Block Medical's Homepumps are convenient and relatively less expensive than PCAs. However, they do not allow extra bolus dosing of analgesics and the flow rate is preset. These devices, as well as PCAs, provide subcutaneous infusion of analgesics as well as other parenteral drugs. (22)

PROFILE NO. 18

18a. **(D)** Propylthiouracil is an antithyroid drug used in treating Graves disease since this disease is characterized by hyperthyroidism. (3)

18b. **(D)** A regimen of chemotherapy known as MOPP is used in the treatment of Hodgkin's disease. Procarbazine (Matulane) and prednisone are given by the oral route on each day of the 14-day schedule. Mechlorethamine (Mustargen) and vincristine (Oncovin) are given intravenously on the first and eighth days of therapy. Combining drugs that have different mechanisms of action increases remission rates and lowers the incidence and severity of side effects. (3)

18c. **(A)** Hepatocellular, renal cell, and thyroid carcinomas have shown poor responses to presently used chemotherapeutic drugs. Ovarian and prostatic carcinomas are moderately responsive, with palliation and probable prolongation of life. Prolonged survival and probably some cures are expected in patients with testicular cancer and Hodgkin's disease. *(5)*

18d. **(A)** The acronym SOAP refers to a plan to evaluate a patient's progress. The letters usually refer to subjective, objective, assessment, and plans. As a group, the health team decides whether the care provided meets the needs of the patient. *(14; 22)*

18e. **(B)** Mechlorethamine is a potent vesicant. Serious localized damage may occur if the drug solution seeps into the area surrounding the infusion site. The thiosulfate ion will react with the nitrogen mustard. Ice compresses will relieve the burning sensation and slow the spread of mechlorethamine. Other solutions that have been infused are normal saline and sodium bicarbonate. *(3)*

18f. **(B)** A 1/6 molar solution of sodium thiosulfate will contain 248 g of chemical in 1 L of solution. A 1/6 mol solution will contain 248/6 or 41 g/L or 4.1g/100 mL. *(3)*

18g. **(B)** Although the official form of sodium thiosulfate contains five waters of hydration, the correct amount of active ingredient can be obtained by using the anhydrous form. Simply subtract 90 (weight of water in the molecule) from 248 to obtain 158 (the weight of anhydrous sodium thiosulfate), then

$$x \text{ g} \qquad\qquad 10 \text{ g}$$

anhydrous sodium $\leftrightarrow$ hydrated sodium
thiosulfate　　　　　thiosulfate
(mol. wt. of 158)　　(mol. wt. of 248)

$$\frac{x \text{ g}}{158} = \frac{10 \text{ g}}{248}$$

$$\therefore x = 6.4 \text{ g.} \qquad (1; 23)$$

18h. **(A)** Many chemotherapeutic drugs, especially the alkylating agents, cause bone marrow

depression, which is characterized by low leukocyte counts with increased susceptibility to infections. The term, nadir, indicates the length of time before the deepest depression occurs. For example, the nadir for a given drug may be 7 to 10 days after the start of therapy, with bone marrow recovery in 14 to 18 days. *(6; 14)*

18i. **(A)** Vincristine as well as the other vinca alkaloids are strong vesicants. The usual method for administration of these drugs is by IV push into the sidearm (Y-site) of a running infusion line. IM injection would likely result in tissue necrosis at the injection site. Intrathecal administration is contraindicated as there have been several deaths attributed to this procedure. *(6; 14)*

18j. **(C)** Epoetin alfa (Epogen) is a stimulant of RBC production. Filgrastim (Neupogen) is a stimulant of granulocyte (leukocyte) production. These are used in patients receiving myelosuppressive drugs such as mechlorethamine. Clopidogrel (Plavix) is an inhibitor of platelet aggregation. *(3)*

18k. **(C)** Cyanocobalamin injection is a pink-colored solution available in strengths of 100 and 1,000 μg/mL. It is administered by either IM or subcutaneous injection, but not IV. The parenteral route offers better bioavailability than oral administration. *(3)*

18l. **(E)** Cetirizine (Zyrtec), desloratidine (Clarinex), and fexofenadine (Allegra) are peripherally selective antihistamines. They cause less drowsiness than nonselective agents. *(3)*

18m. **(C)** Benicar (Olmesartan) is an angiotensin receptor blocker which as a class does not induce coughing. The dosing of the drug is 20 or 40 mg once a day. All of the other choices are ACE inhibitors that may cause coughing in some patients. *(3; 10)*

18n. **(E)** *(3)*

18o. **(E)** The pregnancy category assigned to the ACE inhibitors for the second and third trimesters is D, and category C for the first trimester. However, evidence now indicates that maternal use of these drugs during the first 3 months of pregnancy more than doubles the infant's risk of major birth defects. *(3; 10)*

PROFILE NO. 19

19a. **(B)** A trade name for paclitaxel is Taxol. Taxotere is another popular drug for breast cancer with the generic name of docetaxel. Tazidime (ceftazidime) is a cephalosporin antimicrobial agent used for both gram-negative and gram-positive aerobes as well as for anaerobes. *(3; 10)*

19b. **(A)** Commercial paclitaxel (Taxol) solution is in a nonaqueous vehicle which, when diluted, may be slightly turbid. Therefore, it is a good technique to infuse the solution using an administration set that has an in-line filter. The admixture should be prepared in a glass bottle not PVC plastic bags, which may leach some of the plasticizer, diethylhexyl phthalate (DEHP). Infusion times may be as short as 1 hour. *(10)*

19c. **(A)** Dolasetron mesylate is available under the tradename of Anzemet. It is used to prevent nausea and vomiting during cancer therapy. Both an injection (20 mg/mL) and tablets (50 and 100 mg) are available. The drug is classified as a 5-HT$_3$-receptor antagonist. *(10)*

19d. **(D)** Cisplatin is available as Platinol and Platinol AQ. Paraplatin is a different drug having the generic name of carboplatin. There have been medication errors when these two agents were interchanged with each other. Cisplatin is an alkylating agent used for several types of cancers including ovarian, testicular, and prostate. The incidence of nausea is very high and may be a delayed reaction occurring up to 48 hours after the infusion. *(3; 21)*

19e. **(D)** The medication order calls for 150 mg/m² of BSA, and this patient has a surface area of 1.85 m². Therefore,

$$\frac{150 \text{ mg}}{1} = \frac{x \text{ mg}}{1.85}$$

$$\therefore x = 278 \text{ mg}.$$

Each vial contains 6 mg/mL of drug, thus

$$\frac{6 \text{ mg}}{1 \text{ mL}} = \frac{278 \text{ mg}}{x \text{ mL}} \tag{23}$$

$$\therefore x = 46 \text{ mL}.$$

19f. **(D)** Myelosuppression, or suppression of the bone marrow, usually results in a sharp decrease in white blood cells. This may be life-threatening because of the patient s increased susceptibility to infection. The antineoplastic drug, tamoxifen, is a nonsteroidal antiestrogen used in the treatment of breast cancer. Adverse effects of the drug include nausea, vomiting, hot flashes, vaginal bleeding, hypercalcemia, and thrombocytopenia, but the drug is not noted for causing bone marrow depression. Tamoxifen is available as oral tablets under the tradenames of Nolvadex, Nolvadex-D, and Tamofen. Dosage strengths are 10 and 20 mg plus a 20 mg enteric-coated tablet to reduce GI tract irritation. *(5; 26)*

19g. **(A)** Peripheral neuropathy is a degenerative state of peripheral nerves in which motor, sensory, or vasomotor fibers may be affected. Symptoms may include muscle weakness, numbness, and/or pain. *(16; 27)*

19h. **(D)** The dictionary defines "nadir" as the place or time of deepest depression. When discussing drug chemotherapy, the term usually refers to the length of time before maximum bone marrow depression occurs. Many chemotherapeutic drugs, especially the alkylating agents, cause a depression characterized by low leukocyte counts with increased susceptibility to infection. For example, the nadir for a given drug may be 7 to 10 days after the start of therapy, with bone marrow recovery in 14 to 18 days. *(3; 27)*

19i. **(D)** Patients undergoing therapy with cisplatin should be well hydrated. Usually 12 L of solutions containing dextrose and sodium chloride are infused 8 to 12 hours before the cisplatin infusion. Discontinuing the hydrochlorothiazide will also reduce water loss. *(14; 21)*

19j. **(A)** FUO refers to the presence of a fever of unknown origin, likely due to a systemic infection. The patient will be placed on a broad-spectrum antibiotic until the culture and sensitivity tests indicate the need for a more specific antibiotic. To reduce fever, oral or rectal acetaminophen will likely be prescribed. *(6; 14)*

19k. **(A)** Augmentin is available in oral dosage forms including tablets, capsules, and oral suspensions. However, it is not intended for parenteral administration. From the symptoms provided, it appears that Ms. Hockford may have developed a respiratory tract infection. A possible substitute would be ceftriaxone sodium (Rocephin), which has a broad-spectrum of action and is dosed at 1 or 2 g daily. *(3; 10)*

19l. **(C)** Laboratory culture and sensitivity testing allows identification of antimicrobial activity of common antimicrobial agents against a specific, isolated microorganism. By reviewing the lab report of minimum inhibitory concentrations (MICs), one may choose the drug of choice for an infection. Usually the antibiotic with the lowest MIC should be selected. The targeted peak concentration of the antibiotic is usually four to five times the MIC. *(1; 14)*

19m. **(C)** Vancomycin injection should be infused over a minimum of a 1-hour duration. Otherwise, serious hypotension including shock may occur. Also, a rash known as red man syndrome may occur during or a short time after the infusion has occurred. The rash usually resolves within a few hours. Pseudomembranous colitis may be a result of vancomycin administration but is not an immediate result of rapid infusion. *(3)*

19n. **(E)** A heparin well refers to a short infusion line containing a small storage area (a well) that is placed into the arm of patient for convenient administration of parenterals solutions at set time intervals. To keep the line open (patent) a low dose of heparin is placed into the heparin well. When the nurse is administering an antibiotic solution, a procedure known as SASH is used. Rinse the heparin line with saline, administer the antibiotic, rinse the well once again with saline, then store a few milliliters of heparin solution in the well until it is time for the next infusion. *(21)*

PROFILE NO. 20

20a. **(A)** Hytrin has the generic name of terazosin and is classified as an alpha$_1$-adrenergic blocker. It is indicated for prevention of hypertension either by itself or combined with a diuretic or beta-adrenergic blocking agent. Other drugs in the same class include Cardura, Flomax, and Minipress. *(3)*

20b. **(C)** Terazosin is available under the tradename of Hytrin. It and other drugs in its class causes a marked hypotension, especially postural, in patients for the first few doses. Some patients may experience syncope (fainting). *(3)*

20c. **(D)** Raloxifene (Evista) is available as 60 mg tablets and is intended for the prevention of osteoporosis in the postmenopausal female. It is classified as a selective estrogen receptor modulator since it has estrogen-like effects on bone but lacks estrogen-like activity on either uterine or breast tissues. It is not intended for the premenopausal woman since it is a pregnancy category X drug. *(3; 10)*

20d. **(B)** Ortho-Evra is a transdermal drug delivery patch intended as a contraceptive. A patch is applied once weekly for a total of 3 weeks. Each day, constant amounts of norelgestromin and ethinyl estadiol are released. While the patient may experience some of the adverse effects inherent in the use of hormonal contraceptives, the intensity should be less since there are no bolus amounts of drug released at one time. Choice E is incorrect since Estraderm transdermal is intended to moderate the symptoms of menopause. *(3; 10)*

20e. **(A)** The bulk of *Facts and Comparisons* describes drugs available in the United States. However, it also identifies drugs available in Canada by their generic and trade names. Once the generic name of the drug has been located, comparable products could be located. Martindale is another reference book that allows identification of foreign drug products. Its listings are mainly for European drugs. *(1; 3)*

20f. **(C)** Iodine dissolved in mineral oil has been used as a topical product because the iodine will impart a darker color to the skin and the mineral oil provides emolliency. However, this combination does not filter out ultraviolet rays and, therefore, provides virtually no protection against sunburn. All of the other choices are approved sunscreen agents. *(1; 2)*

20g. **(E)** Haldol, Risperdal, or Seroquel may be tried for schizophrenia. The neuroleptic Seroquel is available as tablets and is considered first-line treatment probably because of the lower incidence of adverse effects. Haldol is available in several dosage forms. Risperdal is available in both tablets and an oral solution. *(10; 16)*

20h. **(B)** Fluphenazine is a good choice of a neuroleptic drug for the management of several psychotic disorders. The decanoate and enanthate esters are formulated into oil solvents thus providing a long duration of action usually 2 to 3 weeks. *(1; 14)*

20i. **(D)** Glycated hemoglobin (A_{1c}) is formed by a reaction between hemoglobin and glucose and reflects the average glucose level in a patient during the past 3- to 4-month period. Home testing for A_{1c} is now possible with the development of an OTC test (Metrika A_{1c} Now), which simply requires a blood sample from the finger. Hemoglobin A_{1c} values should ideally be below 7.0. *(2; 10; 14)*

20j. **(B)** Ascites refers to an accumulation of serous fluid in the peritoneal cavity. First treatment is usually the administration of a diuretic. *(27)*

20k. **(D)** Ankylosing spondylitis is a disease of the connective tissue that resembles rheumatoid arthritis. It usually presents as an inflammation of a large joint and spine. Usually symptoms include recurring episodes of back pain. Treatment involves the use of NSAIDs, especially the COX-2 drugs. *(16)*

20l. **(C)** Although the depressant effects of alcohol may occur at lower blood levels, mental impairment and loss of motor coordination is obvious in most individuals once blood alcohol levels exceed 0.1%. The major problem with alcohol metabolism is the limited supply of enzymes available for the oxidation. Therefore, alcohol metabolism may be described as mainly following zero-order kinetics with limited amounts metabolized each hour. *(3; 17)*

20m. **(A)** Butenafine in Lotrimin Ultra is claimed to possess fungicidal activity rather than just fungistatic properties. Clotrimazole is present in Lotrimin AF cream, lotion, and solution while Lotrimin powder and liquid spray contain miconazole. *(2; 3)*

20n. **(C)** TMP-SMZ is the acronym for the combination of trimethoprim and sulfamethoxazole, now referred to as cotrimoxazole. Brand names of this combination include Bactrim and Septra. The product is effective against UTIs, acute otitis media, traveler's diarrhea, and chronic bronchitis in adults. The ingredient ratio is one part of trimethoprim to every five parts of sulfamethoxazole. *(3)*

20o. **(D)** By placing a cold drop in the eye, the patient is more likely to feel the contact which will assure her that the drop did enter the eye. Since the surface of the eye has limited volume capacity, separating the two drops will assure more of the liquid is deposited. This capacity limit explains why choice III is not good advice.

20p. **(A)** Grapefruit juice appears to inhibit the intestinal CYP3A4 enzyme, thus reducing the metabolism of certain drugs including the statins such as lovastatin and simvastatin. One would then expect higher than normal serum levels. The effect of the juice lasts for 12 to 24 hours. Orange juice does not appear to have similar action when compared to grapefruit juice. *(3; 5)*

20q. **(D)** St. John's wort is an inducer of the CYP3A4 enzyme thus reducing the action of certain drugs including cyclosporine, indinavir, nifedipine, and the tricyclic antidepressants.

PROFILE NO. 21

21a. **(A)** Hypothyroidism (myxedema) is characterized by the slowing of body processes because of a deficiency of thyroid hormone. The classic treatment has been thyroid tablets. Today, this drug has been replaced with L-thyroxine (T4), L-thyronine (T3), and liotrix (a mixture of T4 and T3). Levoxyl is levothyroxine sodium (L-thyroxine). Graves' disease is a form of hyperthyroidism. *(5)*

21b. **(E)** Omission of a single dose of Levoxyl will not have significant effects on the disease state. *(3)*

21c. **(B)** Both Levoxyl and Synthroid are brands of the generic drug levothyroxine. There are a number of strengths of the tablets from 0.025 mg up to 3 mg. Cytomel is a brand of liothyronine and Thyrolar is generically known as liotrix. *(5; 9)*

21d. **(C)** The pharmacist must consider the possibilities of both overusage or underusage of drugs especially by the elderly. The original Levoxyl order on 8/4 was for 30 tablets with directions of one tablet per day, but a refill was not requested until 9/28. Furosemide 40 mg tablets were ordered with the directions of one every other day. Despite the 2-month supply provided on 9/28, the patient is requesting a refill on 10/28. Perhaps she is taking a tablet every day rather than every other day. The digoxin appears to be taken on schedule.

21e. **(A)** Glucosamine and chondroitin combinations are nonprescription dietary supplements used to improve joint flexibility. Usually doses of 500 mg glucosamine and 400 mg chondroitin are used. *(2; 18a)*

21f. **(C)** Although there is some patient-to-patient variation, one of the earliest signs of Alzheimer's disease is the forgetfulness of current events, for example, what one has eaten for lunch. Although gradual, this memory loss becomes progressively worse. *(5)*

21g. **(A)** Selegiline is available as Eldepryl and is used in the treatment of parkinsonism. Donepezil, galantamine, and rivastigmine appear to increase the concentration of brain acetylcholine. Memantine counteracts the effect of gutamate which overstimulates certain brain cells. *(3)*

21h. **(B)** Aspartame and saccharin are artificial sweeteners that are 200 and 400 times sweeter, respectively, than sucrose. These agents are used in many dietary foods and in some pharmaceuticals. The use of saccharin in place of one teaspoonful of sugar saves the consumer 33 calories. Aspartame should be avoided in patients with phenylketonuria. *(3)*

21i. **(C)** The tannins in teas may react with iron to form insoluble iron tannates. It is well established that many antacids combine with iron, thereby reducing its absorption. *(3)*

21j. **(C)** Women, especially postmenopausal women, should increase their intake of calcium to avoid osteoporosis. Tums is available containing 500 mg of calcium carbonate per chewable tablet, 750 mg chewable tablets (Tums E-X), and 1,000 mg chewable tablets (Tums Ultra). Although calcium carbonate can be used in the prevention of gastroesophageal reflux (GERD), there are more effective products on the market. The antacid dosing regimen for GERD would be a dose after each meal as well as at bedtime. *(3)*

21k. **(A)** Many of the elderly have an increase in the relative amount of fat in their bodies, partially because of dehydration and less activity. The corresponding volume of distribution for lipophilic drugs may increase. Renal clearance rates are often lower in the elderly because of impaired kidney function. The plasma albumin levels are sometimes lower than normal, thereby affecting the amount of protein binding. *(3)*

21l. **(C)** If both dosage forms had 100% bioavailability (*F* value of 1.0), the answer would be 5 mL.

$$\frac{0.05 \text{ mg}}{1 \text{ mL}} = \frac{0.25 \text{ mg}}{x \text{ mL}}$$

$$\therefore x = 5 \text{ mL of elixir.}$$

However, the entire dose of the drug is not available as reflected in the *F* values of 0.6 for the tablet and 0.75 for the elixir. Therefore,

$$Q_1 \times C_1 = Q_2 \times C_2$$
$$0.25 \text{ mg} \times 0.6 = x \text{ mg} \times 0.75$$

$$\therefore x = 0.2 \text{ mg of digoxin needed.}$$

Since the elixir contains 0.05 mg per milliliter,

$$\frac{0.05 \text{ mg}}{1 \text{ mL}} = \frac{0.2 \text{ mg}}{x \text{ mL}}$$

$$\therefore x = 4 \text{ mL of elixir.}$$

21m. **(A)** Many elderly persons who exhibit digoxin toxicity experience hazy vision rather than the more classic halo and color vision changes that occur in younger patients. Rather than having an increase in appetite, anorexia often occurs. *(3)*

21n. **(E)** All of the choices decrease digoxin's volume of distribution and renal clearance rate. When these drugs are used with digoxin, it is often necessary to reduce the digoxin dose by 50%. *(3)*

PROFILE NO. 22

22a. **(C)** The term tocolytic refers to a drug that will reduce uterine contractility, thereby preventing premature delivery. *(5)*

22b. **(B)** Terbutaline is available under the trade names of Brethine and Bricanyl. To inhibit preterm labor, it is administered orally, SC, or IV. However, its greatest market is as a bronchodilator. A second agent that has been very successful for tocolytic therapy is ritodrine (Yutopar), which can be given either orally or IV. *(3)*

22c. **(D)** The medication order calls for 25 μg of drug per minute. The pharmacist added 2 mL (2 mg or 2,000 μg) to 250 mL of diluent.

$$\frac{2,000 \text{ μg}}{250 \text{ ml}} = \frac{25 \text{ μg}}{x \text{ ml}}$$

$$\therefore x = 3.125 \text{ mL.}$$

$$\frac{15 \text{ gtt}}{1 \text{ mL}} = \frac{x \text{ gtt}}{3.125 \text{ mL}}$$

$$\therefore x = 46.8 \text{ drops/min.}$$

22d. **(B)** The total amount of drug present is 2,000 μg in 250 mL. It is being administered at a rate of 25 μg/min or 3.125 mL/min.

$$\frac{250 \text{ mL}}{x \text{ min}} = \frac{3.125 \text{ mL}}{1 \text{ min}}$$

$$\therefore x = 80 \text{ min.}$$

22e. **(C)** Ibuprofen is available in a number of nonprescription drug products at a strength of 200 mg. It is used as an analgesic, anti-inflammatory, and to reduce fever. *(2)*

22f. **(D)** REM refers to rapid eye movement. This involves the normal paralysis of muscles during sleep; lack of which may cause the person to act out the dream that is being experienced. The sleeper may kick or strike out at his/her companion especially if the dream is violent.

22g. **(E)** Barium sulfate is best described as a diagnostic agent. It is used to render the intestinal tract opaque for X-rays. A dose of 60 to 250 g is administered as a suspension. Barium sulfate is practically insoluble in water; thus, there is little danger of toxicity from systemic absorption of the chemical. It is administered either orally or rectally, depending on the portion of the GI tract to be X-rayed. *(3)*

22h. **(B)** Atropine is classified as an antimuscarinic/antispasmodic agent used to inhibit salivation and other excessive secretions during surgery. It may also prevent cholinergic effects such as cardiac arrhythmias, hypotension, and bradycardia during surgery. An alternative drug is glycopyrrolate (Robinul), which may be administered 30 minutes prior to surgery for action similar to that of atropine. It is also available as oral tablets (1 and 2 mg) to suppress gastric secretions for the treatment of peptic ulcers. *(3)*

22i. **(B)** The usual adult dose of atropine is 0.4 mg SC, IM, or even IV. Atropine sulfate and chlorpromazine HCl (Thorazine) will be compatible in a syringe. The purpose of chlorpromazine is to relieve presurgical apprehension, and control nausea and vomiting during surgery. *(3)*

22j. **(A)** Because of their sizing and use, urinary catheters bear a federal warning concerning dispensing without a prescription. Ostomy pouches are available in several sizes and designs, but the consumer may purchase them, as well as bandages and dressings, without a prescription. *(3)*

22k. **(B)** An ileostomy results when the entire colon (large intestine) and a portion of the small intestine are removed, and the remaining end of the small intestine is attached to the abdominal wall. Because of the narrow diameter of the small intestine, the wall opening (stoma) is not as large when compared to colostomy stomas. The fecal discharge is watery because there has been limited opportunity for water reabsorption. Also, there are higher concentrations of enzymes present that may irritate the skin. *(1; 22)*

22l. **(C)** The active ingredient in Metamucil and Fibercon is the bulk-forming laxative psyllium. Some psyllium-containing products contain sucrose as a sweetener. A pharmacist may wish to discourage diabetics away from this type of product to one that contains an artificial sweetener such as aspartame (eg, Orange Flavor Metamucil Instant Mix). Mitrolan is an incorrect answer since it and Equalactin contain calcium polycarbophil, another bulk-forming ingredient. *(3)*

22m. **(A)** Bulk-forming agents such as Metamucil should be dispersed in water or a flavored liquid such as orange juice, stirred quickly, then swallowed immediately. Otherwise, the powder will swell, forming a gel that would be difficult to swallow. Metamucil is also available in a capsule dosage form. *(3)*

22n. **(E)** There are several problems for the discharge orders. First, both Prinivil (lisinopril, an ACE inhibitor) and Prosom (estazolam, a benzodiazepine) are pregnancy category D or X drugs and are contraindicated for this patient. Because of its fast onset of action, Sonata (zaleplon) is taken right at bedtime not 2 hours before. Since it belongs to pregnancy category C, it would be more appropriate to prescribe a sedative such as Ambien (zolpidem) which is in category B. *(3; 10)*

22o. **(D)** The centrally acting beta$_2$-agonist methyldopa (Aldomet) is used as an antihypertensive agent during pregnancy. Other alternatives include labetalol (Normodyne or Trandate) or hydralazine (Apresoline). *(3)*

22p. **(B)** An increase in sodium loss (hyponatremia) is a serious problem for ostomy patients especially ileostomies with large water loss and electrolyte loss. While the signs reported by Mr. J are not exact, it is a likely explanation. Failure to compensate for the sodium loss may lead to serious CNS changes such as agitation, confusion, and stupor, which may lead to convulsions. *(6)*

PROFILE NO. 23

23a. **(A)** The active ingredient in Mycelex G is clotrimazole, an antifungal agent effective against *Candida* albicans, which infects the vagina. Mycelex G is available as a vaginal tablet. Many clotrimazole vaginal products are now available OTC. *(10)*

23b. **(B)** With the successful treatment of gonorrhea with either fluoroquinolones or cephalosporins, other causes of sexually transmitted urethritis have emerged. More than 50% of cases of non-gonorrheal urethritis are caused by the obligate intracellular parasite Chlamydia. *(5)*

23c. **(A)** Syphilis is usually transmitted by direct contact with an active lesion containing spirochetes. Although there are several stages and types of syphilis, the drug of choice is still parenteral penicillin G, such as 2.4 million units of benzathine penicillin G. For patients allergic to penicillin, doxycycline is generally used. *(5)*

23d. **(A)** Infections caused by Chlamydia are usually asymptomatic in females, whereas males experience dysuria. Primary treatment will be either doxycycline 100 mg twice a day for 7 days or azithromycin as a single 1,000-mg dose. Alternatives include erythromycin 500 mg q.i.d. or ofloxacin 300 mg b.i.d. for 7 days. Ciprofloxacin has been used but is not as successful as doxycycline. *(5)*

23e. **(D)** Plan B is an emergency contraceptive product. It contains a large dose of levonorgestrel, a progestin. When a dose of Plan B is administered within 72 hours of unprotected sexual intercourse and a second dose is administered 12 hours later, this product is claimed to have a 95% success rate in preventing pregnancy. A spermicidal cream will not likely be effective after intercourse has occurred. Progestasert is an IUD contraceptive device that provides contraceptive action for about 1 year. Evra is a transdermal contraceptive patch. Clomid is an ovulation stimulant. *(10)*

23f. **(D)** White vaseline or any other petrolatum product is not acceptable as a lubricant for either condoms or diaphragms, because small openings will develop due to the solvent characteristics of petrolatum toward rubber. *(5)*

23g. **(C)** The testicular hormone danazol (Danocrine) is given orally in 100- to 200-mg doses to treat endometriosis, a condition characterized by menstrual-like bleeding and localized inflammation and pain, usually within the pelvis. A second drug successful in the treatment of endometriosis is nafarelin acetate (Synarel), which is available as an intranasal spray. *(3)*

23h. **(D)** Myocardial infarctions (MIs) are the leading cause of death in diabetics. The glycosylated products associated with diabetes accelerate the atherosclerotic process. Particularly at risk are patients with hypertension and smokers. (Answer A—incorrect) Diabetic ketoacidosis (DKA) has a high mortality rate for type 1 diabetics. *(5; 6)*

23i. **(C)** Orlistat (Xenical) is a lipase inhibitor used to reduce dietary fat absorption in order to help lose weight. By inhibiting the action of lipase, dietary fats are not absorbed as well and pass out of the body via the colon. If dietary fat restriction is not maintained by the patient, diarrhea and foul smelling stools may result. *(10)*

23j. **(E)** Mr. Woolbright should schedule yearly eye examinations to observe possible development of retinopathy, the noninflammatory degenerative disease of the retina. Patients with long-term diabetes are especially susceptible and are often advised to include lutein in their vitamin supplement. *(6; 27)*

23k. **(A)** Methylphenidate (Ritalin) is classified as a centrally acting sympathomimetic agent. It is used in the therapy of ADHD. *(3)*

23l. **(B)** The benzodiazepines exert their antianxiety effects by potentiation of the inhibitory neurotransmitter GABA. *(3)*

23m. **(B)** The Atkins diet is one which tends to contain low levels of carbohydrate. While it often contains high levels of fat and protein, there is evidence that it may be an effective short-term approach to weight loss. *(3)*

23n. **(D)** Flumazenil (Romazicon) is a specific antidote for benzodiazepine overdose. Naloxone and naltrexone are specific opiate antagonists. *(3)*

23o. **(B)** An approximation of the caloric content of a product serving can be made by recognizing that fats contribute 9 kcal/g while the carbohydrate and protein contribute approximately 4 kcal/g. Therefore, 3 g × 9 kcal/g = 27 kcal, 8 g × 4 kcal/g = 32 kcal, and 1 g × 4 kcal/g = 4 kcal, and 27 + 32 + 4 = 63. *(3)*

23p. **(C)** Infants should be treated only under the supervision of their pediatrician. The mildest laxative of the choices listed is glycerin suppositories, which exert an osmotic effect in the GI tract. *(2)*

23q. **(D)** TENS devices provide transcutaneous electrical nerve stimulation. Electrical impulses are transferred to a body area to block nerve stimulation that is causing pain in the patient. The unit is attached to the body by the use of electrodes. Three variables can be controlled pulse rate, width of the waves, and amplitude of the charge. The devices have been successful in relief of lower back pain, painful knees, and in some arthritic cases. *(1)*

23r. **(B)** Vytorin is an antihyperlipidemic drug with two ingredients each possessing different mechanisms of action. The combination is claimed to be more effective than many of the other drugs in the same category. However, there is still the possibility of muscle pain that may lead to kidney damage. Also, it should not be used during pregnancy or breast-feeding. *(25)*

23s. **(A)** Butyl hydroxyanisole (BHA) and butyl hydroxytoluene (BHT) are two antioxidants approved for use in both foods and pharmaceuticals as antioxidants. They are both oil soluble. *(24; 25)*

PROFILE NO. 24

24a. **(D)** These two microorganisms are major causes of both otitis media and sinusitis. A third microorganism often implicated is Moraxella catarrhalis. *(5)*

24b. **(C)** Other appropriate agents are cefixime, cefaclor, azithromycin, etc. Doxycycline is a tetracycline and should not be used in children younger than 8 years. *(5)*

24c. **(B)** All three drugs possess antipyretic activity. However, Jason is sensitive to salicylates and neither aspirin nor ibuprofen (to which he may also be sensitive) should be dispensed. The newer OTC agents such as naproxen and ketoprofen carry a label warning that they should not be used in young children unless under a physician's supervision. *(3)*

24d. **(C)** Ibuprofen is 2-(p-isobutylphenyl) propionic acid. *(3)*

24e. **(A)** Fever may be the sign of a serious systemic infection. If the fever is masked by the use of an antipyretic, prompt treatment may be delayed. *(3)*

24f. **(A)** Amount of cromolyn needed for Rx is 30 mL × 2.5% = 0.75 g. The amount of the available 4% solution to use is

$$\frac{4\ g}{100\ mL} = \frac{0.75\ g}{x\ mL}$$

$$\therefore x = 19\ mL\ (\text{which is already isotonic}).$$

Therefore, the pharmacist must make only the remaining 11 mL isotonic.

11 mL × 0.9% NaCl = 0.099 g or 99 mg.   *(24)*

24g. **(A)** Removal of bacteria and fungi from extemporaneously prepared solutions may be accomplished by passage through a 0.20- or 0.22-μm filter into a sterile container. *(24)*

24h. **(E)** "OD" is a Latin abbreviation for the right eye. *(1; 23)*

24i. **(B)** Ophthalmic solutions containing cromolyn sodium are effective in the treatment of allergic conjunctivitis. Chronic allergic conjunctivitis patients should also avoid using OTC sympathomimetic decongestants, which may cause rebound vasodilation. *(3)*

24j. **(D)** The patient directions on the prescription will read "two drops in the right eye three times a day"—two drops × three times a day = six drops per day.

$$\frac{6 \text{ gtt}}{x \text{ mL}} = \frac{15 \text{ gtt}}{1 \text{ mL}}$$

$$\therefore x = 0.4 \text{ mL applied per day.}$$

Since the bottle contains 30 mL,

$$\frac{0.4 \text{ mL}}{1 \text{ day}} = \frac{30 \text{ mL}}{x \text{ days}} \qquad (23)$$

$$\therefore x = 75 \text{ days.}$$

24k. **(D)** Use of a child's body surface area will usually result in more accurate dosing than the other methods mentioned in the question. *(1; 23)*

24l. **(D)** Because of the limited capacity of the eye surface, separating the two drops by a few minutes will increase the amount of solution that actually enters and remains in the eye. Blocking the passageway between the eye and nose will reduce the amount of drug lost through the tear duct. *(24)*

24m. **(C)** Tofranil (imipramine) in doses of 25 mg 1 hour before bedtime reduces the incidence of childhood enuresis. If unsuccessful, the dose may be increased up to 75 mg. *(3)*

24n. **(A)** Debrox drops contain carbamide peroxide, which will soften earwax, easing its removal. S.T. 37 is a mouthwash and topical anti-infective with hexylresorcinol as its active ingredient. Anbesol is used in the treatment of cold sores and contains both benzocaine and phenol. *(3)*

24o. **(E)** Tartrazine (F.D. & C. Yellow #5) is included in both solid and liquid products. A small fraction of the general population is sensitive to the dye and may respond with typical allergic responses. There appears to be a high incidence of cross sensitivity in individuals sensitive to aspirin and to tartrazine. *(24)*

24p. **(E)** The ORD (orally dissolving tablet) or RDT (rapidly dissolving tablet) offers the convenience of fast dosing without the need for water. However, the tablets are formulated and packaged to remain dry until used. Contact with moisture including high humidity may cause the tablets to prematurely disintegrate. *(24)*

PROFILE NO. 25

25a. **(B)** Gout is a chronic metabolic disease characterized by hyperuricemia. The uric acid is an end product of protein catabolism. Either uric acid production has increased, or impaired renal clearance is slowing the removal. The immediate concern during an acute attack is to relieve pain. Only after this relief should longer term therapy be initiated. *(5)*

25b. **(E)** To relieve an acute gout attack, an anti-inflammatory drug (NSAID) such as indomethacin or ibuprofen may be used. Another option is the use of colchicine. Colchicine is most effective if given within the first 12 to 36 hours of the acute attack. *(5)*

25c. **(D)** Allopurinol (Zyloprim) and febuxostat (Uloric) are some of the most commonly used agents for long-term control of chronic gout and are the drugs of choice for patients who are overproducers of uric acid. Each of these drugs act by inhibiting xanthine oxidase, an enzyme which converts xanthine to uric acid. Colchicine is only used to treat pain associated with an acute gout attack. *(5)*

25d. **(C)** Sufficient liquid intake of at least 2 L daily is necessary to prevent formation of urate calculi. Acute attacks of gout may occur on initial therapy; therefore, colchicine therapy may be useful during the intial few weeks of allopurinol therapy. Because of possible stomach irritation, it is best to take allopurinol with food. *(3)*

25e. **(A)** Simethicone is a defrothicant, that is, it causes small gas bubbles in the GI to coalesce to form a large bubble that can easily be eliminated. This is useful in treating a patient that is experiencing abdominal pain caused by the accumulation of gas. *(6)*

25f. **(D)** Phazyme and Mylicon are OTC products that contain simethicone. They are used to relieve abdominal pain caused by gas. *(3)*

25g. **(C)** *Facts and Comparisons* contains information concerning commercial products by listing drugs by similar therapeutic categories. However, it does not present color charts of drug products. All three volumes of the USP DI have color charts. *(3)*

25h. **(C)** Minoxidil (Rogaine) is available as 2% and 5% solutions as Rogaine and extra strength Rogaine, respectively, and are indicated for the treatment of alopecia. Finasteride is available as an oral product called Propecia. It is also used to treat alopecia in male patients. *(3)*

25i. **(E)** Nadolol (Corgard) and penbutolol (Levatol) are beta-adrenergic blocking agents. Irbesartan (Avapro), olmesartan (Benicar), and losartan (Cozaar) are angiotensin II antagonists, and trandolapril (Mavik) is an ACE inhibitor. *(10)*

25j. **(B)** Propranolol (Inderal) has the greatest lipophilic activity. It can, therefore, be expected to produce the greatest degree of CNS adverse effects because of its ability to pass through the lipid blood–brain barrier. *(3)*

25k. **(D)** Chronic alcoholics may develop thiamine deficiency because alcohol can interfere with the intestinal uptake of thiamine as well as its utilization. Thiamine deficiency can lead to Wernicke–Korsakoff syndrome, which may, in part, be characterized by peripheral neuropathy. *(3)*

25l. **(B)** Alpha-tocopherol is a form of vitamin E. This vitamin acts as a lipid-soluble antioxidant. *(6)*

25m. **(B)** Rifampin (Rifadin or Rimactane) discolors urine, sweat, and tears. The drug's major use is in the treatment of tuberculosis, usually in combination with isoniazid or pyrazinamide. *(3)*

25n. **(A)** Prophylactic treatment for the recurrence of gout is life-long dosing with a xanthine oxidase inhibitor such as allopurinol. Pain relief with colchicine occurs 18 to 48 hours after dosing. Besides allopurinol, one may use the uricosuric agents such as probenecid or sulfinpyrazone, which compete with uric acid for both secretion and reabsorption at the renal tubule. Some patients will use an NSAID for acute attacks of gout but not aspirin. In fact, all salicylates should be avoided as they tend to reduce uric acid excretion. *(5; 14)*

PROFILE NO. 26

26a. **(D)** Both sertraline (Zoloft) and citalopram (Celexa) are SSRIs indicated for the treatment of depression. Loxapine is an antipsychotic agent, ondansetron (Zofran) is an antiemetic, phenelzine (Nardil) as an MAO inhibitor, and clozapine (Clozaril) is an antipsychotic agent. *(3)*

26b. **(C)** Bupropion HCl (Wellbutrin) is an aminoketone antidepressant agent and is chemically unrelated to other currently available antidepressant drugs. The long-acting form of bupropion HCl (Wellbutrin XL) is indicated for the treatment of seasonal affective disorder. *(3)*

26c. **(B)** Wellbutrin and Zyban both contain bupropion HCl as their active ingredient. Immediate-release bupropion is indicated for the treatment of depression. Sustained-release forms of this drug (Wellbutrin SR and Zyban) are indicated for smoking cessation treatment. *(3)*

26d. **(E)** Patients using lithium carbonate should be advised to consume 8 to 12 glasses of water daily. This will stabilize lithium levels in the blood and prevent lithium toxicity. *(3)*

26e. **(B)** Adverse reactions to lithium rarely occur when serum lithium levels are below 1.5 mEq/L. Mild to moderate toxic reactions may occur at a level of 1.5 to 2.5 mEq/L, and severe toxicity is seen above these levels. *(3)*

26f. **(E)** The addition of hydrochlorothiazide to this patient's regimen is likely to increase serum lithium levels because when sodium is depleted from the body, the body will conserve lithium, thereby resulting in lithium accumulation. *(3)*

26g. **(C)** Blood samples are drawn just prior to taking a dose, because lithium levels will be steady at that time and will represent the true value for lithium. *(3)*

26h. (B)

$$300 \; mg = \frac{(x \; mEq) \, (74)}{2}$$

$$\therefore x = 8 \; \text{mEq.}$$

26i. **(A)** Hydrochlorothiazide is an example of a thiazide diuretic. *(3)*

26j. **(C)** Triazolam (Halcion) is an ultrashort hypnotic with a half-life of 2 to 3 hours. It is the least likely of any of the benzodiazepines to produce a morning hangover; however, it does produce short-term amnesia in some patients. *(3)*

26k. **(E)** Zolpidem (Ambien) has an onset of action of less than 30 minutes and a half-life of 2 to 5 hours. Thus, a patient will fall asleep quickly, and the drug wears off before waking. The other drugs have much longer half-lives. *(3)*

26l. **(D)** Azulfidine (sulfasalazine) is used in the treatment of inflammatory bowel disease and ulcerative colitis. Usually 1 to 2 g of drug is needed daily. *(3)*

26m. **(C)** Sulfasalazine (Azulfidine) is usually administered for ulcerative colitis in doses of 500 mg q.i.d. Mesalamine (Lialda, Pentasa, Rowasa, Asacol) may also be used. It is an anti-inflammatory agent that is an active metabolite of sulfasalazine. It also does not have a sulfonamide component and is, therefore, safer to use than Azulfidine in sulfa-sensitive patients. *(3)*

26n. **(A)** Phenelzine (Nardil) is an MAO inhibitor. Because the use of an MAO inhibitor in combination with a serotoninergic drug such as fluoxetine, fluvoxamine, paroxetine, sertra-

line, or venlafaxine can cause serious adverse effects such as hypertensive crisis, it is important to discontinue the Zoloft at least 2 weeks before the Nardil is started. *(3)*

26o. **(B)** Anticholinergic action such as that caused by diphenhydramine or doxylamine includes constipation and urinary retention. This may exacerbate the restricted urinary flow often experienced in patients with prostatitis. *(3)*

26p. **(A)** PSA refers to the prostate specific antigen, which as a glycoprotein product is almost exclusively produced by prostate epithelial cells. Routine determination of PSA allows comparison of newer values to the individual's baseline value. Increases indicate the possibility of prostate cancer. *(3)*

26q. **(D)** Mitrolan tablets contain calcium polycarbophil, which possesses both laxative and antidiarrheal properties. It quickly binds water in the GI tract and forms a gel, which provides a bulking effect. *(3)*

26r. **(D)** For many years Ex-Lax contained phenolphthalein as its active ingredient. Because phenolphthalein was suspected of being a carcinogen, Ex-Lax and many other products containing phenolphthalein were reformulated. Ex-Lax now contains 15 mg of senna, also a stimulant laxative. *(3)*

PROFILE NO. 27

27a. **(A)** Daypro is the brand name of oxaprozin. All of the choices are NSAIDs. *(3)*

27b. **(D)** NSAIDs have analgesic and antipyretic action, which appears to be related to their ability to inhibit cyclooxygenase activity and prostaglandin synthesis. *(6)*

27c. **(C)** Aleve is a nonprescription brand of naproxen sodium. This drug is usually administered two to three times daily. Antacids may be taken with naproxen sodium to increase GI tolerance to the drug. *(11)*

27d. **(E)** Tums chewable contains calcium carbonate. The product has become popular not only as an antacid but as a source of calcium for individuals who are attempting to reduce their chance of developing osteoporosis. *(11)*

27e. **(A)** Miacalcin contains salmon calcitonin as its active ingredient. It is used primarily in reducing bone resorption in postmenopausal women. It is administered intranasally as a spray, generally alternating nostrils each day. *(3)*

27f. **(E)** Oxaprozin (Daypro) is a relatively long-acting NSAID that requires only a single daily 1,200 mg dose for most patients. *(3)*

27g. **(D)** With the exception of long-acting statins such as atorvastatin (Lipitor) and rosuvastatin (Crestor), all of the statins are generally administered in the evening since most cholesterol synthesis occurs at night. As is the case with all statins, patients should be monitored for the development of muscle pain and, in the extreme case, rhabdomyolysis. All statins are classified in pregnancy category X and should not, therefore, be used in pregnant women. *(3)*

27h. **(C)** Misoprostol is a synthetic prostaglandin analog that has both antisecretory activity and mucosal protective properties. It is employed primarily in preventing NSAID-induced gastric ulcers. *(3)*

27i. **(D)** Misoprostol (Cytotec) is contraindicated for use during pregnancy and is classified as a pregnancy category X drug by the US FDA. *(3)*

27j. **(B)** Tramadol (Ultram) is a centrally acting analgesic agent that can be administered every 4–6 h in treating pain. Because it acts centrally, patients should be advised to expect central adverse effects such as dizziness and fatigue. *(3)*

27k. **(D)** Etanercept (Enbrel) and adalimumab (Humira) are drug products that are used parenterally in the treatment of rheumatoid arthritis. They are not indicated for the treatment of osteoarthritis. *(3)*

PROFILE NO. 28

28a. **(E)** Digoxin is a cardiac glycoside that produces a negative chronotropic effect (slowed heart rate), a positive inotropic effect (greater force of contraction), and a vagomimetic effect on the heart. *(3)*

28b. **(D)** Most patients using digoxin will experience a slowed heart rate (negative chronotropic effect). *(6)*

28c. **(E)** Milrinone lactate, although not a digitalis glycoside, is a positive inotropic agent. *(6)*

28d. **(E)** Lanoxicaps are liquid-filled capsules that contain a solution of digoxin in polyethylene glycol. Because the digoxin is already in solution, the Lanoxicap dosage form provides greater bioavailability of digoxin than is achieved from digoxin tablets. A dose of 0.25 mg (250 µg) of digoxin from a tablet dosage form is equivalent to 0.2 mg (200 µg) from the Lanoxicap dosage form. *(3)*

28e. **(A)** Digoxin toxicity is characterized by nausea and vomiting, diarrhea, disorientation, and ventricular tachycardia. *(6)*

28f. **(B)** If amiloride (Midamor) is substituted for Lasix as a diuretic in this patient's regimen, the patient should no longer receive the potassium supplement Klor-Con because amiloride is a potassium-sparing diuretic, and the administration of the combined agents would likely result in hyperkalemia. *(3)*

28g. **(A)** Normal serum potassium concentration is 3.5 to 5.0 mEq/L. When the serum level of potassium is below this range, the patient is said to be hypokalemic. If above this range, the patient is said to be hyperkalemic. *(14)*

28h. **(E)** Torsemide (Demadex) and furosemide (Lasix) are both loop diuretics. Dyrenium is a potassium-sparing diuretic, and acetazolamide is a carbonic anhydrase inhibitor. *(3)*

28i. **(B)** The patient appears to be noncompliant because he received a month's supply of digoxin but did not get a refill until about 1½ months later. *(3)*

PROFILE NO. 29

29a. **(E)** Diphenhydramine (Benadryl) is an ethanolamine antihistamine with both sedative and antipruritic properties. *(6)*

29b. **(B)** Pyrethrins, one of the active ingredients in RID, is a parasite neurotoxin that is used for the treatment of human lice and scabies. Piperonyl butoxide is an agent also present in RID. It does not have pesticidal properties but it does increase the effectiveness of the pyrethrins. *(11)*

29c. **(B)** When RID Shampoo is used, it is essential that the product does not come in contact with the eyes because it can cause significant irritation. RID should not be used on the face or on open cuts or excoriated areas of the body. *(3)*

29d. **(C)** The term *"pediculus"* refers to lice. *Pediculus capitis* refers to head lice, whereas *Pediculus pubis* refers to pubic lice. *Sarcoptes scabiei* is the organism that causes scabies. The term *"Tinea"* refers to a type of fungal organism. *(14)*

29e. **(A)** RID Shampoo is generally administered once. After working it thoroughly into the shampooed and dried hair, it remains in place for 10 minutes and is then worked into a lather with water. It is then rinsed well from the hair, and the hair is towel-dried and combed to ensure the removal of any remaining nit shells. Retreatment may occur after 7 days if there is still evidence of living lice at that time. *(11)*

29f. **(B)** Diprosone cream contains 0.05% betamethasone dipropionate in a hydrophilic emollient base. *(3)*

29g. **(D)** Betamethasone dipropionate cream, or any other potent corticosteroid topical product, should not be used on areas of the skin that are infected by bacteria, fungi, or a virus because the corticosteroid will inhibit the body's defense mechanisms and potentially cause spreading of the infection. Corticosteroids are useful in the treatment of psoriasis because they slow down the rate of skin cell replication. *(3)*

29h. **(C)** Both Nix (permethrin) and A-200 Pyrinate (pyrethrins, piperonyl butoxide, and petroleum distillate) are available for OTC use. Eurax (crotamiton) is available only by prescription. *(3)*

29i. **(A)** People with ragweed allergy should avoid pyrethrin-containing products because pyrethrins are plant derivatives that may precipitate a hypersensitivity reaction in such patients. *(3)*

29j. **(D)** Scabies is a skin condition caused by the mite *Sarcoptes scabiei*. The mite burrows into the skin and causes severe itching and excoriation of the affected area. Lindane and crotamiton are effective drugs for the treatment of scabies. *(14)*

29k. **(E)** Treatment of psoriasis is generally aimed at reducing the rate of skin cell turnover and reducing pruritis, which can lead to scratching that would exacerbate the disease. Corticosteroids such as Synalar cream will slow down skin cell replication. Acitretin (Soriatane) is a retinoid product that likely slows the turnover rate of skin cells and has been successfully used to treat psoriasis. Ustakinumab (Stelara) is a monoclonal antibody that inhibits interleukin-12 and interleukin-23, proteins that are believed to be involved in plaque psoriasis. *(3)*

PROFILE NO. 30

30a. **(B)** Naloxone is a pure narcotic antagonist that, when administered parenterally, rapidly reverses the effects of opioid narcotic agents such as heroin. Because it has no agonist action of its own, there is no danger in administering this agent to an unconscious patient even if the source of drug toxicity is unknown. *(6)*

30b. **(A)** Heroin is diacetylmorphine. Codeine is methylmorphine, whereas dionin is ethylmorphine. *(6)*

30c. **(C)** *Pneumocystis carinii* pneumonia (PCP) is a condition seen commonly in AIDS patients. It is an opportunistic infection that emerges when the immune system of a patient is suppressed by disease or drugs. *(14)*

30d. **(C)** Zidovudine or azidothymidine (AZT) is a nucleoside reverse transcriptase inhibitor (NRTI) antiviral agent commonly used in the management of patients with HIV infection who have evidence of impaired immunity. The drug is available as the brand name Retrovir. *(3)*

30e. **(A)** Patients on Retrovir are at risk of developing granulocytopenia or anemia that may require discontinuation of the medication or blood transfusions. It is therefore important to monitor the patient's hematologic status closely while on Retrovir therapy. *(3)*

30f. **(A)** Ritonavir (Norvir) is the only choice that is a protease inhibitor. The other choices are NRTIs. *(3)*

30g. **(A)** Acetaminophen use may competitively inhibit the glucuronidation of zidovudine (Retrovir). This may increase the blood levels of zidovudine and increase the likelihood of granulocytopenia. *(3)*

30h. **(D)** Pentamidine isethionate (Pentam, Nebu-Pent) is an agent that is useful in the treatment of PCP. It is available as an injectable product that may be administered intravenously or intramuscularly, and as an aerosol solution administered by inhalation using a nebulizer. *(3)*

30i. **(E)** Patients receiving pentamidine must be monitored for a variety of serious adverse effects, including sudden, severe hypotension that may occur after a single parenteral dose. Other adverse effects include hypoglycemia, bronchospasm, and cough. *(3)*

30j. **(D)** Robitussin DM is an OTC product used for the treatment of cough. It contains guaifenesin, an expectorant, and dextromethorphan HBr, a cough suppressant. *(11)*

30k. **(A)** Lamivudine (Epivir) is an NRTI that may cause lactic acidosis accompanied by hepatic steatosis in some patients. *(10)*

30l. **(E)** Ritonavir (Norvir) is protease inhibitor that has been found to be a potent inhibitor of cytochrome P450 3A (CYP3A) both in vitro and in vivo. Drugs that are extensively metabolized by this enzyme and are involved in significant first-pass metabolism may be most severely affected. This interaction can increase the AUC of these drugs by more than threefold, thereby necessitating a corresponding reduction in the dose of these interacting drugs. All of the drugs listed have this potentially serious drug interaction with ritonavir. *(3)*

Frequently Dispensed Drugs

Pharmacists should be familiar with commonly pre-scribed drug products. If given the generic name, he/she should be able to identify the following in-formation:

1. Brand or tradename
2. Dosage forms that are available
3. Strengths of dosage forms
4. General pharmacological category or use
5. Names of other drug products with identical or similar ingredients

Although it is impossible to memorize all of the above information for all commercially available products, those products most frequently dispensed are most likely to be included on the NAPLEX. The list on the following pages represents compilations from "Top 200 Drugs" lists published every year in several pharmacy journals. Drugs included on the "Top 200" lists vary. Some lists are based on number of prescriptions dispensed while others are based on dollar volume. Thus, the following table contains drug products that the community pharmacist may not be familiar with. Being acquainted with the trade name and generic names of the drugs will be a good starting point for answering questions. The names of companies manufacturing a specific drug have not been included since the NAPLEX seldom questions such information. However, one should recognize that a number of popular drugs are no longer protected by patents and have the generic versions among the top 200. These drugs are indi-cated by the designation of "GENERIC" along with the most popular trade name.

Other useful information included is a brief de-scription of pharmacological categories, common dosage forms, and strengths. Again, it is impossible to memorize all of this information, but familiarity with some will be useful. Note especially when a product is available in a sustained-release dosage form or as an injectable.

This table is also useful when reviewing phar-macology for the NAPLEX. If the candidate is not familiar with a specific drug, review it in one of the standard references such as the *Remington, Facts and Comparisons,* or even the PDR. At the same time, investigate closely related drugs so that you can picture how each drug fits into its specific category. Abbreviations used in the table include:

Drug Abbreviations

APAP	acetaminophen
ASA	aspirin
HCTZ	hydrochlorothiazide
HC	hydrocortisone
NSAID	nonsteroidal anti-inflammatory drug
PE	phenylephrine

TABLE OF FREQUENTLY DISPENSED DRUGS

Generic Name	Trade Name	Category or Use	Dosage Forms & Strengths
Acetaminophen + Codeine	Tylenol or Empracet with codeine GENERIC	Analgesic	APAP 300 mg with 7.5, 15, 30, or 60 mg codeine
Acyclovir sodium	GENERIC Zovirax	Treatment of herpes	Inj. (600 mg vial), cap (200 mg) oint. 5%, tab (800 mg); susp.
Adapalene	Differin	Retinoid-like agent	Cream, gel, solution (0.1%) for acne
Albuterol	GENERIC Proventil Ventolin Volmax ProAir HFA	Bronchodilator	Tab (2 and 4 mg); repetabs; inhalation aerosol; syrup; nebulizer sol., extended release tab (4 and 8 mg)
Albuterol + Ipratropium	Combivent DuoNeb	Bronchodilator	Aerosol inhalation solution
Alendronate	Fosamax		Tab (5, 10, 30, & 70 mg
Alendronate + Cholecalciferol	Fosamax Plus D	Treat and prevent osteoporosis and Paget's disease	Tab (5, 10, 35 and 70 mg) Tab 70 mg with either 5,600 or 2,800 IU vitamin D
Allopurinol	GENERIC Zyloprim	Treatment of gout (hyperuricemia)	Tab (100 and 300 mg)
Alprazolam	GENERIC Xanax	Anxiolytic	Tab (0.25, 0.5, 1, and 2 mg)
Amlodarone	Cordarone	Antiarrhythmic	Tab (100, 200, and 400 mg); inj.
Amitriptyline	GENERIC Elavil	Antidepressant	Tab (10, 25, 50, 75, 100, and 125 mg); inj.
Amlodipine	Norvasc	Antihypertensive	Tab (2.5, 5, and 10 mg)
Amlodipine + Benazepril	Lotrel	Anxiolytic	Tab (2.5 + 10; 5 + 10; 5 + 20 mg)
Amoxicillin	GENERIC Amoxil, Moxatag, Trimox, Wymox		
Amoxicillin " + Clavulanate K	GENERIC Augmentin XR	Broad-spectrum antibiotic	Cap (250 and 500 mg); susp. Tab (250 and 500 mg + 125 mg clavulanate); susp.
Amphetamine salts	Adderall XR	CNS stimulant	Mixture of salts totaling 5, 7.5, 10, 12.5, 15, 20, and 30 mg; also XR totaling 10, 20, and 30 mg
Anastrozole	Arimidex	Antineoplastic (breast cancer)	Tablet (1 mg)
Aripiprazole	Abilify	Antipsychotic	Dismelt (ODT) 10 and 15 mg IM Inj; Tab 5, 10, 15, 20, 30 mg
Atenolol	GENERIC Tenormin	Antihypertensive	Tab (25, 50, and 100 mg)
Atomoxetine	Strattera	Psychotherapeutic agent for ADHD	Cap (10, 18, 25, 40, and 60 mg)
Atorvastatin	Lipitor	Antihyperlipidemic	Tab (10, 20, 40, and 80 mg)
Azelastine	Astelin Optivar	Antihistamine	Intranasal sol.; ophth. sol.
Azithromycin	GENERIC Zithromax	Macrolide antibiotic	Tab (250, 500, and 600 mg); Tri-Pak; Z-Pak; suspension
Baclofen	Lioresal	Skeletal muscle relaxant	Tab (10 and 20 mg); intrathecal inj.
Benazepril	GENERIC Lotensin	Antihypertensive (ACE inhibitor)	Tab (5, 10, 20, and 40 mg)

(continued)

TABLE OF FREQUENTLY DISPENSED DRUGS (cont.)

Generic Name	Trade Name	Category or Use	Dosage Forms & Strengths
Bimatoprost	Lumigan	Treat glaucoma	Ophth. sol. 0.03%
Brimonidine tartrate	Alphagan P	Reduce intraocular pressure (glaucoma)	Ophth. sol. (0.1 and 0.15%)
Bupropion HCl	GENERIC Wellbutrin SR Zyban	Antianxiety, aid in smoking cessation	Tab (5, 10, 75, and 100 mg) SR (100, 150, and 200 mg)
Buspirone HCl	BuSpar generic	Antianxiety agent	Tab (5, 7.5, 10, 15, and 30 mg)
Calcitonin salmon	Fortical Miacalcin	Postmenopausal osteoporosis	Nasal spray
Carbidopa/Levodopa	GENERIC Sinemet	Antiparkinson	Tab of several strengths (10 + 100 mg up to 50 + 200 mg)
Candesartan	Atacand	Antihypertensive (angiotensin II receptor blocker)	Tablet (4, 8, 16, and 32 mg)
Capecitabine	Xeloda	Antineoplastic for breast CA	Tablet (150 and 500 mg) chewable tab. (100 and 200 mg)
Cephalexin HCl	GENERIC	Antibiotic	Tab and cap (250 and 500 mg); suspension
Cetirizine + Pseudoephedrine	Zyrtec D	Seasonal or allergic rhinitis	Tablet (5 and 10 mg); syrup (5 mg/5 mL); chewable tab. (5 and 10 mg)
Cetuximab	Erbitux	Treat colorectal cancer	Inj. (100 mg in 50 mL vial)
Cinacalcet	Sensipar	Treat hypercalcemia and hyperparathyroidism	Tablet (30, 60, 90 mg)
Ciprofloxacin	GENERIC Cipro Proquin XR	Broad-spectrum antibiotic	Tab (250, 500, and 750 mg); antibiotic inj.
Ciprofloxacin + Dextromethasone	Ciprodex Otic	Treat ear infections (otitis media and external)	Otic suspension (0.3% + 0.1%) Ophth. sol. 0.5%
Citalopram	GENERIC Celexa	Antidepressant	Tab (20 and 40 mg)
Clindamycin + Benzoyl peroxide	Benzaclin	Treat facial acne	Gel (1% and 5%)
Clonazepam	GENERIC Klonopin	Treat petit mal and panic attacks	Tab (0.5, 1, and 2 mg)
Clonidine	GENERIC Catapres	Antihypertensive	Tab (0.1, 0.2, and 0.3 mg) Transdermal patch (Catapres TTS)
Conjugated estrogens and Medroxyprogesterone	Prempro	Treat symptoms of menopause	Tablet (several strengths)
Cyclobenzapine	GENERIC Flexeril	Skeletal muscle relaxant	Tab 10 mg
Cyclosporine	Restasis, Gengraf, Neoral, Sandimmune	Immunosuppressant	Cap. 25, 50, and 100 mg; inj. 50 mg/mL Ophth. emulsion 0.05%; oral sol. 100 mg/mL
Darbepoetin	Aranesp	Treat anemia associated with chronic renal failure (increased RBC production)	Inj. and prefilled syringes (25–100 μg)
Darifenacin	Enablex	Cholinergic blocking agent (treat overactive bladder)	Ext. release tab (7.5 and 15 mg)
Desloratadine	Clarinex	Antihistamine	Tab 5 mg

(continued)

TABLE OF FREQUENTLY DISPENSED DRUGS (cont.)

Generic Name	Trade Name	Category or Use	Dosage Forms & Strengths
Dexmethylphenidate	Focalin XR	CNS stimulant (treat ADHD)	Tablet (2.5, 5, and 10 mg) ER cap (2.5, 5, and 10 mg)
Diazepam	GENERIC Valium	Antianxiety	Tab (2, 5, and 10 mg)
Digoxin	GENERIC Lanoxin Digitek	Cardiovascular agent	Tab (0.125, 0.25, and 0.5 mg); pediatric elixir; inj.
Diltiazem	GENERIC Cartia XT Cardizem, Dilacor XR Tiazac	Antianginal agent (calcium channel blocker)	Tab (30, 60, 90, and 120 mg); SR cap (60, 90, and 120 mg) Extended-release cap (120, 180, 240, 300, 360, and 420 mg)
Donepezil	Aricept	Treat mild to moderate dementia (Alzheimer's)	Tab (5, 10 and 23 mg)
Dorzolamide HCl + Timolol maleate	Cosopt	Reduce intraocular pressure (glaucoma)	Ophth. sol (20 + 5 mg/mL in 5 and 10 mL bts.)
Doxycycline	Doryx GENERIC Vibramycin	Antibiotic	Cap and tab (50 and 100 mg); susp.; inj.
Dronabinol	Marinol	Appetite stimulant (treat anorexia); antiemetic	Capsule (2.5, 5, and 10 mg)
Dutasteride	Avodart	Treat BPH	Tablet 0.5 mg
Efavirenz	Sustiva	Antiviral	Cap. (50, 100, 200 mg) Tab. (300 and 600 mg)
Efavirenz + Emtricitabine + Tenofovir	Atripla	Combination of antiretroviral agents (HIV-1 infections)	Tab (600/200/300 mg)
Eletriptan	Relpax	Antimigraine	Tab. (24.2 and 48.5 mg) equivalent
Enalapril	GENERIC Vasotec Vaseretic	Antihypertensive	Tab. (2.5, 5, 10, and 20 mg) Tab (5 and 10 mg + HCTZ (12.5 or 25 mg)
Enfuvirtide	Fuzeon	Antiretroviral fusion inhibitor	Powder for inj. 100 mg
Enoxaparin	Lovenox	Low molecular weight heparin	Inj. (several strengths–30 and 150 mg); prefilled syringe
Erlotinib	Tarceva	Lung and pancreatic cancer	Tablet (25, 50, and 100 mg)
Esomeprazole	Nexium	Treatment of GERD	Delayed-release cap (20 and 40 mg); inj.
Eszopiclone	Lunesta	Sedative/hypnotic	Tab (1, 2, and 3 mg)
Ethinyl estradiol + Drospirenone	Yasmin 28	Monophasic oral	Tab (0.03 mg + 3 mg)
Ethinyl estradiol + Drospirenone	Yaz	Oral contraceptive	Tablet (0.02 mg + 3 mg)
Ethinyl estradiol + Etonogestrel	Nuva Ring	Contraceptive device	Vaginal ring with 11.7 + 2.7 mg
Ethinyl estradiol + Norethindrone + Ferrous fumarate	Loestrin FE	Oral contraceptive	Tab. (20 mcg + 1 mg + 75 mg Fe)
Exenatide	Byetta	Antidiabetic	Inj. (5 or 10 μg per dose in prefilled pens)
Ezetimibe	Zetia	Antihyperlipidemic	Tab. (10 mg)
Famciclovir	Famvir	Antiviral	Tab. (125, 250, and 500 mg)
Fenofibrate	Tricor	Reduce cholesterol	Tab (48 and 145 mg)
Fentanyl	Duragesic GENERIC Fentora Actiq	Narcotic analgesic	Transdermal patch (12.5, 25, 50, 75, and 100 μg/h) Tab. (100, 200, 300, 400, 600, and 800 mg) Transmucosal lozenges (200–1,600 μg)

(continued)

Generic Name	Trade Name	Category or Use	Dosage Forms & Strengths
Ferrous sulfate	GENERIC Feosol Slow FE	Iron deficiency	Tab, syrup, drops
Fexofenadine Fexofenadine + Pseudoephedrine	Allegra Allegra D 12 and 24	Antihistamine Antihistamine + decongestant	Cap 60 mg, tab (30, 60, 180 mg) (60 + 120; 180 + 240 mg)
Fish oil (Omega-3 fatty acids)	Lovaza	Reduce triglycerides Prevent heart disease	Cap 1,000 mg
Fluconazole	GENERIC Diflucan	Antifungal	Tab (50, 100, 150, and 200 mg); pwd. For susp.; inj.
Fluticasone	Flovent Flonase Flovent HFA	Corticosteroid Seasonal and perennial allergic rhinitus Glucocorticoid for asthma	HFA inhalation aerosol (44, 110, and 200 mg) Nasal spray Aerosol and nasal spray
Fluoxetine	GENERIC Prozac	Antidepressant	Pulvules and cap. (10, 20, and 40 mg); liq.; cap. (90 mg)
Folic acid	GENERIC	Treat megaloblastic anemia	Tab (0.4, 0.8, and 1 mg) Inj. (5 mg/mL)
Furosemide	GENERIC Lasix	Loop diuretic	Tab (20, 40, and 80 mg) Oral sol.; inj.
Gabapentin	GENERIC Neurontin	Anticonvulsant	Cap (100, 300, and 400 mg)
Gentamicin	GENERIC	Broad-spectrum antibiotic	Oint., cream, inj., ophth. sol. and oint.
Glipizide	GENERIC Glucotrol XL	Antihyperglycemic	Tab (5 and 10 mg), XL (extended release—5 and 10 mg)
Glyburide	GENERIC Micronase Diabeta Glynase	Antidiabetic	Tab (1.25, 2.5, and 5 mg) Prestab (3 and 6 mg)
Hydrochlorothiazide (HCTZ)	GENERIC	Antihypertensive Diuretic	Tab (25 and 50 mg)
Hydrocodone bitartrate + APAP	GENERIC Vicodin Zydone	Narcotic, analgesic, antitussive	Tab (5 + 500 mg); ES (7.5 + 750) Tab (5, 7.5, and 10 mg + 400 mg APAP)
Hydrocodone + Chlorpheniramine Polistirex	Tussionex	Relief of cough and upper respiratory symptoms	ER suspension (10 mg + 8 mg) in Pennkinetic System
Hydroxyzine	GENERIC Vistaril	Antianxiety	Tab (10, 25, 50, and 100 mg) Syrup, inj, cap, suspension
Ibandronate	Boniva	Prevent osteoporosis	Inj. (3 mg every 3 months) Tab. 2.5 mg (once daily) Tab. 150 mg (once monthly)
Imiquimod	Aldara	Treat actinic keratosis and misc. skin cancers	Cream 5%
Insulin	Humalog Humulin N NovoLog	Antidiabetic	Regular; Mix 75/25 Regular; 70/30 Mix 70/30
Insulin Detemir	Levemir	Antidiabetic	Inj (vials, PenFill, prefilled syringes)
Insulin glargine	Lantus	Antidiabetic	Inj.; Solostar
Insulin Lispro	Humalog	Antidiabetic	Inj.
Interferon alpha-2b	Rebetron	Antineoplastic (treat hepatitis C)	Inj.

(continued)

TABLE OF FREQUENTLY DISPENSED DRUGS (cont.)

Generic Name	Trade Name	Category or Use	Dosage Forms & Strengths
Interferon beta-1a	Avonex Rebif	Treat multiple sclerosis, hepatitis, brain tumor	Powder for inj.
Irbesartan	Avapro	Antihypertensive	Tab (75, 150, and 300 mg)
Irbesartan HCTZ	Avalide		Tab (150 or 300 mg + 12.5 mg HCTZ)
Isosorbide dinitrate	Isordil	Treat angina pectoris	Oral tab (5 and 10 mg); chewable tab; sublingual tab (5 and 10 mg); titradose (5, 10, 20, 30, and 40 mg)
Isosorbide mononitrate	GENERIC	Coronary vasodilator	Ext. release tab (30, 60, and 120 mg; tab (30, 60, and 100 mg)
Isotretinoin	Accutane	Prevent and treat acne	Tab (10, 20, and 40 mg)
Lamotrigine	Lamictal Lamictal XR	Anticonvulsant	Tab (25, 100, 150, and 200 mg) extended release, enteric coated
Lamivudine + Zidovudine	Combivir	Antiviral for HIV infections	Tablet (150 and 300 mg)
Lansoprazole	Prevacid	Proton pump inhibitor	Delayed-release cap (15 and 30 mg)
Latanoprost	Xalatan	Reduce intraocular pressure	Ophth. sol. 0.005%
Letrozole	Femara	Antineoplastic agent	Tab. 2.5 mg
Levalbuterol	Xopenex	Reverse bronchospasms	Sol. for Inhalation (0.31, 0.63, and 1.25 mg) Sol. for Inhal. Concentrate (1.25 mg/0.5 mL)
Levofloxacin	Levaquin	Fluoroquinolone antibiotic	Tab (250 and 500 mg); inj.
Levothyroxine	Levoxyl Levo-T Synthroid Eltroxin Levothroid Unithroid	Management of thyroid	Tab. (various strengths from 0.025 to 0.3 mg)
Lidocaine	Lidoderm	Local anesthetic	Transdermal patch 5%
Linezolid	Zyvox	Antimicrobial (for nosocomial pneumonia and serious skin infections)	Tab (400 and 600 mg); inj.
Lisinopril	GENERIC Prinivil Zestril	Antihypertensive	Tab (2.5, 5, 10, 20, and 40 mg)
Lopinavir + Ritonavir	Kaletra	Antiretroviral	Tab. (100 + 25; 200 + 50 mg) Sol. 80 + 20 mg/mL
Lorazepam	Ativan Generic	Antianxiety agent	Tab (1, 2, and 5 mg); inj.
Losartan	Cozaar	Antihypertensive (angiotensin II blocker)	Tab (25, 50, and 100 mg)
Lubiprostone	Amitiza	Treat chronic constipation	Cap. (8 and 24 μg)
Meclizine	GENERIC Antivert Bonine	Treat motion sickness and vertigo	Tab (12.5, 25, and 50 mg)
Memantine	Namenda	Treat Alzheimer's disease	Tab (5 and 10 mg); oral sol. 2 mg/mL
Mesalamine	Asacol Pentasa Rowasa Lialda	Anti-inflammatory	Cap (250 and 500 mg) Rectal enema (4 g/60 mL) Supp. (500 and 1,000 mg) Delayed release tab 400 mg

(continued)

Generic Name	Trade Name	Category or Use	Dosage Forms & Strengths
Metformin	GENERIC Glucophage Glucophage XR	Antidiabetic	Tab (500, 750, 850, and 1,000 mg)
Methotrexate	GENERIC	Treat cancer; antipsoriasis	Tab (2.5 mg); inj. (2.5, 10, and 25 mg/mL)
Methylphenidate	GENERIC Concerta Ritalin	Treat attention-deficit disorder (ADD or ADHD)	Tab (5, 10, and 20 mg) SR 20 mg; ext. release tab (18, 36, and 54 mg)
Metoclopramide	GENERIC Reglan	Antinauseant; stimulate GI tract motility	Tab 10 mg; syrup; inj. (10 mg/2 mL)
Metoprolol	GENERIC Lopressor Toprol XL	Antihypertensive	Tab (50 and 100 mg); inj. Extended-release tab (50, 100, and 200 mg)
Mirtazapine	GENERIC Remeron	Antidepressant	Tab (15, 30, and 45 mg)
Modafinil	Provigil	CNS stimulant; analeptic	Tab (100 and 200 mg)
Mometasone	Nasonex Asmanex Twisthaler	Anti-asthmatic	Nasal spray Powder for inhalation
Montelukast	Singulair	Anti-asthmatic	Tab 10 mg; chewable tab 5 mg
Morphine	GENERIC MS Contin Oramorph Duramorph Kadian Avinza	Narcotic analgesic	Tab, cap CR (15, 30, and 100 mg) Inj. Cap (10–50 mg) Ext. rel. pellets (30, 60, 90, and 120 mg)
Moxifloxacin HCl	Avelox Vigamox	Antibiotic	Inj. 400 mg; tab 400 mg; ophth. sol. 0.05% in Alcon's Drop-tainer dispensing system
Mycophenolate	Cellcept	Immunosuppressant	Cap 250 mg; tab 500 mg; Pwd for inj.
Nabumetone	GENERIC Relafen	NSAID	Tab (500 and 750 mg)
Naproxen	GENERIC Naprosyn Aleve Anaprox Naprelan	Anti-rheumatic	Tab (250, 375, and 500 mg) Controlled release (375 and 500 mg) Suspension
Niacin	Niaspan	Antihyperlipidemic	Extended release tab (500, 750, and 1,000 mg)
Nifedipine " ER	GENERIC Procardia Adalat Adalat CC Procardia XL	Antihypertensive	Cap (10 and 20 mg); ext. release and sustained release (30, 60, and 90 mg)
Nitroglycerin	GENERIC Nitro-Dur Nirostat	Treatment of angina	Sublingual tab (0.15, 0.4, and 0.6 mg); Cap 2.5 mg; prolonged release 6.5 mg; oint 2%; inj. transdermal patches
Nystatin	GENERIC Mycostatin	Antifungal	Tab 500,000 units; susp.; vaginal sup.; cream; ointment
Olmesartan	Benicar	Antihypertensive	Tab (5, 20, and 40 mg) also with HCTZ

(continued)

Generic Name	Trade Name	Category or Use	Dosage Forms & Strengths
Omeprazole	GENERIC Prilosec	Short-term treatment of active duodenal ulcers	Sustained release cap (20 mg)
Oseltamivir	Tamiflu	Antiviral	Cap. (30, 45, and 75 mg) Pwd. for susp. (12 mg/mL)
Oxaliplatin	Eloxatin	Treat advanced colorectal cancer	Inj.
Oxycodone	GENERIC OxyContin	Narcotic analgesic	Tab. (10, 20, 30, and 80 mg)
Oxycodone + APAP	GENERIC Percocet-5 Roxicet; Tylox Endocet	Analgesic; antipyretic	Tab. (several strengths) (5, 7.5, 10 mg + 325, 500, and 600 mg APAP)
Paliperidone	Invega	Antipsychotic	Tab. (1.5, 3, 6, and 9 mg)
Pantoprazole	GENERIC	Treatment of GERD	Tab (20 and 40 mg)
Pegfilgrastim	Neulasta	Hematopoietic stimulant	Inj. 6 mg
PEG Interferon alpha 2a	Pegasys	Immunomodulator	Inj. 180 μg/mL
Penicillin V Pot. (pot. phenoxymethyl penicillin)	GENERIC Beepen VK V-Cillin K Pen-Vee K Veetids	Antibiotic for gram-positive microbes	Tab and suspension (several strengths)
Phenobarbital	GENERIC	Sedative, hypnotic, antiepileptic	Tab (15, 30, 60, and 100 mg)
Phenytoin extended	GENERIC Dilantin	Anticonvulsant	Cap (30 and 100 mg)
Pioglitazone HCl	Actos	Antidiabetic	Tab (15, 30, 60, and 45 mg)
Pioglitazone HCl + Metformin	Actoplus Met	Antidiabetic	Tab (15 + 500; 15 + 850 mg)
Potassium chloride	GENERIC Klor-Con 10 K-Tab, K-Lor Slow-K, Micro-K	Potassium supplement	Tab, pwd., liquid (various strengths)
Prednisone	GENERIC	Adrenal corticosteroid	Tab. (2.5, 5, 10, 20, and 50 mg)
Pramipexole	Mirapex	Antiparkinson	Tab. (0.125, 0.25, 0.5, 1, and 1.5 mg)
Pramipexole	Miraplex ER	Antiparkinson	Tab. (0.375, 0.75, 1.5, 3 and 4.5 mg)
Pregabalin	Lyrica	Anticonvulsant, analgesic	Cap. (25–300 mg); oral liq. (20 mg/mL)
Promethazine HCl	GENERIC Phenergan	Antiemetic, antihistamine	Tab. (12.5 and 25 mg); supp. (25 and 50 mg)
Propranolol	GENERIC Inderal	Treat angina, arrhythmias, etc	Tab (10, 20, 40, 60, and 80 mg) LA cap (80, 120, and 160 mg)
Quetiapine fumarate	Seroquel Seroquel XR	Antipsychotic	Tab (25, 100, and 200 mg) Sust. rel. (200, 300, and 400 mg)
Quinapril	Accupril	Antihypertensive	Tab (5, 10, 20 and 40 mg)
Rabeprazole	Aciphex	Treat GERD, duodenal and Zollinger–Ellison syndrome	Delayed release tab 20 mg
Raloxifene HCl	Evista	Prevent osteoporosis	Tab. 60 mg
Raltegravir	Isentress	Antiretroviral	Tab. 400 mg
Ramipril	Altace	Antihypertensive	Cap (1.25, 2.5, 5, and 10 mg)
Risedronate	Actonel	Prevent osteoporosis; treat Paget's disease	Tab (5 and 35 mg)
Risperidone	Risperdal Consta	Schizophrenia; bipolar diseases	ER (long acting) inj. (12.5, 25, 37.5, and 50 mg/vial)

(continued)

Generic Name	Trade Name	Category or Use	Dosage Forms & Strengths
Rizatriptan	Maxalt Maxalt-MLT	Migraine therapy	Tab (5 and 10 mg); ODT (oral dissolving tab—5 and 10 mg)
Ropinirole	Requip	Antiparkinson, teat restless leg syndrome	Tab (0.25, 0.5, 1, 2, 3, 4, and 5 mg)
Rosuvastatin	Crestor	Antihyperlipidemic agent	Tab (5, 10, 20, and 40 mg)
Salmeterol + Fluticasone	Advair Diskus	Respiratory inhalant	50 µg salmeterol + fluticasone (100, 250, and 500 µg)
Sertraline	Zoloft	Antidepressant	Tab (50 and 100 mg)
Sildenafil	Viagra	For erectile dysfunction	Tab (25, 50, and 100 mg)
Simvastatin	Zocor	Antihyperlipidemic	Tab (5, 10, 20, and 40 mg)
Sitagliptin	Januvia	Antidiabetic	Tab (25, 50, 100 mg)
Sitagliptin + Metformin	Janumet	Antidiabetic	Tab. (50/500 and 50/1,000 mg)
Sumatriptan	Imitrex	Treatment of migraine	Tab. (25 and 50 mg); nasal generic spray; SQ inj. (12 mg)
Solifenacin	Vesicare	Cholinergic blocking agent (treat urinary incontinence)	Tablet (5 and 10 mg)
Tadalafil	Cialis	Treat erectile dysfunction	Tab (5, 10, and 20 mg)
Tamoxifen	GENERIC Nolvadex	Anti-estrogen (reduce incidence of breast CA)	Tab 10 mg
Tamsulosin HCl	Flomax	Treat benign prostatic hyperplasia (BPH)	Cap 0.4 mg
Telmisartan	Micardis	Antihypertensive	Tab. (20, 40, and 80 mg)
Telmisartan + HCTZ	Micardis HCT	Antihypertensive (angiotensin II receptor blocker)	Tablet (40/12.5, 80/12.5, 80/25 mg)
Temazepam	GENERIC Restoril	Sedative/hypnotic	Cap (15 and 30 mg)
Tenofovir	Viread	Antiretroviral agent	Tab 300 mg
Terazosin	Hytrin	Antihypertensive; treat BPH	Tab (1, 2, 5, and 10 mg)
Teriparatide	Forteo	Treat osteoporosis	Inj. (250 µg/mL)
Testosterone	AndroGel	Anabolic steroid (treat hypogonadism)	Gel 1%
Tetracycline HCl	GENERIC Sumycin	Broad-spectrum antibiotic	Cap (250 and 500 mg); susp.
Tramadol	GENERIC Ultram	Analgesic	Tab 50 mg; ext. release (100, 200, 300 mg)
Trazodone	GENERIC	Antidepressant	Tab (50 and 100 mg)
Triamcinolone acetonide	GENERIC Kenalog Nasacort AQ	Anti-inflammatory	Cream, ointment, and topical aerosol Intranasal spray
Triamterene + HCTZ	GENERIC Dyazide	Antihypertensive diuretic	Cap (37.5 + 25 mg)
Trimethoprim + Sulfamethoxazole	GENERIC Bactrim Septra	Antibacterial for urinary tract infections	Tab (80 + 400 mg); (Co-Trimoxazole; TMP-SMZ) DS = double strength Infusion solution
Valacyclovir	GENERIC Valtrex	Antiviral	Tab (500 and 1,000 mg)
Varenicline tartrate	Chantix	For smoking cessation	Tablet (0.5 and 1 mg)
Venlafaxine	Effexor Effexor XR	Antidepressant	Tab (25, 37.5, 50, 75, and 100 mg); ext. release cap (37.5, 75, and 100 mg)

(continued)

TABLE OF FREQUENTLY DISPENSED DRUGS (cont.)

Generic Name	Trade Name	Category or Use	Dosage Forms & Strengths
Verapamil	GENERIC Calan	Antihypertensive	Tab (40, 80, and 120 mg) SR 240 mg; inj.
Verapamil XR	Isoptin Verelan Covera HS		Tab (180 and 240 mg)
Warfarin	GENERIC Coumadin	Anticoagulant	Tab (2, 2.5, 5, 7.5, and 10 mg)
Zaleplon	Sonata	Nonbenzodiazepine Sedative	Tab (5 and 10 mg)
Zolpidem	Ambien Ambien CR	Nonbenzodiazepine hypnotic, sedative	Tab (5 and 10 mg) CR (6.25 and 12.5 mg)

Brand Names (Trade Names) Versus Generic Names

NOTE: This compilation contains additional drugs not included in "Most Frequently Dispensed Drugs" lists.

Brand Names (Trade Names)	Generic Names
Abelcet	Amphotericin B Lipid-based
Abilify	Aripiprazole
Accolate	Zafirlukast
Accupril	Quinapril
Accutane	Isotretinoin
Aciphex	Rabeprazole
Actiq	Fentanyl
Actonel	Risedronate
Actoplus	Pioglitazone + metformin
Actos	Pioglitazone
Adalat CC	Nifedipine
Adderall	Amphetamine salts
Adipex-P	Phentermine
Advair	Salmeterol + fluticasone
Advil	Ibuprofen
Aggrenox	Dipyridamole + ASA
Aldactone	Spironolactone
Aldara	Imiquimod
Aldoril	Methyldopa + HCTZ
Alesse	Ethinyl estradiol + levonogestrel
Allegra D	Fexofenadine + pseudoephedrine
Aleve	Naproxen
Alphagan P	Brimonidine
Altace	Ramipril
Amaryl	Glimepiride
Ambien	Zolpidem
Amcil	Ampicillin
AmBisome	Amphotericin B lipid-based
Amitiza	Lubiprostone
Amphotec	Amphotericin lipid-based
Anaprox	Naproxen
AndroGel	Testosterone

Brand Names (Trade Names)	Generic Names
Ansaid	Flurbiprofen
Antivert	Meclizine
Anzemet	Dolasetron
Apri	Ethinyl estradiol + desogestrel
Aranesp	Darbepoetin
Arava	Leflunomide
Aricept	Donepezil
Arimidex	Anastrozole
Asacol	Mesalamine
Asmanex	Mometasone
Astelin	Azelastine
Atacand	Candesartan
Atenolol	Tenormin
Ativan	Lorazepam
Atripla	Tenofovir + efavirenz + emtricitabine
Atrovent	Ipratropium
Augmentin XR	Amoxicillin + clavulanate K
Avalide	Irbesartan + HCTZ
Avandia	Rosiglitazone
Avandamet	Rosiglitazone + metformin
Avastin	Bevacizumab
Avelox	Moxifloxacin
Avinza	Morphine
Avodart	Dutasteride
Avonex	Interferon beta-1a
Axid	Nizatidine
Azmacort	Triamcinolone acetonide
Bactroban	Mupirocin
Bactrim	Trimethoprim + sulfamethoxazole
Beconase	Beclomethasone dipropionate
Benicar	Olmesartan

Brand Names (Trade Names)	Generic Names	Brand Names (Trade Names)	Generic Names
Benzaclin	Clindamycin + benzoyl peroxide	Concerta	Methylphenidate
		Copaxone	Glatiramer
Benzamycin	Erythromycin + benzyl peroxide	Coreg	Carvedilol
		Cordarone IV	Amiodarone
Betapace	Sotalol	Corgard	Nadolol
Betaserone	Interferon beta-1b	Cortisporin	Polymyxin B, neomycin, gramicidin, and hydrocortisone
Betimol	Timolol		
Biaxin	Clarithromycin		
Blocadren	Timolol	Cosopt	Dorzolamide + timolol
Boniva	Ibandronate		
Brethine	Terbutaline	Coumadin	Warfarin
Budeprion SR	Bupropion	Covera HS	Verapamil
Bumex	Bumetanide	Cozaar	Losartan
Buspar	Buspirone	Crestor	Rosuvastatin
Byetta	Exenatide	Crixivan	Indinavir
		Cymbalta	Duloxetine
Caduet	Amlodipine + atorvastatin	Cytotec	Misoprostol
Calan	Verapamil		
Camptosar	Irinotecan	Dalmane	Flurazepam
Cancidas (AS)	Caspofungin	Darvocet N	Propoxyphene + acetaminophen
Capoten	Captopril		
Carafate	Sucralfate	Daypro	Oxaprozin
Cardizem	Diltiazem	DDAVP	Desmopressin
Cardura	Doxazosin	Deltasone	Prednisone
Cartia XT	Diltiazem	Depakene	Valproic acid
Casodex	Bicalutamide	Depakote	Valproic acid
Catapres	Clonidine	Desogen	Ethinyl estradiol
Ceclor	Cefaclor	Desyrel	Trazodone
Ceftin	Cefuroxime	Detrol	Tolerodine
Celebrex	Celecoxib	Diabeta	Glyburide
Celexa	Citalopram	Differin	Adapalene
Cellcept	Mycophenolate	Diflucan	Fluconazole
Chantix	Varenicline	Digitek	Digoxin
Cialis	Tadalafil	Dilacor XR	Diltiazem
Cipro	Ciprofloxacin	Dilantin	Phenytoin
Ciprodex Otic	Ciprofloxacin + dexamethasone	Dimetapp	Brompheniramine maleate
Clarinex	Desloratadine	Diovan	Valsartan
Claritin	Loratadine	Ditropan XL	Oxybutynin
Cleocin	Clindamycin	Doryx	Doxycline
ClimaraPro	Estradiol + levonorgestrel	Dovonex	Calcipotreine
Clinoril	Sulindac	DuoNeb	Albuterol + ipratropium
Clozaril	Clozapine	Duragesic	Fentanyl
Cogentin	Benztropine	Duricef	Cefadroxil
Combivent	Ipratropium + albuterol	Dyazide	Triamterene + HCTZ
Combivir	Lamivudine + zidovudine	Dynacin	Minocycline
Compazine	Prochlorperazine	DynaCirc	Isradipine

Brand Names (Trade Names)	Generic Names	Brand Names (Trade Names)	Generic Names
Effexor XR	Venlafaxine	Glucovance	Metfomin + glyburide
Elavil	Amitriptyline	Glynase	Glyburide
Eldepryl	Selegiline	Gyne-Lotrimin	Clotrimazole
Elocon	Mometasone		
Eloxatin	Oxaliplatin	Halcion	Triazolam
Enablex	Darifenacin	Haldol	Haloperidol
Enbrel Surclik	Etanercept	Haltran	Ibuprofen
Endocet	Oxycodone + APAP	Herceptin	Trastuzumab
Epivir	Lamivudine	Humulin N 70/30	Isophane insulin
Epogen	Epoetin alpha	Humalog	Insulin lispro
Eprex	Epoetin alpha	Humira	Adalimumab
Epzicom	Abacavir + lamivudine	HydroDIURIL	Hydrochlorothiazide
Erbitux	Cetuximab	Hytrin	Terazosin
ERY-TAB, ERYC	Erythromycin	Hyzaar	Losartan + HCTZ
Eskalith	Lithium carbonate		
Estrace or Estraderm	Estradiol	Imitrex	Sumatriptan
		Imodium	Loperamide
Estratest Tab	Esterified estrogens + methyltestosterone	Inderal	Propanolol
		Indocin	Indomethacin
Evista	Raloxifene	Intal	Cromolyn
		Integrilin	Eptifibatide
Famvir	Famciclovir	Invega	Paliperidone
Feldene	Piroxicam	Isentress	Raltegravir
Femara	Letrozole	Isoptin	Verapamil
Fentora	Fentanyl	Isordil	Isosorbide dinitrate
Feosol	Ferrous sulfate		
Fiorecet	Butalbital, APAP, and caffeine	Janumet	Sitagliptin + metformin
Fiorinal with coedine	Butalbital, ASA, caffeine, and codeine	Januvia	Sitagliptin
		K-Lor	Potassium chloride
Flagyl	Metronidazole	K Lyte	Potassium bicarbonate and citrate
Flexeril	Cyclobenzaprine		
Flomax	Tamsulosin	K-Tab	Potassium chloride
Flonase	Fluticasone	Kadian	Morphine sulfate
Flovent	Fluticasone	Keflex	Cephalexin
Floxin	Ofloxacin	Kenalog	Triamcinolone acetonide
Focalin	Dexmethylphenidate	Klonopin	Clonazepam
Forteo	Teriparatide	Klor-Con	Potassium chloride
Fosamax	Alendronate	Kytril	Granisetron
Fosamax Plus D	Alendronate + cholecalciferol		
Fuzeon	Enfuvirtide	Lamictal	Lamotrigine
		Lamisil Oral	Terbinafine
Gemzar	Gemcitabine	Lanoxin	Digoxin
Gengraf	Cyclosporine	Lantus	Insulin glargine
Geodon	Ziprasidone	Lasix	Furosemide
Gleevec	Imatinib	Lescol	Fluvastatin
Glucotrol	Glipizide	Levaquin	Levofloxacin
Glucophage	Metformin		

Brand Names (Trade Names)	Generic Names
Levemir	Insulin detemir
Levitra	Vardenafil
Levo-T	Levothyroxine
Levothroid	Levothyroxine
Levoxyl	Levothyroxine
Lexapro	Escitalopram
Lidex	Fluocinonide
Lidoderm	Lidocaine
Lioresal	Baclofen
Lipitor	Atorvastatin
Lodine	Etodolac
Loestrin-Fe	Ethinyl estradiol + norethindrone
Lomotil	Diphenoxylate + atropine
Lo-Ovral 28	Ethinyl estradiol + norgestrel
Lopid	Gemfibrozil
Lopressor	Metoprolol
Lortab	Hydrocodone bitartrate + APAP
Lotensin	Benazepril
Lotrel	Amlodipine + benazepril
Lotrisone	Clotrimazole + betamethasone
Lorelco	Probucol
Lovaza	Omega-3-acid ethyl esters
Lozol	Indapamide
Lovenox	Enoxaparin
Lumigan	Bimatoprost
Lunesta	Eszopiclone
Lupron Depot	Leuprolide
Luvox	Fluvoxamine
Lyrica	Pregabalin
Macrobid	Nitrofurantoin
Macrodantin	Nitrofurantoin
Marinol	Dronabinol
Maxalt	Rizatriptan
Medrol	Methylprednisolone
Meridia	Sibutramine
Mevacor	Lovastatin
Micro-K	Potassium chloride
Micardis HCT	Telmisartan
Minipress	Prazosin
Minocin	Minocycline
Mirapex	Pramipexole
Mircette	Desogestrel + ethinyl estradiol
Miscalcin	Calcitonin-salmon

Brand Names (Trade Names)	Generic Names
Monistat	Miconazole
Monopril	Fosinopril
Monurol	Fosfomycin
Motrin	Ibuprofen
MS Contin	Morphine sulfate
Mycelex G	Clotrimazole
Mycostatin	Nystatin
Nalfon	Fenoprofen
Namenda	Memantine
Naprelan	Naproxen
Naprosyn	Naproxen
Nasacort AQ	Triamcinolone
Nasalcrom	Cromolyn
Nasonex	Mometasone
Necon	Ethinyl estradiol + norethindrone
Neoral	Cyclosporine
Neosporin	Neomycin, polymyxin B, and bacitracin
Neulasta	Pegfilgrastim
Neupogen	Filgrastim
Neurontin	Gabapentin
Nexium	Esomeprazole
Niaspan	Niacin
Nitrodur II	Nitroglycerin
Nitrostat	Nitroglycerin
Nizoral	Ketoconazole
Nolvadex	Tamoxifen
Noroxin	Norfloxacin
Norvasc	Amlodipine
Norvir	Ritonavir
Novo Log Mix	Insulin
Novolin	Insulin
NuvaRing	Etonogestrel + ethinyl estradiol
Ogen	Estropipate
Omnaris	Ciclesonide
Omnicef	Cefdinir
Opana ER	Oxymorphone
Ortho-Cyclen	Norgestimate + ethinyl estradiol
Ortho Evra	Ethinyl estradiol + norelgestromin
Ortho-Tri-Cyclen + Lo	Ethinyl estradiol + desogestrel

Brand Names (Trade Names)	Generic Names	Brand Names (Trade Names)	Generic Names
Ovcon	Ethinyl estradiol + norethindrone	Prozac	Fluoxetine
		Pulmicort	Budesonide
Oxycontin	Oxycodone	Pulmozyme	Dornase alfa
Oxytrol	Oxybutynin		
		Questran	Cholestyramine
Pamelor	Nortriptyline		
Paraplatin	Carboplatin	Rebetron	Ribavirin + interferon alfa 2b
Patanol	Olopatadine	Rebif	Interferon beta-1a
Paxil	Paroxetine	Reglan	Metoclopramide
PCE	Erythromycin	Relafen	Nabumetone
Pediazole	Erythromycin + sulfisoxazole	Relpax	Eletriptan
Pegasys	Peginterferon alfa 2a	Remeron	Mirtazapine
Pepcid	Famotidine	Remicade	Infliximab
Percocet	Oxycodone HCL + APAP	Renagel	Sevelamer
Percodan	Oxycodone + ASA	ReoPro	Abciximab
Peridex	Chlorhexidine gluconate	Requip	Ropinirole
Persantine	Dipyridamole	Restasis	Cyclosporine
Pen-Vee K	Pot. phenoxymethyl penicillin	Restoril	Temazepam
Phenergan	Promethazine	Retin-A	Tretinoin
Plavix	Clopidogrel	Revlimid	Lenalidomide
Plendil	Felodipine	Reyataz	Atazanavir
Pravachol	Pravastatin	Rheumatrex	Methotrexate
Premarin	Conjugated estrogens	Rhinocort	Budesonide
Prempro	Conjuated estrogens	Risperdal	Risperidone
Prevacid	Lansoprazole	Ritalin	Methylphenidate
Prevpac	Lansoprazole, amoxicillin, + clarithromycin	Rituxan	Rituximab
		Rocephin	Ceftriaxone
Prilosec	Omeprazole	Rogaine	Minoxidil
Primaxin	Imipenem + cilastatin	Roxicet	Oxycodone + APAP
Principen	Ampicillin		
Prinivil	Lisinopril	Septra	Trimethoprim + sulfamethoxazole
ProAir HFA	Albuterol		
Procan SR	Procainamide	Sensipar	Cinacalcet
Procardia	Nifedipine	Serax	Oxazepam
Procrit	Epoetin alfa	Serevent	Salmeterol
Prograf	Tacrolimus	Seroquel	Quetiapine
Pronestyl	Procainamide	Serostim	Somatropin
Propacet	Propoxyphene + APAP	Serzone	Nefazodone
Propecia	Finasteride	Sinemet	Carbidopa + levodopa
Propine	Dipivefrin	Sinequan	Doxepin
Propofol	Diprivan	Singulair	Montelukast sodium
Proquin XR	Ciprofloxacin	Skelaxin	Metaxalone
Proscar	Finasteride	Slow-K	Potassium chloride
Protonix	Pantoprazole	Slo-Phyllin	Theophylline
Proventil	Albuterol	Solodyn	Minocycline
Provera	Medroxyprogesterone	Soma	Carisoprodol
Provigil	Modafinil	Sonata	Zaleplon

Brand Names (Trade Names)	Generic Names	Brand Names (Trade Names)	Generic Names
Spiriva	Tiotropium	Trizivir	Abacavir, lamivudine, & zidovudine
Sporanox	Itraconazole	Truvada	Tenofovir + emtricitabine
Stadol NS	Butorphanol	Tussionex	Hydrocodone + chlorpheniramine
Strattera	Atomoxetine		
Suboxone	Buprenorphine + naloxone	Tylenol	APAP
Sumycin	Tetracycline	Tylox	Oxycodone HCL + APAP
Suprax	Cefixime		
Sustiva	Efavirenz	Ultracet	Tramadol + APAP
Symbicort	Budesonide + formoterol	Ultram	Tramadol
Synagis	Palivizumab	Unasyn	Ampicillin + sulbactam
Synthroid	Levothyroxin		
		Valcyte	Valganciclovir
Taclonex	Calcipotriene + betamethazone	Valium	Diazepam
		Valtrex	Valacyclovir
Tagamet	Cimetidine	Vasotec	Enalapril
Tamoxifen	Nolvadex	Vaseretic	Enalapril + HCTZ
Tamiflu	Oseltamivir	Ventolin	Albuterol
Tarceva	Erlotinib	Veramyst	Fluticasone
Taxol	Paclitaxel	Verelan	Verapamil
Tegretrol	Carbamazepine	VESicare	Solifenacin
Temodar	Temozolomide	Viagra	Sildenafil
Tenormin	Atenolol	Vibramycin	Doxycycline
Terazole	Terconazole	Vibratab	Doxycycline
Tessalon	Benzonate	Vicodin	Hydrocodone + APAP
Thalomid	Thalidomide	Vicoprofen	Hydrocodone + ibuprofen
Theo-24	Theophylline, anhydrous	Vigamox	Moxifloxacin
Tiazac	Diltiazem	Viracept	Nelfinavir
Tigan	Trimethobenzamide	Viramune	Nevirapine
Tilade	Nedocromil	Viread	Tenfovir disoproxil fumarate
Timoptic	Timolol		
TobraDex	Tobramycin + dexamethasone	Vistaril	Hydroxyzine pamoate
		Vivelle	Estradiol patches
Topamax	Topiramate	Voltaren	Diclofenac
Toprol	Metoprolol	Vytorin	Ezetimibe + simvastatin
Toradol	Ketorolac	Vyvanse	Lisdexamfetamine
Transderm Nitro	Nitroglycerin		
Transderm Scop	Scopolamine	Welchol	Colesevelam
Trasylol	Aprotinin	Wellbutrin SR	Bupropion
Tranxene	Chlorazepate		
Trental	Pentoxifylline	Xalatan	Latanoprost
Tricor	Fenofibrate	Xanax	Alprazolam
Trileptal	Oxcarbazepine	Xeloda	Capecitabine
TriNessa	Ethinyl estradiol + norgestimate	Xenical	Orlistat
		Xigris	Drotrecoqin
Trivoral	Ethinyl estradiol + levonorgestrel	Xopenex	Levalbuterol

Brand Names (Trade Names)	Generic Names	Brand Names (Trade Names)	Generic Names
Yasmin 28	Ethinyl estradiol + drospirenone	Zocor	Simvastatin
		Zofran	Ondansetron
Yaz	Ethinyl estradiol + drospirenone	Zoladex	Goserelin
		Zoloft	Sertraline
		Zometa	Zoledronic
Zantac	Ranitidine	Zomig	Zolmitriptan
Zerit	Stavudine	Zosyn	Piperacillin + tazobactam
Zestoretic	Lisinopril + HCTZ	Zovirax	Acyclovir
Zestril	Lisinopril	Zyban	Bupropion
Zetia	Ezetimibe	Zydone	Hydrocodone + APAP
Ziac	Bisoprolol + HCTZ	Zyloprim	Allopurinol
Ziagen	Abacavir	Zyprexa	Olanzapine
Zinacef	Cefuroxime	Zyrtec	Cetirizine
Zithromax	Azithromycin	Zyvox	Linezolid